1990
YEAR BOOK OF
OPHTHALMOLOGY®

The 1990 Year Book® Series

Year Book of Anesthesia®: Drs. Miller, Kirby, Ostheimer, Roizen, and Stoelting

Year Book of Cardiology®: Drs. Schlant, Collins, Engle, Frye, Kaplan, and O'Rourke

Year Book of Critical Care Medicine®: Drs. Rogers and Parrillo

Year Book of Dentistry®: Drs. Meskin, Ackerman, Kennedy, Leinfelder, Matukas, and Rovin

Year Book of Dermatology®: Drs. Sober and Fitzpatrick

Year Book of Diagnostic Radiology®: Drs. Bragg, Hendee, Keats, Kirkpatrick, Miller, Osborn, and Thompson

Year Book of Digestive Diseases®: Drs. Greenberger and Moody

Year Book of Drug Therapy®: Drs. Hollister and Lasagna

Year Book of Emergency Medicine®: Dr. Wagner

Year Book of Endocrinology®: Drs. Bagdade, Braverman, Halter, Horton, Kannan, Korenman, Molitch, Morley, Odell, Rogol, Ryan, and Sherwin

Year Book of Family Practice®: Drs. Rakel, Avant, Driscoll, Prichard, and Smith

Year Book of Geriatrics and Gerontology®: Drs. Beck, Abrass, Burton, Cummings, Makinodan, and Small

Year Book of Hand Surgery®: Drs. Dobyns, Chase, and Amadio

Year Book of Hematology®: Drs. Spivak, Bell, Ness, Quesenberry, and Wiernik

Year Book of Infectious Diseases®: Drs. Wolff, Barza, Keusch, Klempner, and Snydman

Year Book of Infertility: Drs. Mishell, Paulsen, and Lobo

Year Book of Medicine®: Drs. Rogers, Des Prez, Cline, Braunwald, Greenberger, Wilson, Epstein, and Malawista

Year Book of Neonatal and Perinatal Medicine: Drs. Klaus and Fanaroff

Year Book of Neurology and Neurosurgery®: Drs. Currier and Crowell

Year Book of Nuclear Medicine®: Drs. Hoffer, Gore, Gottschalk, Sostman, Zaret, and Zubal

Year Book of Obstetrics and Gynecology®: Drs. Mishell, Kirschbaum, and Morrow

Year Book of Occupational and Environmental Medicine: Drs. Emmett, Brooks, Harris, and Schenker

Year Book of Oncology: Drs. Young, Longo, Ozols, Simone, Steele, and Weichselbaum

Year Book of Ophthalmology®: Drs. Laibson, Adams, Augsburger, Benson, Cohen, Eagle, Flanagan, Nelson, Reinecke, Sergott, and Wilson

Year Book of Orthopedics®: Drs. Sledge, Poss, Cofield, Frymoyer, Griffin, Hansen, Johnson, Springfield, and Weiland

Year Book of Otolaryngology—Head and Neck Surgery®: Drs. Bailey and Paparella

Year Book of Pathology and Clinical Pathology®: Drs. Brinkhous, Dalldorf, Grisham, Langdell, and McLendon

Year Book of Pediatrics®: Drs. Oski and Stockman

Year Book of Plastic, Reconstructive, and Aesthetic Surgery: Drs. Miller, Bennett, Haynes, Hoehn, McKinney, and Whitaker

Year Book of Podiatric Medicine and Surgery®: Dr. Jay

Year Book of Psychiatry and Applied Mental Health®: Drs. Talbott, Frances, Frances, Freedman, Meltzer, Schowalter, and Yudofsky

Year Book of Pulmonary Disease®: Drs. Green, Loughlin, Michael, Mulshine, Peters, Terry, Tockman, and Wise

Year Book of Speech, Language, and Hearing: Drs. Bernthal, Hall, and Tomblin

Year Book of Sports Medicine®: Drs. Shephard, Eichner, Sutton, and Torg, Col. Anderson, and Mr. George

Year Book of Surgery®: Drs. Schwartz, Jonasson, Peacock, Shires, Spencer, and Thompson

Year Book of Urology®: Drs. Gillenwater and Howards

Year Book of Vascular Surgery®: Drs. Bergan and Yao

Richard P. Wilson, M.D.

Attending Surgeon, Glaucoma Service, Wills Eye Hospital; Associate Professor of Ophthalmolgy, Jefferson Medical College of Thomas Jefferson University, Philadelphia, Pennsylvania

Editorial Assistant
Helen Yurkow

1990

The Year Book of
OPHTHALMOLOGY®

Wills Eye Hospital Editorial Board

Editor-in-Chief
Peter R. Laibson, M.D.

Associate Editors
Raymond E. Adams, M.D.
James J. Augsburger, M.D.
William E. Benson, M.D.
Elisabeth J. Cohen, M.D.
Ralph C. Eagle, Jr., M.D.
Joseph C. Flanagan, M.D.
Leonard B. Nelson, M.D.
Robert D. Reinecke, M.D.
Robert C. Sergott, M.D.
Richard P. Wilson, M.D.

Mosby
Year Book

St. Louis   Baltimore   Boston   Chicago   London   Philadelphia   Sydney   Toronto

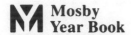
**Mosby
Year Book**

Dedicated to Publishing Excellence

Editor-in-Chief, Year Book Publishing: Nancy Gorham
Sponsoring Editor: Gretchen C. Templeton
Manager, Medical Information Services: Edith M. Podrazik
Senior Medical Information Specialist: Terri Strorigl
Assistant Director, Manuscript Services: Frances M. Perveiler
Assistant Managing Editor, Year Book Editing Services: Wayne Larsen
Production Coordinator: Max F. Perez
Proofroom Supervisor: Barbara M. Kelly

Editorial Office:
Mosby-Year Book, Inc.
200 North LaSalle St.
Chicago, IL 60601

International Standard Serial Number: 0-8151-5266-3
International Standard Book Number: 0084-392X

Table of Contents

The material covered in this volume represents literature reviewed through December 1989.

Journals Represented

Mosby Year Book subscribes to and surveys nearly 850 U.S. and foreign medical and allied health journals. From these journals, the Editors select the articles to be abstracted. Journals represented in this YEAR BOOK are listed below.

Acta Ophthalmologica
American Journal of Ophthalmology
American Orthopedic Journal
Annals of Neurology
Annals of Ophthalmology
Archives of Ophthalmology
Australian and New Zealand Journal of Ophthalmology
British Journal of Ophthalmology
Cancer Research
CLAO Journal
International Ophthalmology Clinics
Investigative Ophthalmology and Visual Science
Journal of Cataract and Refractive Surgery
Journal of Pediatric Ophthalmology and Strabismus
New England Journal of Medicine
Ophthalmic Plastic and Reconstructive Surgery
Ophthalmic Surgery
Ophthalmology
Orbit
Refractive and Corneal Surgery
Retina Journal of Retinal and Vitreous Diseases
Survey of Ophthalmology
Transactions of the American Ophthalmological Society

STANDARD ABBREVIATIONS

The following terms are abbreviated in this edition: acquired immunodeficiency syndrome (AIDS), central nervous system (CNS), cerebrospinal fluid (CSF), computed tomography (CT), electrocardiography (ECG), and human immunodeficiency virus (HIV).

1   Cataract

Cataract 1989: Cause and Composition

RAYMOND E. ADAMS, M.D.
Wills Eye Hospital, Philadelphia, Pennsylvania

The development of lens and retina diseases might reflect the independent or combined effects of such factors as excessive light exposure over years; an inefficient constitutional antioxidant system, such as enzyme superoxide dismutase; dietary antioxidant deficiency of vitamin A, E, or C; and damaging effects of oxidation-potentiating factors, such as dietary psoralens or use of certain drugs.

Historically, cataracts are incidental with diabetes mellitus, corticosteroids, uveitis, ocular trauma, ocular radiation, myotonic dystrophy, lens subluxation, glaucoma, and family trait of cataracts. The following topics highlight the current literature on why cataracts develop from clear lenses.

Congenital cataract (CC) may be associated with multisystem disorders, may be part of an ocular malformation disorder, or may be isolated. Isolated CC often is inherited as a familial trait. Autosomal dominant transmission with complete penetrance seems to be the most common type.

Chromosome mapping indicates that the loci for embryonic and fetal nuclear stationary cataracts are on chromosome 1, the locus for the embryonic nuclear cataract is on chromosome 2, and the loci for posterior polar cataract and progressive familial nuclear cataract are on chromosome 16 (1).

Maternal varicella infection during the second trimester of pregnancy may result in congenital varicella syndrome. Besides systemic abnormalities, ocular findings include congenital cataract, chorioretinitis, atrophy and hypoplasia of the optic nerves, and Horner's syndrome. Children with congenital varicella syndrome should be examined by an ophthalmologist to exclude ocular abnormalities (2).

An association may exist between **age-related macular degeneration** (AMD) and opacifying lens disease. Suggested are a common etiologic (exposure) factor, a common susceptibility element, and common disease-modulating risk factors. Cataract and AMD are weakly associated statistically, possibly reflecting the difficulty of visualizing maculae in eyes with dense cataract.

However, a strong association between AMD and aphakia suggests that a sudden increase in light transmittance after cataract removal may reinitiate and dramatically accelerate progression to frank macular degeneration. This speculation supports the trend toward routine implantation of ultraviolet-blocking intraocular lenses.

The association between lens and macular disease independent of age is consistent with the theory of **ultraviolet/near-ultraviolet light** damage to the eyes. The cheapest and most effective public health measure may be to encourage use of protective eyewear at early ages (3).

In a study of watermen of the Chesapeake Bay of Maryland, Taylor found cortical cataracts increased as exposure to **ultraviolet B** (wavelength, 320–290 nm) increased. The highest level of ambient ultraviolet B varies markedly during the day (it is highest in summer between 10 A.M. and 1 P.M., the time when sunburn is most likely to occur).

Exposure to ultraviolet B can be minimized to half by wearing a hat with a brim, and wearing ordinary glasses with plastic lenses may reduce it to about 5%. Ultraviolet B-absorbing lenses may reduce this even further (4).

Data from the World Health Organization (National Eye Institute, Bethesda, Md.) Tibet Eye Study found the prevalence of age-related cataract to be 0.2% among persons aged 20–39 years, 11.8% among persons aged 40 years old or more, and 50% for persons aged 70 years or more. **Cortical cataracts** were the most common type of cataract diagnosed. This study involved people living at one of the highest inhabited regions of the world (4,000 m), where ultraviolet radiation exposure is greater.

Brilliant, quoted in an article by Hu and associates, qualified that **sunlight** was blocked from reaching higher altitudes by neighboring mountains, and speculated that the reduction in sunlight offset the theoretic gain in ultraviolet exposure in higher altitudes. Persons in sites with an average of 12 hours of sunlight exposure (lower elevations) had almost 4 times as many cataracts as those in sites with 7 hours of sunlight (5).

Certain nutrients also may be involved in **antioxidant defense** of senile cataract formation. Persons with high plasma levels of 2 or more of those vitamins thought to influence antioxidant status (vitamin E, vitamin C, and carotenoids) appear to have a reduced risk of cataract (6).

An unknown mechanism of cataract prevention may be involved with the amino acid **lysine** or bendazac lysine, or both. In rat studies, amino acid content was less in cataractous lenses than in clear lenses. Clinical reversal of cataracts (anterior subcapsular, water-clefts and spokes, wedge-shaped and nuclear) shows that the increase in light scattering over time (i.e., opacification) at the anterior capsule, anterior cortex, and nuclear levels is less in the group given lysine (7, 8).

A study done in Raipur, India, suggested that about 38% of visually disabling cataracts may be attributed to life-threatening **dehydration** associated with diarrheal disease. Similar statistics were noted in another study in central India of the risk of presenile cataract. The risk of cataract is increased with exposure to severe life-threatening diarrheal disease and to heatstroke (9).

Bochow (10) found a significant association between ultraviolet B exposure and posterior subcapsular cataracts (PSC). An association between **low educational level** and the presence of cataracts may result from increased light exposure during manual labor or other outdoor occupations that do not require a high level of education. Also, **blue eyes** appeared more susceptible to formation of PSCs.

The lens has served historically as a kind of **"biologic dosimeter"** for radiation exposure in situ. Recent studies have clarified that accelerated heavy ions have a higher relative biologic effectiveness for production of cataracts than low linear energy transfer x-rays (11). **Microwaves** most commonly cause anterior or posterior subcapsular lenticular opacities, or both, theoretically because of deformation of heat-labile enzymes (glutathione peroxide) or thermoelastic expansion damage to the lens cells. Ionizing radiation is associated with damage to the lens cell membrane or to the lens cell DNA. Mechanical shielding from these radiations is the only recommended means of minimizing the development of cataract (12).

A significant increased risk of pure nuclear opacities was associated with **cigarette smoking** in the study of watermen on the eastern shore of Maryland. This dose-response relationship is measured by comparing the cumulative numbers of pack-years smoked with the severity of the opacity. Conversely, the risk was decreased independently of dose smoked for persons who quit smoking compared with current smokers. Nuclear cataracts were not related to history of diabetes, ultraviolet B exposure, or use of diuretic or cardiac medications (13).

Nuclear cataract is a common type of senile cataract characterized by an increased turbidity, **yellow to brown pigmentation** of the nucleus, and myopic refractive shift. Increases in the water-insoluble and the urea-insoluble protein fractions cause these changes. This insoluble protein–water relationship consists of high-molecular-weight protein aggregates large enough to scatter light. Hence, the positive glare testing in these eyes (14).

Abnormalities in **galactose** pathway enzymes galactokinase and galactose-1-phosphate uridyl transferase may predipose to development of presenile cataracts. For affected people, clinical treatment is possible through dietary restriction of dairy products or by using aldose reductase inhibitors to prevent or reverse cataract formation (15).

The nature of the osmolytes in diabetic eyes is unclear, although both **glucose and sorbitol** have been ruled out. The presence of an osmotic regulatory mechanism in the eye is implied (16).

Development of cataracts has been delayed through the reduction in activity of **aldose reductase.** The search for more effective inhibitors of aldose reductase on sugar cataracts to delay or prevent cataracts in human beings continues. A study showed that compound E-0772 was a more potent inhibitor of aldose reductase than sorbinil. Sorbinil has been found to inhibit diabetes-related changes in many tissues and galactose-induced alterations in the lens (17).

Kinoshita hypothesized that the initiator of lenticular changes in the diabetic rat is an increase in osmolarity of the lens. The **osmolarity change** is caused by the accumulation of sugar alcohol, which is formed by the action of the enzyme aldose reductase (AR) on sugar. Garadi and colleagues found, not that enzyme activity plays a significant role, but rather that the hyperglycemic condition in combination with existing enzyme levels is sufficient to cause cataractous changes (18).

AL01576 is an AR inhibitor of high potency with respect to the inhibition of **naphthalene cataract** development. One drop a day in Brown-Norway rats delayed but did not prevent cataract formation. Four drops per day resulted in no changes in the transparency of the lenses caused by naphthalene treatment (19).

An investigation of the Mediterranean coast of Turkey (Cukurova) found a 33% incidence of red blood cell glucose 6-phosphate dehydrogenase deficiency (**G6PD**) in patients with cataracts vs. 8.2% in those with clear lenses. Color blindness and hemophilia A are well documented with this X-chromosome inheritance pattern (20).

Study of **regional water** lens content of clear and cataractous lenses showed the cortex has significantly higher overall water content than the nucleus has. Similarly, regional biochemical activity is highest in cortical and equatorial regions. Cortical or nuclear cataracts in persons aged 74–82 years had a 10% greater weight. Further hardening of the lens nucleus with greater age is not reflected by a respective decrease in water content. Conversely, PSCs had lower total weight despite their accumulating water in the posterior cortex. **Clear lenses weigh about 200 mg** (21).

The glucocorticoid-induced cataract in the chick embryo is interpreted as a **protein-water phase separation** that occurred during lens opacification (22).

Structural lenticular changes with increased amounts of high-molecular-weight **protein aggregates** accompany the process of opacification in the cortex of the human cataractous lens (23).

The lens capsule is a **typical basement membrane.** Changes in lens capsule characteristics occur with aging in patients with cataracts and in those with diabetes mellitus. The most characteristic change in long-term diabetic persons is the thickening of basement membranes. The bound water as percentage of the total water is increased with the degree of glycosylation of the bovine lens capsules. Glycosylation increases the stiffness and thermal stability (24).

The calcium content of the lens and its possible imbalance in cataract development have been studied for decades. A marked increase in **calcium** is found in the mature senile cataract as well as in the hypocalcemic cataract. This increase has led investigators to conclude that calcium deposition is secondary to lens injury rather than a primary factor in the development of lenticular opacities. The cataract patients unexpectedly had an increase in aqueous humor concentration of magnesium relative to their serum concentrations (25).

Oxidative **inhibition of Ca-ATPase** by low levels of hydrogen peroxide (H_2O_2) may permit accumulation of intracellular calcium, which undoubtedly is deleterious to lens function and perhaps causes lens opacification. The intracellular lens calcium may alter lens metabolism by interacting with cytoplasmic proteins, activating proteases or lipases, or calmodulin-activated pathways (26).

Studies have shown for the first time that both lens fiber and epithelial cell membranes had **beta-adrenergic receptors**. Aqueous humor catecholamines may affect lens development (27).

A decrease in the ability of the lens epithelium to detoxify H_2O_2 subjects the interior of the lens to oxidative insult and could be a major contributor in the development of senile cataracts. Elevated levels of H_2O_2 have been found in the aqueous of cataract patients and lead to opacities in the rabbit lens in organ culture. An age-related decrease in the activity of catalase has been proposed because **catalase** is thought to play an important role in H_2O_2 detoxification (28).

Oxidative stress affects both rat and monkey lenses by similar mechanisms; however, lenses from monkeys are more resistant to these effects because they have better endogenous antioxidant defenses. The rat aqueous has very little H_2O_2, whereas monkeys and human beings have much higher levels. Rats are nocturnal animals, in contrast to monkeys and humans (29).

Long-term restriction of dietary sodium completely prevented the development of cataractous lesions in the Dahl salt-sensitive rat. This finding suggests that cataract formation is not dependent on elevated **blood pressure**, but rather results from the extracellular fluid volume state (30).

Human lens cells and erythrocytes are highly specialized cells, with limited metabolism and many structural and biochemical similarities. **Spectrin** initially was thought to be specific for erythrocytes. These protein structures are important for erythrocyte membrane flexibility and cellular life span. The concept of a spectrin gene family recently has emerged from the finding that the human lens contains both erythroid and nonerythroid (fodrin) spectrin transcripts in abundance (31).

Spectrin is a major protein of the red cell membrane exoskeleton and contributes to erythrocyte membrane elasticity and integrity. Erythrocytes must alter their shapes to pass through the microcirculation. Lens cells are **similar to erythrocytes** in that they have no nuclei or mitochondria. The vertebrate lens is a highly specialized organ whose main function is to refract light. To maintain retinal focus, lens cells must deform their shape to accommodate light beams of varying incidence. One could argue that the lens could deform more easily if lens cells were supported by fiberlike proteins such as spectrin and fodrin (31).

Electron microscopic results indicate that the cortex and nucleus of the bovine eye are quite different, both in terms of morphology and the distribution of membrane specializations. **Large square arrays** are found primarily in the nucleus of the lens, whereas the cortex has **gap junctions** (thick symmetric membrane pairs) containing packed intramembrane particles. The function of these structures needs further study (32).

Many innovations for the treatment of cataract were introduced in 1989. However, none can compare with the Dr. William O. Coffee and his **absorption cure** for cataracts. Doctor Coffee may not have been a reliable researcher; however, he was certainly an advertising entrepreneur. His ad, "I treat eyes free," is the basis for current marketing techniques. In 1935, the U.S. Post Office Department recommended issuance of a fraud order against the Dr. W. O. Coffee Company, 8 years after Dr. Coffey's death (33).

References

1. Marner E, Rosenberg T, Eiberg H: Autosomal dominant congenital cataract morphology and genetic mapping. *Acta Ophthalmol* 67:151–158, 1989.
2. Lambert SR, Taylor D, Kriss A, et al: Ocular manifestations of the congenital varicella syndrome. *Arch Ophthalmol* 107:52–56, 1989.
3. Liu IY, White L, LaCroix AZ: The association of age-related macular degeneration and lens opacities in the aged. *Am J Public Health* 79:765–769, 1989.
4. Taylor HR, West SK, Rosenthal FS, et al: Effect of ultraviolet radiation on cataract formation. *N Engl J Med* 319:1429–1433, 1988.
5. Hu T-S, Zhen Q, Sperduto RD, et al: Age-related cataract in the Tibet Eye Study. *Arch Ophthalmol* 107:666–669, 1989.
6. Jacques PF, Chylack LT, McGandy RB, et al: Antioxidant status in persons with and without senile cataract. *Arch Ophthalmol* 106:337–340, 1988.
7. Brown RA: Persons communication. April 5, 1989.
8. Hockwin O, Laser H, DeGregorio M, et al: Bendazac lysine in selected types of human senile cataract. *Ophthalmic Res* 21:141–154, 1989.
9. Minassian DC, Mehra V, Verrey J-D: Dehydrational crises: A major risk factor in blinding cataract. *Br J Ophthalmol* 73:100–105, 1989.
10. Bochow TW, West SK, Azar A, et al: Ultraviolet light exposure and risk of posterior subcapsular cataracts. *Arch Ophthalmol* 107:369–372, 1989.
11. Worgul BV: Accelerated heavy particles and the lens. *Ophthalmic Res* 20:143–148, 1988.
12. Lipman RM, Tripathi BJ, Tripathi RC: Cataracts induced by microwave and ionizing radiation. *Surv Ophthalmol* 33:200–210, 1988.
13. West S, Munoz B, Emmett EA, et al: Cigarette smoking and risk of nuclear cataracts. *Arch Ophthalmol* 107:1166–1169, 1989.
14. Palmquist B-M, Philipson B, Fagerholm P: Nuclear cataract: A microradiographic study. *Acta Ophthalmol* 66:671–677, 1988.
15. Stevens RE, Datiles MB, Srivastava SK, et al: Idiopathic presenile cataract formation and galactosaemia. *Br J Ophthalmol* 73:48–51, 1989.
16. Xiong H, Cheng H: Aqueous/vitreous tonicity in "sugar" cataracts. *Ophthalmic Res* 21:292–296, 1989.
17. Unakar N, Tsui J, Johnson M: Aldose reductase inhibitors and prevention of galactose cataracts in rats. *Invest Ophthalmol Vis Sci* 30:1623–1632, 1989.
18. Garadi R, Lou MF: Aldose reductase in early streptozotocin-induced diabetic rat lens. *Invest Ophthalmol Vis Sci* 30:2370–2375, 1989.
19. Hockwin O, Muller P, Krolczyk J, et al: Determination of AL01576 concentration in rat lenses and plasma by bioassay for aldose reductase activity measurements. *Ophthalmic Res* 21:285–291, 1989.
20. Yuregir G, Varinli I, Donma O: Glucose 6-phosphate dehydrogenase deficiency both in red blood cells and lenses of the normal and cataractous native population of Cukurova, the southern part of Turkey. *Ophthalmic Res* 21:155–157, 1989.
21. Deussen A, Pau H: Regional water content of clear and cataractous human lenses. *Ophthalmic Res* 21:374–380, 1989.
22. Mizuno A, Nishigori H, Iwatsuru M: Glucocorticoid-induced cataract in chick embryo monitored by raman spectroscopy. *Invest Ophthalmol Vis Sci* 30:132–137, 1989.
23. Kodama T, Wolfe J, Chylack L, et al: Quantitation of high molecular weight protein aggregates in opaque and transparent parts from the same human cataractous lens. *Jpn J Ophthalmol* 33:114–119, 1989.
24. Popdimitrova N, Bettelheim FA: Bound water content of bovine lens capsules. *Ophthalmic Res* 21:352–359, 1989.

25. Ringvold A, Sagen E, Bjerve KS, et al: The calcium and magnesium content of the human lens and aqueous humour. *Acta Ophthalmol* 66:153–156, 1988.
26. Borchman D, Paterson CA, Delamere NA: Oxidative Inhibition of Ca2+-ATPase in the Rabbit Lens. *Invest Ophthalmol Vis Sci* 30:1633–1637, 1989.
27. Ireland ME, Jacks LA: Initial characterization of lens beta-adrenergic receptors. *Invest Ophthalmol Vis Sci* 30:2190–2194, 1989.
28. Mancini MA, Unakar NJ, Giblin FJ, et al: Histochemical localization of catalase in cultured lens epithelial cells. *Ophthalmic Res* 21:369–373, 1989.
29. Zigler JS Jr, Lucas VA, Du X: Rhesus monkey lens as an in vitro model for studying oxidative stress. *Invest Ophthalmol Vis Sci* 30:2195–2199, 1989.
30. Rodriguez-Sargent C, Berrios G, Irrizarry JE, et al: Prevention and reversal of cataracts in genetically hypertensive rats through sodium restriction. *Invest Ophthalmol Vis Sci* 30:2356–2360, 1989.
31. Yoon S-H, Skalka H, Prchal JT: Presence of erythroid and nonerythroid spectrin transcripts in human lens and cerebellum. *Invest Ophthalmol Vis Sci* 30:1860–1866, 1989.
32. Costello MJ, McIntosh TJ, Robertson JD: Distribution of gap junctions and square array junctions in the mammalian lens. *Invest Ophthalmol Vis Sci* 30:975–989, 1989.
33. Ferry AP: Dr. William O. Coffee and his absorption cure for cataract. *Ophthalmology* 96:1257–1266, 1989.

Long-Term Evolution of Astigmatism Following Planned Extracapsular Cataract Extraction

Parker WT, Clorfeine GS (Southern California Permanente Med Group, San Diego)

Arch Ophthalmol 107:353–357, March 1989   1–1

What is the course of astigmatism after planned extracapsular cataract extraction with a posterior chamber intraocular lens? Sixty-six eyes were followed up for 3 years after cataract surgery when 10-0 nylon sutures were used for wound closure. All suture cutting was completed 3 months postoperatively. The sutures were oriented radially and passed at a depth of 75% to 90% of corneal thickness. Sutures were cut selectively after 7 and 8 weeks if necessary to minimize astigmatism.

Induced astigmatism measured at 3 months was not stable, but shifted 0.69 diopter toward against-the-rule astigmatism. It was not possible to consistently induce with-the-rule astigmatism, but permanent against-the-rule induced astigmatism could be produced. The number of intact sutures did not influence the trend toward more against-the-rule astigmatism.

It is not possible consistently to induce permanent with-the-rule astigmatism using this wound closure method, probably because nylon deteriorates and loses its structural integrity 1 to 2 years after surgery. Attempts to influence the course of astigmatism by surgery such as keratotomy, at the time of cataract surgery or afterward, probably are imprudent.

Long-Term Corneal Astigmatism Related to Selected Elastic, Monofilament, Nonabsorbable Sutures

Cravy TV (Santa Maria, Calif)
J Cataract Refract Surg 15:61–69, January 1989

1–2

The course of surgically induced corneal astigmatism was studied in 395 patients having planned extracapsular cataract extraction. Limbal or scleral pocket incisions of 60–140 degrees were made. Limbal incisions were closed with a full-thickness shoelace technique using 9-0 or 10-0 nylon, 10-0 polypropylene (Prolene), or 10-0 polyester (Mersilene). Scleral pocket incisions were closed using a modified shoelace technique (Fig 1–1).

Nylon sutures had significant hydrolysis starting as soon as 5 months after operation. The use of 10-0 nylon was eliminated when scleral pocket closure was done, but hydrolysis of 9-0 nylon sutures led to excessive late astigmatism in patients without normal healing. No hydrolysis was evident with Prolene or Mersilene sutures, but elastic Prolene resulted in more against-the-rule change than was desired.

The author now uses Mersilene routinely in both cataract surgery and keratoplasty. Running closure provides uniform wound tension and a low rate of suture removal. Studies with miniature incisions would be of interest.

► These articles (Abstracts 1–1 and 1–2) describe long-term refractive instability in cataract wounds, toward against-the-rule astigmatism, when nylon suture material is used for wound closure. This instability may be related to the biodegradation of nylon over 2 to 4 years. Polydioxanone (PDS, Ethicon) is an absorbable 9-0 suture material with acceptable wound stability after an initial lag of 7 to 8 weeks. It may offer better long-term refractive stability than nylon,

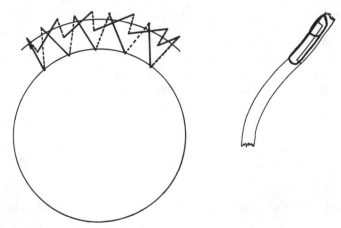

Fig 1–1.—Modified shoelace closure used for scleral pocket incisions. **Left,** *dashed lines* represent intrascleral suture path; *solid lines* represent the surface course of the suture. **Right,** suture penetration and depth are shown in cross section. (Courtesy of Cravy TV: *J Cataract Refract Surg* 15:61–69, January 1989.)

because PDS causes more tissue reaction. I find PDS suture very acceptable in regard to refractive stability when phacoemulsification is combined with a scleral *tunnel* wound; also, it eliminates cutting and removing sutures.—R.E. Adams, M.D.

Visual Results Following Vitreous Loss and Primary Lens Implantation
Spigelman AV, Lindstrom RL, Nichols BD, Lindquist TD (Univ of Minnesota)
J Cataract Refract Surg 15:201–204, March 1989   1–3

Use of an intraocular lens after vitreous loss remains controversial. The outcomes for 20 patients having vitreous loss and primary implantation of a posterior chamber lens, 14 of whom were followed up longer than 6 months, were reviewed. Six other patients received anterior chamber lens implants. All had either planned extracapsular cataract extraction or phacoemulsification. Inadvertent rupture of the posterior capsular membrane took place with vitreous loss, and vitrectomy was done to preserve the remaining posterior capsule and remove as much vitreous as possible from the posterior segment.

All patients given posterior chamber lens implants had improvement in acuity of 20/40 or better. Four of the 6 with anterior chamber lens implants had such acuity, and 2 had 20/50 acuity at 6-month follow-up. One patient had a retinal detachment.

Vitreous loss at cataract surgery has been viewed as a disaster, partly because of cystoid macular edema. However, if a meticulous anterior vitrectomy is done, a good outcome is possible. Cystoid macular edema is more likely if vitreous remains incarcerated in the wound. The risk of retinal detachment is higher than in uncomplicated cases.

▶ Anterior chamber lenses are not good primary intraocular lenses, especially after torn posterior capsules. In-the-bag intraocular lens (IOL) placement can be used in small openings, but large breaks require IOL sulcus-fixation or no-capsule-suture fixation. Plan ahead for this complication by preserving as much anterior capsule as possible to assist IOL sulcus placement.—R.E. Adams, M.D.

A Comparison of Retrobulbar and Periocular Anesthesia for Cataract Surgery
Weiss JL, Deichman CB (Mary Imogene Bassett Hosp, Cooperstown, NY)
Arch Ophthalmol 107:96–98, January 1989   1–4

Periocular anesthesia is being used increasingly because of rare but significant complications from retrobulbar anesthesia. A prospective comparison was undertaken in 79 consecutive cataract extractions with intraocular lens implantation. Forty patients received retrobulbar injections, and 39 received periocular injections. A 5-mL volume of a 50:50 mixture of 2% lidocaine and 0.75% bupivavaine with 1:200,000 epinephrine was used in all cases. Hyaluronidase was added to the mixture.

A Honan pressure balloon set at 30 mm Hg was placed immediately after anesthesia and was left in place for 10 minutes.

There were no significant group differences in lid or globe akinesia or globe anesthesia. Chemosis was more prominent with periocular anesthesia. Comfort ratings were good in both groups, and comparable numbers of patients needed supplemental anesthesia.

Low-volume periocular anesthesia is as effective as retrobulbar anesthesia for cataract surgery. The risks of damaging the globe and of intrathecal injection are avoided. Anesthetic is injected slowly with a 1.6-cm needle outside the muscle cone and diffuses into the cone. A single injection suffices.

▶ Periocular local anesthesia may be safer than retrobulbar, but prolonged orbital pressure and hyaluronidase are necessary. In general, those endorsing periorbital anesthesia have failed to convince the average ophthalmologist that periocular is worthwhile.—R.E. Adams, M.D.

Protective Effect of the Anterior Lens Capsule During Extracapsular Cataract Extraction: Part II. Preliminary Results of Clinical Study
Patel J, Apple DJ, Hansen SO, Solomon KD, Tetz MR, Gwin TD, O'Morchoe DJC, Daun ME (Med Univ of South Carolina, Charleston)
Ophthalmology 96:598–602, May 1989   1–5

There is experimental evidence that a largely intact anterior lens capsule protects the corneal endothelium during removal of lenticular material. A small anterior capsulotomy, therefore, might be clinically beneficial.

Sixty-one eyes had cataract extraction with phacoemulsification and implantation of a posterior chamber intraocular lens. A round 7-mm can opener anterior capsulotomy was done in 38 eyes, and an intercapsular capsulotomy was done in 23. The latter technique involves a 3- to 4-mm midperipheral curvilinear capsulotomy extending from the 10-o'clock to the 12-o'clock position.

Mean endothelial cell loss was 3.9% with the intercapsular anterior capsulotomy and 10.1% with the can opener capsulotomy technique. Longer ultrasound time was correlated with the degree of endothelial cell loss in the latter group but not when the intercapsular technique was used. In 3 eyes where an anterior capsular tear complicated the intercapsular procedure, cell loss averaged 15.6%.

Sparing of the anterior lens capsule appears to limit endothelial cell loss in cataract extraction. The capsule may dampen the ultrasonic shock waves and lower aqueous turbulence. A small anterior capsulotomy, combined with use of a viscoelastic agent, will help make safer, less traumatic cataract surgery possible.

▶ The "protective effect" of the anterior capsule is a fine suggestion; it is helpful in *soft* cataract phacoemulsification. This would be advantageous in common *dense* nuclear cataracts. In reality, however, hard lenses often tear the capsulotomy, reducing the protective effect.— R.E. Adams, M.D.

The Effect of Hyaluronidase on Akinesia During Cataract Surgery

Abelson MB, Paradis A, Mandel E, George M (Harvard Med School; Lawrence Gen Hosp, Boston)
Ophthalmic Surg 20:325–326, May 1989   1–6

It has been assumed that hyaluronidase is as effective in promoting akinesia as in shortening the induction time for retrobulbar anesthesia. Retrobulbar block with and without hyaluronidase was compared in 40 consecutively seen patients having cataract surgery. Hyaluronidase or saline was added to the mixture of lidocaine and bupivacaine, and the injections were given in a blind manner. Extraocular movements were recorded with a Honan cuff inflated to 30 mm Hg.

Akinesia was achieved in 92.5% of patients, and it was complete in 70% of the patients given hyaluronidase and 40% of those given saline. Mean akinesia scores were significantly higher in the hyaluronidase group in 4 of 6 sectors.

These findings suggest that hyaluronidase be added to retrobulbar anesthesia mixtures when these are used for outpatient ophthalmic surgical procedures.

▶ Time management of the surgical operating suite (read "turnover") is key for increased hospital efficiency. Hyaluronidase enhances the local anesthetic, particularly in peribulbar blocks. For me, the key for happier people is providing comfort during surgery with this old agent.— R.E. Adams, M.D.

Axial Length and the Average Ophthalmologist: Is Biometry Worthwhile?

Story PG, Wiesner PD (Montrose, Colo)
Ophthalmic Surg 20:327–331, May 1989   1–7

Most studies indicate that biometric data from ultrasound and keratometry, combined with lens power formulas, are better than simply implanting standard-power intraocular lenses (IOLs). Past studies show that 84% of eyes have refractive errors within 1.25 D of the predicted error, and 95% have errors within 2 D. The present series included 477 eyes, most having extracapsular cataract extraction with posterior IOL implantation. A lens power of +20.00 D was selected for posterior chamber lenses and a power of +18.50 D for anterior chamber lenses. Refractions were done at least 6 months after surgery (Fig 1–2).

Eighty percent of eyes required postoperative cylindrical corrections of 1.50 D or less, and 90% corrections of 1.75 D or less. All eyes with final cylindrical corrections exceedingt 4.00 D had these cylinders before surgery. The overall average difference between the desired and actual final postoperative refraction obtained with the calculated lenses was 0.66 D. With

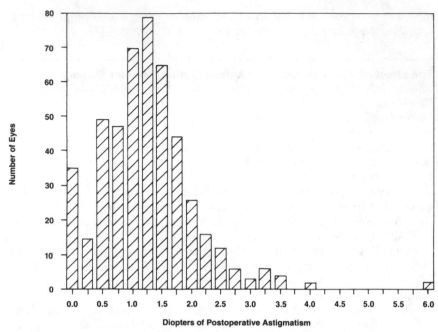

Fig 1–2.—Refractive cylinders 6–12 months postoperatively of all 477 eyes. (Courtesy of Story PG, Wiesner PD: *Ophthalmic Surg* 20:327–331, May 1989.)

standard lens implants the average difference would have been 1.19 D. The average power of the calculated posterior chamber implant was 21 D, and that of the anterior chamber implant was 17 D.

An estimated 40% of eyes with calculated lenses might be expected to see reasonably well at distance without glasses. A large number of eyes will have a postoperative refraction within 1.25 D of that predicted, and virtually all will stabilize within 2.00 D when biometric data and a lens formula are used.

Intraocular Lens Power Calculation: A Retrospective Analysis of Its Practical Value
Rouhiainen HJ (Univ Central Hosp of Kuopio, Finland)
Acta Ophthalmol (Copenh) 67:79–82, 1989   1–8

Although 80% of eyes have postoperative refraction within 2.00 D of predicted with various methods of predicting intraocular lens (IOL) power, the refraction sometimes deviates markedly from the predicted value. These eyes are characterized by a relatively short axial length.

Lens power predicted with the SRK method was analyzed in 202 consecutive IOL implantations. In this regression formula, power = A − 2.5 × AL − 0.9 × K, where the A-constant is 115 for anterior chamber lenses and 117 for posterior chamber lenses. Refractions were measured by retinoscopy a mean of 4.7 months postoperatively. The standard lens was 18 D for the anterior chamber and 20 D for the posterior chamber.

Errors in prediction were within 2 D in 84% of eyes and within 1 D in 59%. The mean difference between actual and predicted refractions was 0.59 D. The difference exceeded 3 D in 7% of eyes. The mean axial length was 23.2 mm; no 3-D errors occurred in 7 eyes with measured values exceeding 25 mm.

Preoperative IOL measurements serve to detect eyes where the IOL power needed to obtain emmetropia is not within the "normal" range. The risk of obtaining a high error is considerable when high astigmatism is measured preoperatively. Similar results could have been obtained in the present material by implanting standard-power lenses, and at present, these may be used unless a high refractive error not included by the cataractous lens is present.

▶ If these articles (Abstracts 1–7 and 1–8) are right, the IOL manufacturers should consider postponing the release of multifocal intraocular lenses. These IOLs require greater power accuracy because of incongruous focal ranges. Our current system of IOL power selection lacks sophistication to cope with multifocal lenses. Factors that induce postoperative refractive errors are preoperative data (biometry, keratometry, and AC depth measurement), position of the IOL in the eye (bag, sulcus, or combination bag-sulcus), manufacturing differences, and others.—R.E. Adams, M.D.

Atonic Pupil After Cataract Surgery
Lam S, Beck RW, Hall D, Creighton JB (Univ of South Florida, Tampa)
Ophthalmology 96:589–590, May 1989   1–9

A dilated, atonic pupil is an uncommon postoperative complication of cataract surgery. Seven patients with atonic pupils after cataract extraction were described.

The patients, 2 men and 5 women aged 55 to 75 years, had undergone uneventful extracapsular cataract extraction with implantation of an intraocular lens (IOL). All 7 patients had normal findings on preoperative pupil examinations. Six patients were given retrobulbar anesthesia with bupivacaine 0.75% and hyaluronidase, and 1 patient received lidocaine 4% and bupivacaine 0.75%. During surgery, all patients received sodium hyaluronate and acetylcholine chloride. After surgery, each patient was given a short course of topical corticosteroid therapy, and 3 patients were given topical antibiotics. None of the patients used cycloplegic drops.

One patient had a dilated pupil on the first postoperative day. The other 6 patients had normal pupils at the initial postoperative follow-up examination, but had atonic pupils after an average follow-up of 52.3 days or a median of 20.5 days. The atonic pupil was round and measured 5–7 mm in diameter. Testing with cycloplegic drops yielded normal pupil dilation, and no adhesions of the lens to the iris were noted. The lens was slightly decentered in 1 patient, but all other patients showed normal lens positions. Four patients underwent testing with pilocarpine 1% drops, which resulted in only slight or no pupillary constriction. One patient underwent fluorescein angiography, but the findings were normal.

That the pupils did not constrict with pilocarpine 1% suggests that the iris sphincter muscle itself, rather than a neurogenic cause, was responsible for the complication. However, the cause for the development of an atonic pupil after cataract extraction has not yet been identified. Operation in the treatment of postoperative atonic pupil is not indicated. This complication may be more common than was previously assumed.

▶ Iatrogenic iris trauma seems the most logical cause for a postoperative atonic pupil. Yet several colleagues have told me of a case of dilated pupil without iris trauma. This is a mystery.—R.E. Adams, M.D.

The Effect of Treatment With Topical Nonsteroidal Anti-Inflammatory Drugs With and Without Intraoperative Epinephrine on the Maintenance of Mydriasis During Cataract Surgery
Gimbel HV (Univ of Calgary, Alta)
Ophthalmology 96:585–588, May 1989   1–10

Maintaining mydriasis during extracapsular cataract extraction (ECCE) is essential to a successful outcome. Surgical trauma caused by manipulation of the iris is thought to release prostaglandins that constrict the iris sphincter independent of cholinergic or adrenergic receptors. Because nonsteroidal anti-inflammatory drugs (NSAIDs) inhibit prostaglandin synthesis, a study was done to determine whether preoperative treatment with topical NSAIDs can prevent or reduce surgically induced miosis.

The study population consisted of 216 patients who were undergoing uncomplicated ECCE with intraocular lens (IOL) implantation. Patients were randomly assigned to 1 of 6 treatment regimens, including preoperative flurbiprofen or indomethacin, with or without concurrent intraoperative epinephrine, epinephrine alone, or placebo alone. Pupil diameters were measured just before entering the anterior chamber and immediately after phacoemulsification and cortex aspiration.

The treatment groups that were given placebo, flurbiprofen, or indomethacin without epinephrine had average percentage decreases in pupil diameter ranging from 19% to 24%, whereas all epinephrine-treated groups had average percentage decreases ranging only from 0.75% to 2.6%. Thus, the main effect of epinephrine treatment was significant, regardless of NSAID pretreatment. The main effect of NSAID pretreatment was also significant in that indomethacin-treated patients had significantly less miosis than did placebo-treated patients. The group given flurbiprofen alone had no less miosis than did the placebo-treated group. However, when flurbiprofen was used in conjunction with epinephrine, an additive effect was noted, as the actual proportion of cases with any miosis was reduced. In addition, a larger proportion actually dilated further. Thus, the use of intraoperative epinephrine was by far the most effective factor in reducing progressive miosis, regardless of whether NSAIDs were used.

Either epinephrine continues to affect directly the adrenergic receptors while the effect of preoperative NSAIDs dissipates, or epinephrine exerts its effects by another mediator. Although the differences were small, the findings confirm an interaction between NSAIDs and epinephrine.

▶ Intraocular epinephrine in the irrigating fluid has been a significant factor in phacoemulsification. I routinely use preoperative NSAIDs to assist in maintenance of the mydriasis.—R.E. Adams, M.D.

Vitreous Loss Rates in Extracapsular Cataract Surgery by Residents
Pearson PA, Owen DG, Van Meter WS, Smith TJ (Univ of Kentucky; VA Hosp, Lexington, Ky)
Ophthalmology 96:1225–1227, August 1989   1–11

Vitreous loss as a complication of cataract operations is associated with an increased incidence of postoperative cystoid macular edema, corneal decompensation, retinal detachment, uveitis, and glaucoma. Previous surveys have shown that vitreous loss rates are increased in patients operated on by residents learning to perform extracapsular cataract extraction (ECCE). This retrospective review was done to evaluate the effectiveness of implementing a more rigid education program for ophthalmic surgery residents. Only operations in which a second- or third-year resident was the primary surgeon were included in the survey.

Between 1982 and 1988, 24 resident surgeons performed 936 ECCE procedures. Vitreous loss occurred in 64 cases, yielding an overall incidence of 6.8%. Before the educational program was revised in 1985, 13 surgeons performed 474 ECCE procedures of which 49 (10.3%) were complicated by vitreous loss. After 1985, 13 surgeons performed 462 operations, of which 15 (3.2%) resulted in vitreous loss. The difference was statistically significant.

When vitreous loss rates were tabulated for second-year residents only, the incidence of vitreous loss was 10.8% before 1985, 2.1% after 1985, and 6.7% for the overall 6-year period. The difference between vitreous loss rates of second- and third-year residents was statistically not significant.

Residents now practice surgery on cadaver eyes with an attending surgeon before performing their first operation on patients. In addition, residents now are given graded responsibility, that is, they are introduced more gradually to cataract operations by doing only small parts of the intraocular procedures during their first year, and by being given unlimited time for performing a cataract operation during their second year.

An educational program that includes practice surgery and graded responsibility can reduce dramatically the incidence of vitreous loss as a complication of ECCE among resident ophthalmic surgeons.

▶ In this day of quality assessment and peer review committees, this article presents reasonable percentages for vitreous loss. It is gratifying to read that education can improve technique and lessen surgical complications. I do not believe a "Weck-Cel" anterior vitrectomy is adequate to prevent postoperative cystoid macular edema or retinal detachment. A SITE or Outcome vitrectomy is my preference when faced with vitreous loss.—R.E. Adams, M.D.

Advanced Versus Immature Cataracts: A Preliminary Report
John ME, Edsell TD (John-Kenyon Eye Research Found, Jeffersonville, Ind)
Ann Ophthalmol 21:222–224, June 1989   1–12

A prospective clinical trial was carried out to determine whether extracapsular cataract extraction (ECCE) of cataracts that had reached an advanced state would be technically more difficult than the removal of immature cataracts, and if so, how this would affect postoperative outcome.

During 1985, ECCE was carried out in 529 eyes, 479 of which were evaluable. Of the 479 eyes, 63 had advanced cataracts and 416 had immature cataracts. The average preoperative visual acuity was less than 20/400 for the advanced cataract group, and 20/70 for the immature cataract group which served as a control. The average age of patients in the advanced cataract group was 68 years, and in the control group, 72 years. Small pupil size, corneal haze, moderate positive pressure, iris prolapse, zonulysis, capsule rent, vitreous loss, poor visibility, peripheral lacy or adherent cortex, and capsular tags were reasons for being classified as difficult.

Anterior capsulotomy was complete in 92% of eyes in the advanced group and in 98% of eyes in the control group. The difference was statistically not significant. Peripheral lacy cortex was present in 38% of the advanced group and in 1.2% of the control group. Cloudy capsules were found in 70% of the advanced group and in 20% of the control group. In the advanced group, 48% of the cases were considered difficult, compared with 17% of the control group. Vitreous loss occurred in 2 cases in the advanced group and in 1 case in the control group. After operation, 79% of the advanced cases had visual acuity of 20/40 or better, compared with 92% of the control patients. Thus, when removing advanced cataracts, the incidence of cloudy capsules and peripheral lacy cortex is higher, immediate postoperative vision is worse, and the operation is technically more difficult.

▶ Phacoemulsification of an immature ("soft") cataract is generally less traumatic to the eye than an advanced ("hard") cataract. The hard lens required more phaco-time, which increases potential damage to cornea, posterior capsule, or retina (via vitreous loss). Nevertheless, surgery is not to be carried out unless the standard criteria are followed, that is, the cataract interferes with life style or vision is 20/50 or less.   R.E. Adams, M.D.

Traumatic Wound Dehiscence in Pseudophakia

Johns KJ, Sheils P, Parrish CM, Elliott JH, O'Day DM (Vanderbilt Univ Med Ctr; Nashville VA Med Ctr, Nashville, Tenn)
Am J Ophthalmol 108:535–539, November 1989   1–13

Eleven pseudophakic patients were seen after sustaining wound dehiscence secondary to blunt trauma. Nine had undergone planned extracapsular cataract extraction, and 2 had intracapsular extraction. Seven patients had posterior chamber lenses in place at the time of injury, whereas 4 had anterior chamber lenses. Injuries occurred up to a year after surgery. A fall was most often responsible. Nine of the patients had a best corrected acuity of 20/60 or better before injury.

Iris prolapse was a constant finding; in 6 cases the iris was structurally damaged. Four patients had vitreous prolapse, and 3 had retinal detachment. Seven patients had hyphema. In 5 patients the intraocular lens was dislocated. One lens was fractured, and 2 were expulsed. Six patients had a final visual acuity of 20/40 or better. Two others had acuity of less than 20/200 because of retinal detachment.

The altered tensile strength of a limbal cataract wound dispose to dehiscence after blunt ocular trauma. An implant that is fibrosed into position theoretically, can structurally support the open eye. Today a smaller limbal incision is made, and improved suture material and methods are available. An extruded lens should not be replaced, and a fractured lens should be removed. Ophthalmologists must inform their patients about the need to use protective eyewear after cataract surgery, not only shortly after the operation, but whenever there is a threat of ocular injury.

▶ Wearing safety glasses or a shield is the single most important factor in preventing wound dehiscence. The second may be wound placement and size. Phacoemulsification, small scleral pocket wound, anterior entry into the anterior chamber, and running sutures would be my guess as important preventive steps. Theoretically, in third place may be the soft intraocular lens (silicone or other). This IOL may bend or flex under external pressure or blows better than a rigid PMMA lens. No statistics are available at this time. Wounds always will undergo dehiscence in certain groups, such as the 250+-LB truck driver after lifting lumber from a flatbed truck or the poorly nourished alcoholic patient who falls frequently. For those who thrive on calamity, we have those who are promoting the "1-stitch" or "no-stitch" wound closures!—R.E. Adams, M.D.

Heparin Surface Modified Intraocular Lenses Implanted in the Monkey Eye

Fagerholm P, Björklund H, Holmberg Å, Larsson R, Lydahl E, Philipson B, Selén G (Karolinska Inst, Stockholm; Pharmacia Ophthalmics AB, Uppsala, Sweden)
J Cataract Refract Surg 15:485–490, September 1989   1–14

There is evidence that polymethyl methacrylate (PMMA) is less inert than initially thought and that some degree of foreign body reaction consistently occurs after lens implantation. A new type of PMMA lens had heparin bound covalently to the lens surface; the surface is hydrophilic and does not readily accept cell attachment in vitro. One-piece lenses were placed in the anterior and posterior chambers of adult cynomolgus monkey eyes and the animals killed after 12 weeks.

Very little inflammation was present a day after lens implantation. Significantly more cellular precipitate was present on the optic of control lenses than on heparin surface-modified lenses at 3 weeks and thereafter. Synechia formation generally was more prominent in control cases. The histologic findings confirmed the clinical observations. The local cellular reaction around the haptics was similar in both groups of animals.

The heparin surface-modified intraocular lens appears to limit accumulation of inflammatory precipitate on the lens surface, as well as synechia formation. The hydrophobic nature of normal PMMA might promote better cellular attachment on the lens surface, enhancing synechia formation. It is likely that the modified lenses will prove useful for limiting problems after cataract surgery and intraocular lens implantation.

▶ Intraocular lens surface modifications and ultraviolet blockers are difficult issues to determine their "true" benefits; more so when manufacturers suggest their lenses are better because of it. Although this article does not imply this, I have yet to be convinced of any value.—R.E. Adams, M.D.

Legal Blindness Can Be Compatible With Safe Driving

Fonda G (St Barnabas Low Vision Ctr, West Orange, NJ)
Ophthalmology 96:1457–1459, October 1989   1–15

Legal blindness is a best-corrected acuity of 20/200 in the better eye or a field of vision 20 degrees or less in maximal field. Evidence that this condition is compatible with safe driving was sought in a study of 8 patients, 3 of them visually impaired by Stargardt's disease. If acuity was not 20/200 without correction it was blurred to this level by spectacles with convex lenses. The subjects approached traffic sign symbols while driving on a clear day. They recognized the symbols at a distance within which—according to the standards of the U.S. Bureau of Public Roads— a vehicle traveling at 40 mph can stop safely.

Drivers with subnormal levels of central visual acuity are able to drive safely, as is recognized by several states. The literature does not demonstrate that more accidents occur with drivers having 20/200 vision than with those having acuity of 20/40. The present study found that a person with 20/200 acuity can recognize the average stop sign at 228 feet. Yellow signs are recognized from farther away than red signs.

▶ The driving requirement of 20/40 or 20/50 for daytime to obtain a private vehicle operators license is an arbitrary standard. As ophthalmologists, we should push for the addition of glare testing as part of the motor vehicle visual testing. This examination is simple and practical. It would uncover visual problems relative to eye disease, especially cataract. Drivers who pass the usual vision test may have real-life vision of 20/400 or 20/200 when exposed to glare.—R.E. Adams, M.D.

Is Padding Necessary After Cataract Extraction?

Laws DE, Watts MT, Kirkby GR, Lawson J (Birmingham and Midland Eye Hosp, England)
Br J Ophthalmol 73:699–701, 1989   1–16

Because eye pads are used routinely after cataract surgery, eyes dressed only with a cartella shield were prospectively compared with those dressed with petroleum jelly mesh, a gauze pad, and a shield. Forty-two consecutively seen patients scheduled for extracapsular cataract extraction with intraocular lens implantation participated in the study.

Discharge was less frequent in unpadded eyes. One padded patient had a slight wound leak that closed spontaneously, and 1 in the unpadded group had a small corneal abrasion. Lid and conjunctival cultures showed little difference in the prevalence of commensals postoperatively in the 2 groups. With 1 exception, pathogens were eliminated by antibiotic prophylaxis.

It is possible that the moist atmosphere beneath a gauze pad provides an ideal culture medium. A plastic shield alone provides as good mechanical protection as a gauze pad and shield.

▶ I believe it is better to pad the operative eye because the patch "reminds" the patient to keep their fingers out of the operative eye by trapping the excessive tearing. However, continued padding after 24 hours may increase the risk of an ocular infection, especially in diabetic patients. Finally, not using eye pads at surgery is most unsettling to the patients' relatives.—R.E. Adams, M.D.

Warfarin and Cataract Extraction

Robinson GA, Nylander A (Univ Hosp of Wales, Cardiff)
Br J Ophthalmol 73:702–703, September 1989   1–17

Can warfarin therapy safely be continued in patients undergoing cataract extraction? Ten patients treated with anticoagulation therapy were operated on, 6 under general and 4 under local anesthesia. Eight patients had extracapsular cataract extraction, 6 with posterior chamber lens implantation. Two others had endocapsular extraction and received a posterior chamber lens. Indications for anticoagulation included cardiac valve replacement, thrombosis, and atrial fibrillation.

None of the 4 patients receiving local anesthesia had retrobulbar hemorrhage. Three hyphemas occurred, but none of the 3 diabetic patients developed hyphema. Hyphema did not occur in 3 cases where corneal sections were used.

Warfarin frequently is withheld before and after ocular surgery, but serious systemic complications can result. Two of the 3 hyphemas that occurred in the present series were mild and did not compromise the final outcome. Local anesthesia could be modified to avoid retrobulbar injection in these cases. In addition, iridectomy and iris suture can be avoided, sodium hyaluronate used, and lens loops placed in the capsular bag to prevent erosion into the ciliary sulcus.

▶ This is a topic of recurring interest for which more data are desirable. The authors are unclear as to type of wound that bled (limbal or scleral?). I find hyphema rates are around 5% with scleral (pocket) wounds. Also, it is my impression that British surgeons perform clear corneal wounds more than Americans do. Instead of using a corneal wound, I stop coumadin therapy 3 to 5 days before surgery and resume it on postoperative day 5. If this is medically inadvisable, the patient is admitted 48 hours before surgery, coumadin treatment is stopped, and heparin therapy is started and then stopped the night before. A final bleeding time measurement is repeated before surgery. If the time is normal, surgery proceeds; if it is prolonged, the case is placed at the end of the schedule or postponed to the next day. Postoperatively the patient is held 24 to 48 hours to reestablish the coumadin level. This sounds complicated, but it is routine for the interest.—R.E. Adams, M.D.

2 Cornea

Cornea and External Disease

Elisabeth J. Cohen, M.D.
Cornea Service, Wills Eye Hospital, Philadelphia, Pennsylvania

Three aspects of corneal and external disease that deserve emphasis in a review of 1989 are ocular infections associated with sexually transmitted diseases, computer-assisted corneal topography, and contact lens–associated microbial keratitis. Although the cornea is not the usual ocular target of infections in AIDS patients, sexually transmitted diseases are receiving increased attention. Computerized corneal topography systems provide interesting information about corneal shape in various diseases and after surgery. Clinical applications of topographic analysis are evolving but lag behind research usefulness. The long-awaited studies sponsored by the Contact Lens Institute on the relative risk and incidence of contact lens–associated ulcerative keratitis among wearers of extended-wear versus daily-wear cosmetic soft lenses have been published. The increased risk of extended wear is not a surprise, but the lack of statistical significance of lens hygiene is a bit unexpected.

Sexually Transmitted Diseases

A major change in the management of external ocular infections has occurred in the treatment of adult gonococcal conjunctivitis. Until recently, standard treatment was a 5-day course of intravenous penicillin or, more recently, intramuscular or intravenous ceftriaxone. A single dose of ceftriaxone, 1 g intramuscular, recently has been shown to be adequate therapy for non-neonatal gonococcal conjunctivitis (1, 2; Abstract 2–6). The Centers for Disease Control now recommend this regimen for adults (in U.S. Government Printing Office Publication no. 1990-732-160).

This treatment regimen allows for the possibility of outpatient treatment of adults with gonococcal conjunctivitis without corneal infiltrates. One must be sure, however, that patients receiving treatment as outpatients will return the next day for necessary follow-up examination and cultures. If patient reliability is a concern, inpatient therapy is preferable.

People with corneal involvement should be hospitalized and receive ceftriaxone intramuscularly for the previously standard 5-day course. Neonates also need a 7-day course of parenteral ceftriaxone or cefotaxime. Topical antibiotic therapy is inadequate and unnecessary. However, it seems reasonable to give patients with conjunctivitis topical antibiotics such as erythromycin or bacitracin. Patients with corneal ulcers should be given fortified antibiotics.

Oral norfloxacin (1,200 mg) for 1 to 3 days also has been shown to be effective for adult gonococcal keratoconjunctivitis (3). This, however, is not standard treatment in the United States. Soon, an increasing role for norfloxacin and other quinolones may evolve in the treatment of external ocular infections.

It is interesting that neonatal ocular prophylaxis with erythromycin or tetracycline ointment was not shown to be more effective than silver nitrate in preventing ophthalmia neonatorum caused by chlamydia (4; Abstract 2–1). Once again, well-designed studies are necessary to determine optimal therapy. The *New England Journal of Medicine* remains useful reading for ophthalmologists.

It is interesting that herpes simplex keratitis in AIDS patients is more like primary than recurrent epithelial infections with regard to having a prolonged course, peripheral location, and the absence of stromal involvement (5; Abstract 3–8). Atypical presentation of common diseases as well as uncommon infections should make one consider the possibility of systemic immunocompromise. Depression of immunoresponsiveness is associated with reduced inflammatory manifestations of herpes simplex keratitis that result in scarring and loss of vision.

That an alcohol wipe is sufficient to disinfect tonometer tips of HIV and HSV viruses is reassuring (6; Abstract 2–21). It is important to know that simply wiping the tonometer tip with gauze is ineffective. We must perform this simple but necessary step routinely before or after examining all patients, or both.

Corneal Topography

Corneal topographic analysis provides interesting information about irregular astigmatism associated with diseases and after surgery. Computerized systems provide impressive color-coded maps, but it is not clear how much the practicing clinician will benefit from these sophisticated and expensive systems compared with simpler photokeratoscopes (or corneoscopes). The computerized systems may remain research tools while the simpler corneoscopes are used increasingly to aid clinical practice.

Corneoscope photographs can be used for patient education. It is helpful to show corneoscope photos to keratoconus patients. One can explain that the photos are analogous to contour maps and that where the lines are closer together the cornea is steeper and where the lines are further apart, the cornea is flatter. Use of corneoscope photos can make it easier for patients to understand why glasses cannot be expected to correct vision maximally and why a rigid gas contact lens is necessary to create a regular spherical surface.

Corneoscopy or keratoscopy is helpful in selective removal of sutures after penetrating keratoplasty (7; Abstract 2–17). I think that it is helpful to combine various sources of information in decision making, including visual acuity, manifest refraction keratometry, and corneoscopy. Corneoscopy is particularly helpful when the visual acuity cannot be improved by manifest refraction and the keratometry mires are irregular. However, when the manifest refraction and keratometry measurements are clear and consistent they can provide information sufficient to suggest the meridian for suture removal. Careful slit lamp biomicroscopy also can help to determine which suture or sutures along a particular meridian are tight. Corneoscopy may show irregular topography despite good visual acuity. In the absence of visual complaints, sutures should be left in place. However, visual complaints despite good visual acuity may be caused by irregular topography. It would be interesting to correlate visual acuity, topographic analysis, and the results of contrast sensitivity and glare testing, especially when the visual acuity is good.

Contact Lens—Associated Microbial Keratitis

Studies supported by the Contact Lens Institute show that people using cosmetic extended-wear soft lenses overnight have approximately a 10 times greater risk of corneal ulcers than people using daily wear lenses on a daily basis (8; Abstract 2—11). The increased risk begins with the first night of overnight wear and increases progressively. One cannot conclude that overnight wear is safe up to 7 days and unsafe thereafter, despite the manufacturers' and FDA's recommendation to limit extended wear to 7 days. People wearing cosmetic soft lenses need education about the relative risks so that they can make informed decisions. The incidence figures appear low, but because of the millions of people wearing cosmetic soft contact lenses, they represent an annual estimate of 12,000 corneal ulcers per year among these people (9; Abstract 2—12).

It is interesting that lens hygiene was only almost significant in the relative risk study. Poor lens hygiene is widespread among lens wearers with and without ulcers (8, 10). One hopes disposable lenses will be safer than conventional extended-wear lenses, but this remains unproven. Ulcers have been associated with disposable lenses and have been seen by us (11). The risk associated with overnight wear remains for people wearing disposable lenses despite the advantages of reduced lens care and problems of contaminated solutions.

Acanthamoeba keratitis remains an uncommon nightmare. The epidemiology of just more than 200 cases shows that soft lens wear and use of homemade saline are associated with most but not all cases (12; Abstract 2—7). Treatment remains extremely problematic without major new breakthroughs. Prevention is the best approach to the problem. Elimination of tap water rinsing of contact lenses seems appropriate but is controversial.

References

1. Ullman S, Rousel TJ, Calbertson WW, et al: *Neisseria gonorrhoeae* keratoconjunctivitis. *Ophthalmology* 94:524, 1987.
2. Haimovici R, Rousel TJ: Treatment of gonococcal conjunctivitis with single-dose intramuscular ceftriaxone. *Am J Ophthalmol* 107:511, 1989.
3. Kestelyn P, Bogaerts J, Stevens AM: Treatment of adult gonococcal keratoconjunctivitis with oral norfloxacin. *Am J Ophthalmol* 108:516, 1989.
4. Hammerschlag MR, Cummings C, Roblin PM, et al: Efficacy of neonatal ocular prophylaxis for the prevention of chlamydial and gonococcal conjunctivitis. *N Engl J Med* 320:769, 1989.

5. Young TL, Robin JB, Holland GN, et al: Herpes simplex keratitis in patients with acquired immune deficiency syndrome. *Ophthalmology* 96:1476, 1989.
6. Pepose JS, Linette G, Lee SF, et al: Disinfection of Goldmann tonometers against human immunodeficiency virus type 1. *Arch Ophthalmol* 107:983, 1989.
7. Harris DJ, Waring GO III, Bank LL: Keratography as a guide to selective suture removal for the reduction of astigmatism after penetrating keratoplasty. *Ophthalmology* 96:1597–1607, 1987.
8. Schein OD, Glynn RJ, Poggio EC, et al: The relative risk of ulcerative keratitis among users of daily wear and extended wear soft contact lenses. A case control study. *N Engl J Med* 321:773, 1989.
9. Poggio EC, Glynn RJJ, Schein OD, et al: The incidence of ulcerative keratitis among users of daily wear and extended wear soft contact lenses. *N Engl J Med* 321:779, 1989.
10. Bowden FW III, Coheen EJ, Arentsen JJ, et al: Patterns of lens care practices and lens product contamination in contact lens-associated microbial keratitis. *CLAO J* 15:49, 1989.
11. Dunn JR Jr, Mondino BJ, Weissman BA, et al: Corneal ulcers associated with disposable hydrogel contact lenses. *Am J Ophthalmol* 108:113, 1989.
12. Stehr-Green JK, Bailey TM, Visvesvara GS: The epidemiology of *Acanthamoeba* keratitis in the United States. *Am J Ophthalmol* 107:331, 1989.

Efficacy of Neonatal Ocular Prophylaxis for the Prevention of Chlamydial and Gonococcal Conjunctivitis

Hammerschlag MR, Cummings C, Roblin PM, Williams TH, Delke I (State Univ of New York, Brooklyn)
N Engl J Med 320:769–772, March 23, 1989   2–1

The altered epidemiology of neonatal conjunctivitis invites the question of whether silver nitrate still is adequate. The efficacy of erythromycin and tetracycline ophthalmic ointments was compared with that of silver nitrate drops in a large urban population of infants.

Gonococcal ophthalmia occurred in 8 of 12,431 infants born during the study. Differences in the various prophylaxis groups were not significant. Seven of the 8 infants were born to women who had not received prenatal care. Cervical cultures for *Chlamydia* were positive for 8% of 4,357 women screened in a 2-year period. Among the 230 infants evaluated for chlamydial conjunctivitis, incidences were 20% with silver nitrate prophylaxis, 14% with erythromycin ointment, and 11% with tetracycline ointment.

All these prophylactic regimens appear to be effective. The most important way of preventing neonatal gonococcal ophthalmia may well be prenatal screening and treatment of maternal gonorrhea. Similarly, chlamydial ophthalmia may be controlled most effectively by screening and treatment of pregnant women. The choice of prophylaxis rests in part on cost and the desire to avoid chemical conjunctivitis.

▶ Because chlamydia infection is responsive to systemic treatment with tetracycline and erythromycin, one would have thought that prophylaxis of newborns with these antibiotics would be much more effective than silver nitrate against *Chlamydia*. It is apparent from this large study, however, that none of these agents entirely prevents ophthalmia neonatorum caused by *Chlamydia*. Screening and appropriate systemic treatment of pregnant women is necessary to eliminate ophthalmia neonatorum caused by *Chlamydia* and gonococcal infection.   E.J. Cohen, M.D.

The Use of Contact Lenses After Keratoconic Epikeratoplasty
Lembach RG, Lass JH, Stocker EG, Keates RH (Ohio State Univs, Columbus; Case Western Reserve Univ; Univ Hosps of Cleveland)
Arch Ophthalmol 107:364–368, March 1989   2–2

Keratonic epikeratoplasty is a possible alternative for keratoconic patients who are intolerant of contact lenses. Thirty-one such patients had 33 epikeratoplasties, 32 of which succeeded anatomically in producing a clear lenticule and a flatter cornea. In 1 case the lenticule developed a persistent epithelial defect requiring its removal; later, penetrating keratoplasty was done successfully.

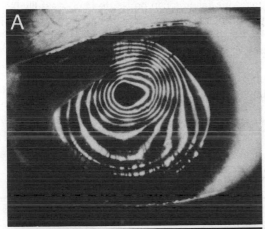

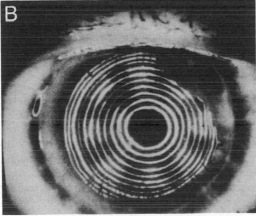

Fig 2–1.—A, preoperative photokeratoscopic photograph demonstrating irregular astigmatism. B, 2-month postoperative photokeratoscopic photograph of same patient demonstrating correction of irregular astigmatism. (Courtesy of Lembach RG, Lass JH, Stocker EG, et al: *Arch Ophthalmol* 107:364–368, March 1989.)

Twenty of the anatomically successful eyes achieved satisfactory visual improvement, requiring either no correction or spectacle lenses (Fig 2–1). Twelve other eyes were refitted successfully with contact lenses for anisometropic refractive error or, in 1 instance, residual irregular astigmatism. Three patients have since had penetrating keratoplasty to gain further improvement in vision. In the contact lens wearers the lens base curve flattened significantly after operation, but lens power did not change significantly.

In the minority of keratoconic epikeratoplasty patients who fail to achieve satisfactory visual results unaided or with spectacles, contact lens wear may be resumed effectively. Presumably, the altered corneal curvature provides a more suitable surface for contact lens fitting. The single major complication in this series was a persistent epithelial defect of the lenticule.

▶ The role of epikeratoplasty for keratoconus is uncertain. Rigid contact lenses are successful in more than 90% of keratoconus patients. Even the majority of people who are considered contact lens failures can be refitted successfully by experienced fitters. Penetrating keratoplasty for keratoconus has a greater than 95% success rate with excellent visual results. Keratoconus patients must have intolerance of contact lenses with no central scarring to be candidates for epikeratoplasty. On the basis of data presented to the FDA, the Ophthalmic Device Panel recommended approval for epikeratoplasty for keratoconus only when contact lenses fail and penetrating keratoplasty is contraindicated. Further study of epikeratoplasty for keratoconus is needed to determine its place in management.— E.J. Cohen, M.D.

Drug Binding of Ophthalmic Viscoelastic Agents
McDermott ML, Edelhauser HF (Med College of Wisconsin, Milwaukee)
Arch Ophthalmol 107:261–263, February 1989   2–3

When viscoelastic agents containing hyaluronate are used in anterior segment surgery, some material often remains in the eye, and various intracameral or topical drugs may bind to the polyanionic hyaluronate molecule. Because this may lead to altered therapeutic efficacy or drug toxicity, in vitro drug-binding studies were done on 3 viscoelastic agents.

Aliquots of Amvisc, Healon, and Viscoat were mixed with radiolabeled D-threo-chloramphenicol, dexamethasone, L-epinephrine, and pilocarpine, and the mixtures were dialyzed for 24 hours against isotonic phosphate buffer. Drug binding by the viscoelastic agents ranged from zero to 1.5%. Epinephrine was the drug most bound by all the viscoelastic agents.

It seems unlikely that any significant interaction between ophthalmic drugs and viscoelastic agents occurs in the postoperative eye. The viscoelastic drugs also do not prevent equilibrium, meaning that the drugs diffuse freely through the viscoelastic polymer network.

▶ Use of viscoelastic agents has improved the safety of intraocular surgery, especially involving intraocular lenses. It is important to evaluate interactions of these commonly used substances with other agents used during eye surgery. That this study suggests significant drug interactions do not occur is encouraging.—E.J. Cohen, M.D.

Immunohistologic Findings and Results of Treatment With Cyclosporine in Ligneous Conjunctivitis
Holland EJ, Chan C-C, Kuwabara T, Palestine AG, Rowsey JJ, Nussenblatt RB
(Univ of Minnesota; Natl Eye Inst, Bethesda, Md; Univ of Oklahoma)
Am J Ophthalmol 107:160–166, February 1989   2–4

Ligneous conjunctivitis is a rare chronic disorder of recurrent membranous lesions, usually starting in childhood. Treatment generally has been ineffective. Conjunctival lesions from 2 patients were examined immunohistochemically and, after other treatment had failed, excisional biopsy and topical cyclosporine were tried.

The lesions (Fig 2–2) had a significant immune reaction with activated T lymphocytes and the focal accumulation of both plasma cells and B lymphocytes. Immunofluorescence study showed that immunoglobulin G (IgG) was a prominent component of the amorphous hyaline material in the lesions. One patient had a dramatic response to treatment; the other had significant improvement. In the latter case small, slow-growing recurrences replaced the extensive, rapidly occurring ones seen before cyclosporine therapy. Inflammatory infiltration was less marked after treatment, and T lymphocytes—especially suppressor–cytotoxic cells—were less numerous than before.

Ligneous conjunctivitis may be caused partly by an exaggerated inflammatory response to conjunctival epithelial injury. The hyaline material may result from release of IgG by plasma cells or IgG in serum leaking from neovascularization. Cyclosporine acts by interfering with T lymphocyte activation.

▶ Ligneous conjunctivitis is an uncommon problem that tends to be refractory to available treatment. Cyclosporine has been used systemically for a variety of immunologic problems, including prevention of organ transplant rejection. It is interesting to note that topical cyclosporine was helpful in treatment of 2 cases of ligneous conjunctivitis. In the future, topical cyclosporine may prove beneficial in a variety of inflammatory ocular diseases.—E.J. Cohen, M.D.

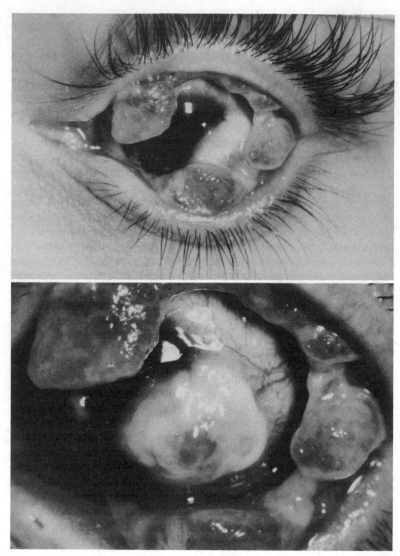

Fig 2–2.—Patient before cyclosporine treatment. **Top,** extensive ligneous lesions of the superior and inferior palpebral conjunctiva. **Bottom,** ligneous lesion of the bulbar conjunctiva extending over the lateral third of the cornea. (Courtesy of Holland EJ, Chan C-C, Kuwabara T, et al: *Am J Ophthalmol* 107:160–166, February 1989.)

Patterns of Lens Care Practices and Lens Product Contamination in Contact Lens Associated Microbial Keratitis

Bowden FW III, Cohen EJ, Arentsen JJ, Laibson PR (Wills Eye Hosp, Philadelphia)

CLAO J 15:49–54, January 1989   2–5

Microbial keratitis remains a serious complication of contact lens use, especially for those using daily or extended-wear soft lenses. In a prospective study of 24 patients with culture- or histopathology-proved microbial keratitis, bacterial cultures were done for lenses, lens cases, and solutions and the patients were asked in detail about lens care practices.

Only 3 of the 24 patients complied fully with standard recommendations for contact lens care. Bacterial contamination of the lens, case, or solutions was found in 20 instances. Fifteen patients used solutions more than 3 months old. Seven of 8 cosmetic users of extended-wear lenses used old solutions, and 6 of the 8 had contaminated solutions. *Pseudomonas* was the most frequently isolated organism. Some patients apparently believed that enzymatic cleaning constituted disinfection. Often patients had continued to use their lenses despite ocular injection and discomfort in the past.

Improper lens care and contaminated lens care products were prominent factors in microbial keratitis in this prospective study. The use of solutions more than 3 months old was prevalent. Perhaps labels should advise limiting solution use to 2 to 8 weeks after opening. Persons who persistently are noncompliant should be encouraged to stop wearing soft contact lenses.

▶ Improper lens care and contamination of contact lens solutions likely are predisposing factors in corneal ulcers among people wearing contact lenses. Use of solutions that have been open more than 3 months probably increases the likelihood of exposure to contaminated solutions and should be discouraged. Ophthalmologists should educate their lens-wearing patients about proper lens care and the possibility of serious infection.—E.J. Cohen, M.D.

Treatment of Gonococcal Conjunctivitis With Single-Dose Intramuscular Ceftriaxone

Haimovici R, Roussel TJ (Univ of Miami)
Am J Ophthalmol 107:511–514, May 1989   2–6

Ocular infection by *Neisseria gonorrhoeae* can lead to ulcerative keratitis and perforation unless promptly treated. Single-dose intramuscular (IM) injections of ceftriaxone, a third-generation cephalosporin, were used to treat 13 consecutive adult patients with culture-proved *N. gonorrhoeae* conjunctivitis. A single conjunctival saline lavage was carried out, and follow-up conjunctival cultures were made 6 and 12 hours after treatment. The dose was 1 gm, or 50 mg/kg in patients weighing less than 20 kg.

The patients had purulent discharge, conjunctival injection and chemosis, and lid edema. Four had punctate corneal epithelial erosions, but no patient had infiltration of the corneal stroma. Three of the isolates produced penicillinase. All 13 patients had responses to treatment, and all posttreatment cultures were negative for *N. gonorrhoeae.*

A single IM injection of ceftriaxone reliably cures non-neonatal gonococcal conjunctivitis. Repeated IM or IV antibiotic injections, conjunctival saline lavage, and topical antibiotics are not necessary, nor is hospitalization beyond 24 hours necessary or cost-effective. Most patients probably can be treated on an outpatient basis. Those with corneal stromal infiltration, however, should be admitted and receive more intensive treatment.

▶ This study recommends that the management of gonococcal conjunctivitis in adults without corneal involvement be changed significantly away from inpatient intravenous antibiotics treatment for 5 days and toward outpatient treatment with a single injection of ceftriaxone. One must be cautious about changing management because gonococcal conjunctivitis can evolve rapidly into a perforated corneal ulcer and because patients with venereal diseases may not always be reliable in their follow-up care.

In this study, patients were admitted overnight, and I think this practice should probably be continued to ensure that patients are evaluated after treatment and are responding well. The revised recommendations of the Centers for Disease Control for the treatment of gonococcal conjunctivitis in adults, to be published in the fall of 1989, will include a single IM injection of 1 of ceftriaxone.

It is also important to remember to screen gonococcal conjunctivitis patients for other sexually transmitted diseases, including chlamydia, syphilis, and HIV infection.—E.J. Cohen, M.D.

The Epidemiology of *Acanthamoeba* Keratitis in the United States
Stehr-Green JK, Bailey TM, Visvesvara GS (Ctrs for Disease Control, Atlanta)
Am J Ophthalmol 107:331–336, April 1989   2–7

Acanthamoeba keratitis has been associated with penetrating corneal injury and exposure to contaminated water, but contact lens wear now is associated most commonly with this disease. The authors explored the epidemiology of this form of keratitis by surveying the Ocular Microbiology and Immunology Group and reviewing laboratory requests at the CDC.

Cases of *Acanthamoeba* keratitis totaled 208. The number increased gradually from 1981 to 1984 and then increased dramatically starting in 1985. Forty-one percent of infected patients lived in California, Texas, Florida, or Pennsylvania (Fig 2–3). All but 15% of patients wore contact lenses, mainly daily-wear or extended-wear soft lenses. About two thirds of evaluable patients used saline prepared by dissolving salt tablets in distilled water. A history of trauma was most frequent among older patients and among males.

Contact lens wear is the chief risk factor for *Acanthamoeba* keratitis in the United States. Wearers may be less meticulous than before in handling their lenses, or they may receive less than adequate instruction in proper lens care. The use of homemade saline solution should be discouraged.

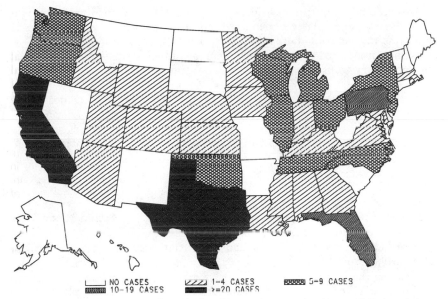

Fig 2–3.—United States *Acanthamoeba* keratitis cases by state of residence, 1973 through June 1988. (Courtesy of Stehr-Green JK, Bailey TM, Visvesvara GS: *Am J Opthalmol* 107:331–336, April 1989.)

▶ *Acanthamoeba* keratitis remains an uncommon but devastating problem. This epidemiologic study by the CDC documents the past and present scope of the problem. There is no question that homemade saline and distilled water should never be used for care of soft contact lenses.   E.J. Cohen, M.D.

The Use of Cyclosporine in High-Risk Keratoplasty
Hill JC (Groote Schuur Hosp, Cape Town; Univ of Cape Town, South Africa)
Am J Ophthalmol 107:506–510, May 1989   2–8

A study of high-risk keratoplasty patients served to compare the effects of topical corticosteroids only, topical and systemic corticosteroids, and systemic cyclosporine added to topical and systemic corticosteroids. Many of the patients previously had rejected corneal grafts, and all had acuity less than 20/200 in the affected eye.

All patients received topical 0.1% dexamethasone drops after surgery. Systemic steroid therapy consisted of 125 mg of methylprednisolone, given intravenously after operation, and 25 mg prednisone for 1 month followed by tapering. Cyclosporine was given orally to maintain a blood level of 250 to 400 µg/L.

Only 2 of 19 grafts in patients given topical corticosteroids only survived, as did 1 of 20 grafts in patients given both topical and systemic steroids. In contrast, 16 of 18 grafts in cyclosporine-treated patients survived. No patient had permanent side effects from cyclosporine therapy.

Systemic cyclosporine has significantly improved corneal graft survival in high-risk keratoplasty patients compared with local or combined local and systemic steroid therapy. Cyclosporine therapy is relatively safe if carefully monitored to detect early liver or kidney damage. It probably is not necessary to use systemic steroids concomitantly.

▶ Cyclosporine may prove to be useful for patients undergoing corneal transplantation who are at high risk for rejection. Multicenter, randomized clinical trials are needed to determine the value of systemic or topical cyclosporine in high-risk graft patients. This treatment represents a new direction in the management of these graft patients, in contrast to studies evaluating the role of HLA-matched tissue.—E.J. Cohen, M.D.

Corneal Topography of Transverse Keratotomies for Astigmatism After Penetrating Keratoplasty

Maguire LJ, Bourne WM (Mayo Found, Rochester, Minn)
Am J Ophthalmol 107:323–330, April 1989   2–9

Transverse keratotomy is a means of correcting postkeratoplasty astigmatism; however, the management of patients with irregular corneal to-

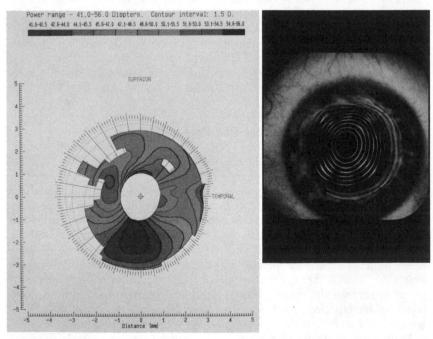

Fig 2–4.—Left, corneal topography contour map, and **right,** keratoscope photograph from which it was generated before corneal relaxing incision. Note how the surface differs from a classic spherocylindrical optical pattern. Steep hemimeridians are not separated by 180 degrees, asymmetry of power exists between the 2 steep areas, and a large area of high power extends superonasally. (Courtesy of Maguire LJ, Bourne WM: *Am J Ophthalmol* 107:323–330, April 1989.)

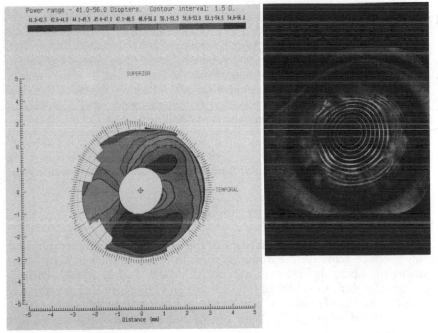

Fig 2–5.—Left, contour map, and **right**, keratoscope photograph 1 day after paired transverse keratotomy. A comparison with the preoperative power map shown in Figure 2–4 shows that power is reduced in the areas where the incisions were placed based on visual inspection of the keratoscope photographs but persists in the superonasal area. (Courtesy of Maguire LJ, Bourne WM: *Am J Ophthalmol* 107:323–330, April 1989.)

pography and high astigmatism may be problematic. The authors used a computer-based analysis system, the Louisiana State University topography system, to measure surface power at hundreds of points on the corneal surface (Figs 2–4 and 2–5). The computer-based system was used to assess 6 patients having high postkeratoplasty astigmatism. All relaxing incisions had been placed by visual inspection of keratoscope mires alone.

Preoperative topography indicated considerable individual variation in the degree of surface irregularity. The steep axis of the graft was best conceived of as 2 steep hemimeridians. In 2 cases these were separated by an angle other than 180 degrees. In 3 cases there was a fairly large change in power from the most central to peripheral areas of the graft. Asymmetry of power between the 2 steep meridians was noted in all cases. Areas of maximal steepening often were present in the peripheral regions of the graft in areas other than the major hemimeridians.

Visual inspection of keratoscope photographs does not demonstrate the surface optics in enough detail to allow reasonable decisions on the placement of incisions, especially in patients with very irregular preoperative topography. It is hoped the regular use of computer-based topographic analysis will reduce refractive variability after the placement of relaxing incisions.

▶ Computerized analysis of corneal topography is providing interesting new information that should aid in planning interventions and evaluating their results in the management of corneal astigmatism and refractive disorders. This new modality is increasing our understanding of corneal topography. It is likely to have many clinically relevant applications in the future.—E.J. Cohen, M.D.

Ophthalmic Solutions, the Ocular Surface, and a Unique Therapeutic Artificial Tear Formulation
Gilbard JP, Rossi SR, Heyda KG (Harvard Med School)
Am J Ophthalmol 107:348–355, April 1989   2–10

Present ophthalmic solutions deplete the conjunctiva of goblet cells and may produce gross surface abnormalities. In rabbit models of keratoconjunctivitis sicca, the changes are noted nearly 1 year before corneal changes develop. Eyes bathed for 12 hours in Hypotears, Tears Naturale, and Refresh had markedly abnormal gross appearances. Goblet cells were depleted substantially. With Unisol and BSS, the changes were less prominent.

An electrolyte solution was developed that preserves normal gross appearances, goblet cell density, and corneal epithelial glycogen levels. An artificial tear formulation was made by adding a demulcent and a buffering system and lowering the osmolarity of the solution to 162 mOsm/L. In a double-blind comparison with Hypotears in 11 patients with dry eye disorders, the new formulation was more effective in reducing tear film osmolarity and rose bengal staining, and it was preferred by most of the patients.

The electrolyte content of ophthalmic solutions is critical for maintaining a healthy ocular surface; it is not enough for a solution to be free of preservatives. More compliant patients who use current solutions for a long time are at risk of their disease becoming worse.

▶ This paper contains reports of a study that unfortunately was discussed in the lay press before most ophthalmologists were able to read it in a scientific journal. The message that reached dry eye patients from their newspapers alarmed many about the safety of artificial tears they were using. Evidence of the toxicity of commercially available brands of artificial tears was obtained in a study performed with rabbits using methods remotely related, at best, to clinical usage. The data obtained for patients were obtained by comparing only 1 brand of commercial artificial tears with the study preparation in only a very small number of patients. Further study in randomized clinical trials is necessary to document the safety and efficacy of various artificial tear preparations.—E.J. Cohen, M.D.

The Relative Risk of Ulcerative Keratitis Among Users of Daily-Wear and Extended-Wear Soft Contact Lenses: A Case-Control Study

Schein OD, Glynn RJ, Poggio EC, Seddon JM, Kenyon KR, the Microbial Keratitis Study Group (Massachusetts Eye and Ear Infirmary, Boston; Harvard Med School)
N Engl J Med 321:773–778, Sept 21, 1989   2–11

The risk of ulcerative corneal infection in wearers of soft contact lenses has been much discussed in both the professional and the popular press. However, estimates of the relative risks of using daily-wear lenses as compared with extended-wear lenses have been only speculative. This multicenter case-control study was done to compare the relative risk of ulcerative keratitis in users of cosmetic extended-wear soft contact lenses with that in users of cosmetic daily-wear soft contact lenses.

The study population consisted of 86 case patients with ulcerative keratitis associated with the use of soft contact lenses, 61 hospital-based controls who wore soft contact lenses but who had acute eye conditions unrelated to lens use, and 410 randomly selected population-based controls who wore soft contact lenses. Each case patient had a corneal epithelial defect with an underlying stromal infiltrate, had undergone corneal scraping for culture, and was receiving ocular antibiotics. Cultures from corneal scrapings were positive for 63% of the case patients.

The relative risk of ulcerative keratitis for extended wear as compared with daily-wear lenses was 3.90 for the population-based controls and 4.21 for the hospital-based controls. In the control groups, 38% of the extended-wear lens users wore their lenses only during the day, and 11% of the daily-wear lens users wore their lenses overnight at least once in a 2-week period. When lens wearers were categorized according to their

TABLE 1.—Estimated Relative Risks of Ulcerative Keratitis According to Lens Type and Level of Overnight Used as Compared With Daily-Wear Lenses Not Worn Overnight

Lens Type and Overnight Use	Relative Risk (95% CI)*	
	Case patients vs. population-based controls	Case patients vs. hospital-based controls
Daily-wear		
No overnight use	1.00†	1.00†
Overnight use	8.96 (4.09–19.63)	9.55 (2.87–31.80)
P value	0.0001	0.0002
Extended-wear		
No overnight use	2.76 (1.06–7.20)	2.57 (0.70–9.51)
P value	0.038	0.156
Overnight use	10.17 (5.29–19.55)	15.04 (5.21–43.43)
P value	0.0001	0.0001

*CI, confidence interval.
†By definition, because risks are relative to the risk for daily-wear lenses with no overnight use.
(Courtesy of Schein OD, Glynn RJ, Poggio EC, et al: *N Engl J Med* 321:773–778, Sept 21, 1989.)

TABLE 2.—Relative Risks of Ulcerative Keratitis for
Extended-Wear Lenses as Compared With Daily-Wear
Lenses Not Worn Overnight, According to the Number of
Consecutive Days Extended-Wear Lenses Are Worn

Days*	RELATIVE RISK (95% CI)†	
	CASE PATIENTS VS. POPULATION-BASED CONTROLS	CASE PATIENTS VS. HOSPITAL-BASED CONTROLS
1	3.6 (1.3–9.7)	2.4 (0.7–9.0)
2–7	6.8 (3.3–14.0)	10.0 (3.1–31.9)
8–14	11.8 (4.7–30.0)	37.9 (3.4–423.2)
≥15	14.5 (5.6–37.9)	45.0 (4.3–467.3)

*Value indicates number of consecutive days the lenses were worn before cleaning.
†CI, confidence interval.
(Courtesy of Schein OD, Glynn RJ, Poggio EC, et al: *N Engl J Med* 321:773–778, Sept 21, 1989.)

overnight use of lenses, the risk for those who used daily-wear lenses and sometimes wore them overnight was estimated to be 8.96 to 9.55 times the risk for those who used the lenses on a strictly daily-wear basis. The risk for those who used extended-wear lenses on an extended-wear basis was estimated to be 10.17 to 15.04 times the risk for those who used daily-wear lenses worn on a strict daily-wear basis (Table 1). For users of extended-wear lenses, the risk of ulcerative keratitis was incrementally related to the extent of overnight wear (Table 2). A lens care index developed to examine the effect of lens care on the risk of ulcerative keratitis showed that more careful lens hygiene would tend to lower the risk.

The data strongly indicate that overnight use of soft contact lenses carries a significantly greater risk for ulcerative keratitis than soft contact lenses worn strictly on a daily-wear basis.

The Incidence of Ulcerative Keratitis Among Users of Daily-Wear and Extended-Wear Soft Contact Lenses

Poggio EC, Glynn RJ, Schein OD, Seddon JM, Shannon MJ, Scardino VA, Kenyon KR (Abt Associates, Cambridge, Mass; Massachusetts Eye and Ear Informary, Boston; Harvard Med School)
N Engl J Med 321:779–783, Sept 21, 1989   2–12

It has been estimated that in 1987, 18.2 million Americans wore contact lenses, of whom 9.1 million were using daily-wear lenses and 4.1 million were using extended-wear lenses approved for overnight use. This prospective, 5-state study was done to estimate the incidences of ulcerative keratitis among users of daily-wear and extended-wear soft contact lenses.

All ophthalmologists practicing in a 5-state area were mailed a survey asking them to identify all cases of ulcerative keratitis diagnosed in their practice during a designated 4-month study period. To estimate the num-

Estimated Annualized Incidence of Ulcerative Keratitis
per 10,000 Cosmetic Wearers and Estimated Relative Risk
of Ulcerative Keratitis*

TYPE OF LENS	INCIDENCE OF ULCERATIVE KERATITIS	RELATIVE RISK†
Daily-wear soft	4.1 (2.9–5.2)	1.00‡
Extended-wear soft	20.9 (15.1–26.7)	5.15 (3.47–7.65)
Hard	2.0 (0–4.4)	0.50 (0.15–1.65)
Rigid gas-permeable	4.0 (0–8.2)	1.00 (0.34–2.89)

*Figures in parentheses are 95% confidence intervals.
†The risk shown is relative to the risk when using daily-wear lenses.
‡The relative risk is by definition 1.00.
(Courtesy of Poggio EC, Glynn RJ, Schein OD, et al: N Engl J Med 321:779–783, Sept 21, 1989.)

ber of persons who wore each type of soft contact lens, 4,178 households were contacted by random-digit dialing.

During the study period, ophthalmologists diagnosed 195 incident cases of ulcerative keratitis in patients who wore contact lenses. Of the 195 patients, 137 wore lenses for cosmetic purposes, 32 wore them for aphakia, and 4 wore contact lenses for therapeutic purposes. The reason was not reported in 22 cases.

The annualized incidence of ulcerative keratitis was estimated at 20.9 per 10,000 for persons wearing extended-wear soft contact lenses for cosmetic purposes, and at 4.1 per 10,000 for those wearing daily-wear soft contact lenses for cosmetic purposes (table). The estimated incidence of ulcerative keratitis among users of extended-wear lenses decreased with age, from 31 per 10,000 for persons aged 12 to 19 years, to 14 per 10,000 for those aged 40 years and more. The estimated incidence for women who used daily-wear lenses was 3.1 per 10,000, and for men, 6.1 per 10,000. The estimated incidence for women who used extended-wear lenses was 20.0 per 10,000 and for men, 22.1.

For comparison, the incidences among wearers of hard and rigid gas-permeable lenses also were estimated. The estimated incidences of ulcerative keratitis among those users were 2.0 per 10,000 for wearers of hard lenses, and 4.0 for wearers of rigid gas-permeable lenses.

Users of soft contact lenses should be made aware of the risks and benefits of daily-wear and extended-wear soft contact lenses, and be instructed to promptly discontinue their use as soon as irritation develops.

▶ It is important that people wearing cosmetic soft contact lenses be informed about the tenfold increased risk of potentially serious corneal ulcers associated with overnight wear compared with daily wear of these lenses. The first study provides valid scientific data to confirm the clinical impression that extended wear is not as safe as daily wear of cosmetic soft lenses. The companion article documents the relatively low incidence of corneal ulcers among people wearing cosmetic soft contact lenses. Because of the low incidence, well-informed patients may choose to use cosmetic soft lenses on an extended-wear basis. It is important that these lens wearers understand that the risk increases with the duration of extended wear. There is nothing magical about the 7-day limit recommended by the FDA. Awareness of the risk of extended wear needs to be coupled with appreciation of the importance of regular disinfection before lens insertion. Otherwise, patients who switch from extended wear to daily wear simply may only exchange the risk associated with extended wear for the risk associated with improper lens care. All ophthalmologists who see patients wearing soft lenses, whether or not they fit lenses, should read these articles in the *New England Journal of Medicine.*—E.J. Cohen, M.D.

Corneal Ulcers Associated With Disposable Hydrogel Contact Lenses
Dunn JP Jr, Mondino BJ, Weissman BA, Donzis PB, Kikkawa DO (Univ of California, Los Angeles)
Am J Ophthalmol 108:113–117, August 1989   2–13

Disposable, extended-wear hydrogel contact lenses are intended to be worn continuously for 1 to 2 weeks, after which they are to be discarded. Advantages of the use of disposable extended-wear contact lenses include the reduction of problems caused by noncompliance with proper lens care, the reduction of risks associated with aging lenses, and the elimination of some of the allergic and toxic complications of contact lens care products. A premarket study of 733 patients who wore extended-wear contact lenses for 8 months showed an overall complication rate of only 5.6%, with corneal ulcers developing in none of the patients.

Four case histories of patients who had corneal ulcers associated with the use of disposable, extended-wear hydrogel contact lenses are reported. All 4 patients were women aged between 22 and 40 years. Three of the women had discarded their lenses after 10 or more days of extended wear, and their corneal ulcers developed toward the end of the wearing cycle. One of these women admitted to wearing the lenses occasionally longer than the recommended 2-week period. She also admitted to infrequent handwashing before handling her lenses, and had long fingernails with which she may have scratched the cornea. The fourth patient removed her lenses every 2 days for cleaning and overnight disinfection and discarded the lenses on a weekly basis.

All 4 patients were treated hourly with topical tobramycin. After discharge, the antibiotic dosage was tapered slowly and administration of the drug was discontinued over a 3-week period. All 4 corneal ulcers responded to antibiotic treatment. Visual acuity returned to normal in 3 patients, but the patient who admitted to improper wear and lens hygiene had a scarred cornea, resulting in a reduced visual acuity to 20/60.

The increased cost of disposable contact lenses may tempt some patients to wear their lenses longer than suggested. In addition, when being worn, any contact lens is subject to contamination from environmental pollutants, cosmetics, and eyedrops. Therefore, the concepts behind the disposability of extended-wear soft contact lenses should not give patients and practitioners a false sense of their safety.

▶ It is hoped that use of disposable extended-wear cosmetic lenses will reduce the problems associated with extended wear. Proper lens care of disposable lenses requires only regularly discarding the lens and not the correct use of various lens care solutions and disinfecting systems. Whether patients will use disposable lenses correctly outside pre–market approval studies remains to be seen. Early case reports show that disposable lenses have not eliminated corneal ulcers associated with extended wear of cosmetic lenses. Additional experience with this modality is needed. Perhaps disposable daily-wear soft contact lenses will become routine in the future.— E.J. Cohen, M.D.

Clinical Indications for and Procedures Associated With Penetrating Keratoplasty, 1983–1988
Brady SE, Rapuano CJ, Arentsen JJ, Cohen EJ, Laibson PR (Wills Eye Hosp, Philadelphia)
Am J Ophthalmol 108:118–122, August 1989   2–14

According to the Eye Bank Association of America, the number of penetrating keratoplasties (PKs) performed in the United States has increased from 15,000 in 1981 to more than 36,000 in 1988. The charts of all patients who underwent PK at 1 hospital between 1983 and 1988 were reviewed to examine the changing trends in indications for performing PK.

During the 6-year study period, 2,299 PKs were performed by 18 surgeons, with 3 surgeons performing 87% of the operations. Pseudophakic bullous keratopathy (PBK) accounted for 22.9% of all the transplants done. Beginning in 1985, the number of PKs performed for PBK was markedly increased. The association of anterior chamber intraocular lenses (IOLs) in eyes with PBK increased from 19 (44%) of 43 cases in 1983 to 79 (73%) of 108 cases in 1988. Iris-fixated IOLs accounted for 19% of the cases, but gradually decreased from 37% in 1983 to 9% in 1988. The incidence of IOL exchanges at the time of PK increased from 14% in 1983 to 58% in 1988.

Other major indications for PK included Fuchs' dystrophy (16%), keratoconus (15%), aphakic bullous keratopathy (14%), and regraft (10%). No significant change was noted in the percentage of regrafts performed per year. Aphakic (20%) and pseudophakic (19%) bullous keratopathy were the most common indications for performing the previous PKs in patients with failed grafts. Viral diseases, which accounted for 4% of the cases overall, decreased in frequency from 6% in 1983 to 3% in 1988. The incidence of triple procedures, comprising PK, cataract extraction, and IOL implantation, increased from 11% in 1983 to 26% in 1988.

▶ During the 1980s, pseudophakic bullous keratopathy became the most common indication for corneal transplantation. Patients who have had implanted closed-loop anterior chamber lenses continue to have corneal decompensation and need transplantation. In considering future modifications of currently highly successful posterior chamber lenses, it is important to remember the long-term sight-threatening consequences of problematic intraocular lenses.—E.J. Cohen, M.D.

Epidemiology of Ocular Herpes Simplex: Natural History in Rochester, Minn, 1950 Through 1982
Liesegang TJ (Mayo Clinic, Rochester, Minn)
Arch Ophthalmol 107:1160–1165, August 1989   2–15

A previous report from this institution reported the incidence and prevalence of primary and recurrent ocular herpes simplex virus (OHSV) infections in a defined population in the United States. The clinical features of OHSV infections in that same population are described.

During the 33-year period between 1950 and 1982, 151 residents of Rochester, Minnesota, had 294 episodes of OHSV infection. Of these 151 patients, 122 had their first episodes of OHSV in 131 eyes; the other 29 patients had recurrences of OHSV. Recurrence rates after the first episode of OHSV as assessed with life-table methods were 9.6% at 1 year, 22.9% at 2 years, 49.5% at 10 years, and 63.2% at 20 years. Recurrence rates seemed to increase after repeated episodes. Eighteen (12%) of the 151 patients had involvement of both eyes or of periocular tissues at some time during the course of their disease.

Of the 122 patients who had their initial episode of OHSV, 54% had conjunctival or lid disease, 63% had corneal-epithelial disease, 6% had corneal-stromal disease, and 4% had uveitis. Most patients had more than 1 symptom during their initial episode. Twenty-eight patients had stromal keratitis.

Eighteen percent of the 122 initial OHSV infections, and 28% of the 172 recurrent OHSV episodes resulted in a visible corneal scar. Twelve patients had indolent or trophic corneal ulcerations. Recurrent corneal erosions developed in 2 patients after previous OHSV without clinical evidence of a clinical herpetic recurrence. OHSV-related cataracts developed in 3 patients. One patient had a corneal perforation after long-term stromal keratitis.

After a mean follow-up of 9 years for 131 eyes at risk, 94 eyes still had 20/20 visual acuity, another 11 eyes had visual acuity of 20/40 or better, and only 3 eyes had visual acuity worse than 20/100. Thus, 90% of 131 eyes in 122 patients who had their primary OHSV infection in Rochester maintained 20/40 or better visual acuity throughout the course of the follow-up.

▶ The recurrence rate of OHSV infection increases with time. The frequency of bilateral disease is greater in this study (12%) than generally recognized. Most patients with OHSV infection in this series retain good visual acuity during a long follow-up period. Patients with lid involvement alone accounted for 21%

of the series. In interpreting the results of this study, it is important to realize that not all patients with ocular herpes simplex had corneal involvement at any time in their disease course.—E.J. Cohen, M.D.

Herpes Simplex Keratitis in Patients With Acquired Immune Deficiency Syndrome

Young TL, Robin JB, Holland GN, Hendricks RL, Paschal JF, Engstrom RE Jr, Sugar J (Univ of Illinois, Chicago; Univ of California, Los Angeles)
Ophthalmology 96:1476–1479, October 1989   2–16

A wide range of systemic and ocular infectious diseases is associated with AIDS. Little is known about herpes simplex virus type 1 (HSV-1) keratoconjunctivitis in patients with AIDS. Six cases of recurrent HSV keratitis in AIDS patients were described.

The herpetic keratitis in these cases was characterized by unilateral dendritic or geographic epithelial keratopathy and predilection for peripheral versus central corneal involvement. The patients had 1 to 3 recurrences in a mean follow-up period of 17 months, with a median dendrite-free interval of 7 months. Their clinical course was moderately prolonged, with a median healing time of 3 weeks using topical antiviral treatments. Only 1 of the patients had stromal infiltrative involvement.

The immunologic abnormalities associated with AIDS may affect the clinical characteristics and course of HSV keratitis. However, more information is needed before any firm associations can be made between HIV and HSV-1. Clinicians must be aware of the unique features of HSV-1 in AIDS patients because its course and management seem to differ from that of immunocompetent patients.

▶ It is interesting that herpetic keratitis in AIDS patients is more like primary herpes infections than the more common typical dendritic keratitis occurring in patients with serum antibody to herpes simplex virus. The immunosuppression associated with AIDS likely contributes to a clinical course more characteristic of primary herpes. Immunosuppression probably is a factor in the relatively frequent infectious recurrences, prolonged course, and lack of stromal involvement. Clinicians should be aware that AIDS patients with herpes may have a different clinical course than usual. In addition, herpes simplex patients with an atypical course perhaps should be evaluated for underlying systemic diseases associated with immunocompromise.—E.J. Cohen, M.D.

Keratography as a Guide to Selective Suture Removal for the Reduction of Astigmatism After Penetrating Keratoplasty

Harris DJ Jr, Waring GO III, Burk LL (Emory Univ, Atlanta)
Ophthalmology 96:1597–1607, November 1989   2–17

Little information has been published on how to use keratography as a guide to selective suture removal. The use of keratography in the postoperative management of eyes after penetrating keratoplasty was described.

Fifty-two consecutive eyes were studied. After penetrating kerato-plasty, keratography refraction and keratometry were used to select appropriate interrupted sutures for removal to decrease astigmatism. All eyes had 1 continuous suture and 12 or 16 interrupted sutures. One hundred seventy-eight keratographs taken between 6 weeks and 6 months after surgery were analyzed and sorted into 6 groups on the basis of similar mire patterns. Removing single sutures associated with 3 patterns reduced astigmatism. The astigmatism was decreased by an average of 0.44 D in the symmetrical oval pattern; by 2.07 D in the D-shaped oval pattern; and by 6.60 D in the focal indentation pattern. The other 3 patterns did not permit quantification of results.

Keratography is a useful guide to selective suture removal in the reduction of astigmatism after penetrating keratoplasty. It is still not known whether the selective removal of interrupted sutures after keratoplasty is more effective and safer than the use of continuous sutures in the long-term reduction of astigmatism.

► Evaluation of corneal topography by keratometry, corneoscopy, and computer modeling systems is providing interesting information that has practical implications. Corneoscopy provides more information than keratometry and is being used increasingly to determine which interrupted sutures to remove selectively after corneal transplantation to reduce astigmatism. This article provides practical information on how to interpret corneoscopy findings and how much astigmatism reduction can be expected after selective suture removal when different patterns are present. Keratometry and refraction still are important measures of central and overall astigmatism. Caution should be used regarding suture removal when all measures of astigmatism are not in general agreement. Results of selective suture removal can be difficult to predict accurately.—E.J. Cohen, M.D.

Cornea Donation Laws in the United States
Lee PP, Stark WJ, Yang JC (Baltimore; New York)
Arch Ophthalmol 107:1585–1589, November 1989   2–18

Penetrating keratoplasty is now one of the most successful and common transplant procedures in the United States. The current laws governing cornea donation and other important issues were discussed.

All 50 states and the District of Columbia have individual variations on the Uniform Anatomical Gift Act (UAGA). The decedent, before death, or the survivors, after death, may voluntarily donate a cornea. The decedent may make the donation by will or another document, such as a donor card witnessed by 2 persons. Survivors may make the donation if they have no knowledge of a decedent's objections to donation. Selling organs and tissue, including corneas, is prohibited in the United States.

The current shortage of corneas for transplantation reflects both the public's hesitancy to make donations and the failure of health care professionals to use the UAGA to obtain tissues. Ambivalence about making donations results from the stress of having to cope with the death, the fear that becoming a donor would result in premature termination of care or a drop in the quality of care, and personal religious beliefs. However, the major obstacle to increasing donations may be health care professionals' unwillingness to fully use the provisions of existing laws. Educational efforts to address the public's fears and the concerns of health care workers may increase the supply of corneas.

Cornea transplants are in many ways the most favored of organ transplants. However, even with limited presumed consent in 18 states, cornea shortages still exist. Measures to increase cornea supplies include educational efforts, better use of required asking laws, and the movement of state laws toward presumed consent and medical examiner's laws.

▶ Required request laws, by which organ donation must be requested from the next of kin of acceptable donors, are a step in the direction of improved availability of donor tissue in states without medical examiner laws. It is important that health care professionals encourage organ donation, whenever appropriate, so that more patients can benefit from transplantation of various organs.—E.J. Cohen, M.D.

Late Endophthalmitis After Transscleral Fixation of a Posterior Chamber Intraocular Lens
Heilskov T, Joondeph BC, Olsen KR, Blankenship GW (Bascom Palmer Eye Inst, Miami)
Arch Ophthalmol 107:1427, October 1989   2–19

Several methods have been used for fixation of an intraocular lens (IOL) in the absence of capsular support, involving both iris and scleral fixation sutures. A disadvantage of the latter technique is the resulting suture passing internally from the hepatic surface externally to the scleral surface, which provides a track for bacteria to enter the eye. A case of late endophthalmitis after transscleral fixation of a posterior chamber IOL was described.

Man, 44, had blunt trauma to the left eye 1 month after secondary implantation of a posterior chamber IOL. A pars plana vitrectomy and retinal detachment repair were done after initial wound repair. Five months later, the patient awoke with pain and severely decreased vision. Vitreous culture yielded *Haemophilus influenzae*. In this patient, the suture ends had eroded through the overlying conjunctiva and provided a track for the organisms into the vitreous cavity.

To avoid this suture track, the prolene suture can be secured to the sclera under an overlying partial-thickness scleral flap. A scleral bite also may be taken posterior to the sclerotomy, and the suture can be tied to itself, directing the free suture ends posteriorly. The haptic sutures also may be used to close the sclerotomy so that the knot is buried in the sclerotomy, thus eliminating exposed suture ends. Finally, 10-0 prolene will produce a slightly smaller suture track than 9-0 prolene.

As transscleral fixation of IOLs becomes more prevalent, clinicians must be aware of the possibility of delayed-onset endophthalmitis. Eyes with exposed transscleral suture ends should be followed up closely. If conjunctival irritation or conjunctivitis occurs, clinicians should consider trimming the exposed suture ends or refixation of the IOL with scleral flaps covering the sutures.

▶ There has been a recent tendency away from use of open loop flexible anterior chamber lenses toward sutured posterior chamber lenses at the time of IOL exchange in the course of penetrating keratoplasty. Suturing of posterior chamber lenses to the ciliary sulcus currently is more popular than suturing these lenses to the iris. However, there have been reports of complications associated with sutured posterior chamber lenses. Good results have been obtained with the use of current generation of open loop anterior chamber lenses. Large series reporting results after use of anterior and posterior chamber lenses for IOL exchange in the absence of capsular support are necessary. As to which approach is best in the management of pseudophakic bullous keratopathy associated with closed loop or rigid anterior chamber and iris fixated IOLs, the answer has not been found.—E.J. Cohen, M.D.

Hydrogen Peroxide Damage to Human Corneal Epithelial Cells In Vitro: Implications for Contact Lens Disinfection Systems
Tripathi BJ, Tripathi RC (Univ of Chicago)
Arch Ophthalmol 107:1516–1519, October 1989   2–20

Exposure to 3% hydrogen peroxide, the concentration used in most disinfection systems for contact lenses, can result in stinging, tearing, hyperemia, blepharospasm, edema, and possibly permanent corneal damage. To determine the extent of cell damage resulting from hydrogen peroxide use and to consider the implications of such damage for peroxide-based contact lens disinfection systems, primary cell cultures of human corneal epithelium were exposed to a single dose of hydrogen peroxide at concentrations of 30 to 100 ppm.

Even at 30 ppm, hydrogen peroxide caused cell retraction and cessation of cell movement and mitotic activity. Membranous vesicle formation preceded cell death occurring within 7 to 8 hours after exposure to 30 ppm. At the concentration of 50 ppm, normal cell activity was stopped almost immediately. Many surface vesicles formed within 1.5 hours of exposure, and the cells died within 4 to 5 hours. The higher concentrations of hydrogen peroxide produced cell death within minutes.

The efficacy of hydrogen peroxide as a contact lens disinfectant is well established, but its margin of safety appears very narrow. More research is needed on the long-term effects of residual peroxide on the cornea.

▶ Hydrogen peroxide is popular for disinfection of hydrogel lenses and can be used for soft contact lenses of various water contents. It is effective against various organisms, including fungi and *Acanthamoeba*, provided exposure times are sufficient (approximately 4 hours). The safety of hydrogen peroxide disinfection is of some concern. Adequate neutralization of hydrogen peroxide is necessary to maximize safety. Potential toxicity of hydrogen peroxide disinfection is a subject of investigation with many unanswered questions (*CLAO J* vol 16, supplement, 1990).—E.J. Cohen, M.D.

Disinfection of Goldmann Tonometers Against Human Immunodeficiency Virus Type 1
Pepose JS, Linette G, Lee SF, MacRae S (Washington Univ, St Louis; Georgetown Univ, Washington, DC; Oregon Health Sciences Univ, Portland)
Arch Ophthalmol 107:983–985, July 1989   2–21

Isolation of HIV-1 from tears, conjunctiva, and contact lenses of AIDS patients has raised concern over possible transmission of infection in the course of routine ophthalmologic examination. A majority of HIV-seropositive persons are ambulatory and asymptomatic. Several regimens of disinfecting Goldmann tonometer tips against HIV-1 and herpesviruses types 1 and 2, all enveloped viruses, were tested.

Tonometer tips were inoculated with 5×10^5 IU of cell-free or cell-associated HIV-1 or 10^4 plaque-forming units of HSV-1 or HSV-2. After 10 minutes of air drying, the instruments were wiped with tissue or sterile gauze, with gauze soaked in 3% hydrogen peroxide, or with a 70% isopropyl alcohol swab. Treatment with peroxide and the alcohol wipe totally disinfected the tonometer tips, but wiping with gauze alone was ineffective.

Wiping tonometer tips with an isopropyl alcohol swab and allowing it to evaporate is an efficient means of disinfecting the instrument against both HIV and herpesviruses. There is evidence that 70% isopropyl alcohol also inactivates hepatitis B virus. Only the tonometer tip itself must be treated.

▶ Routine cleaning of tonometer tips between patients requires use of an alcohol wipe and not just a dry cloth. This should be a standard practice. Disinfection of a tonometer with an alcohol wipe after use rather than before use more readily allows air drying before applanation.—E.J. Cohen, M.D.

3 Glaucoma

Glaucoma Care—1989

RICHARD P. WILSON, M.D.
Glaucoma Service, Wills Eye Hospital, Philadelphia, Pennsylvania

Glaucoma patients frequently complain about visual difficulties. However, when they see 20/30 (6/9) on the Snellen chart in a darkened room with a brightly lit background, our tendency often is to minimize their complaints and tell them how lucky they are to have 20/30 vision. Yet psychophysiologic testing reveals most of these patients have contrast sensitivity loss. Concrete steps and curbs have little contrast when light is not causing shadows. Dusk and conditions of low light provide less contrast, even without the side effects of pilocarpine. These kinds of conditions are difficult for patients with glaucomatous nerve damage.

In explaining lack of contrast sensitivity to patients, I liken their vision to the early days of television when resolution was poor and "snow" was a problem. When glare from a mild media opacity and dim vision from a 1-mm pupil caused by pilocarpine are added to this lack of contrast sensitivity, sympathizing with patients becomes much easier, even though their Snellen acuity may be quite good. An explanation that conditions in the examining room are optimal and their vision in the real world will not be as good often reassures patients that I understand their limitations.

Psychophysiologic testing helps us explain patients' difficulties with vision, but it still does not allow early differentiation of the patient with suspected glaucoma in whom nerve damage is developing. That visual fields are poor evaluators of early glaucoma is commonly agreed upon. Quigley has shown us that up to 50% of optic nerve fibers may be lost before visual field changes are consistently detected with Goldmann perimetry. Efforts to develop a test that will pick up earlier changes are proceeding on several fronts. As Stamper points out in his article that follows (Abstract 3–1), defects in color vision, temporal contrast sensitivity, and spatial contrast sensitivity all are predictive of visual field loss. The problem is the large overlap between healthy persons and those suspected of having disease as well as between those suspected and those definitely with disease. The latter overlap is explainable if the test is reliably detecting the group of suspected patients with early damage. The former overlap is what limits the usefulness of color and contrast sensitivity testing. Psychophysiologic testing apparatuses aimed at the general practitioner are coming to market with claims of effectiveness that must be taken with a large grain of salt. No device yet can separate consistently the glaucoma suspect with early damage from one without it.

For those of us waiting for an effective, topical carbonic anhydrase in-

47

hibitor, it will be early 1992 before MK-927 is introduced into the United States.

The use of postoperative injections of 5-fluorouracil (5-FU) has passed from investigational use into standard practice among glaucoma specialists. During the last year, nearly one third of the patients I operated on were given 5-FU after surgery. My use of shunts between the chamber and external reservoir (Molteno, Schocket) has declined as my enthusiasm for this antifibrosis agent has grown. Shunts are reserved for those patients in whom filtration with 5-FU has failed or those in whom conjunctival scarring prevents raising a conjunctival flap. Almost all patients can have filtration surgery and 5-FU or a shunt.

Cyclodestructive techniques, even though they are being improved rapidly, are reserved for those whose poor vision does not justify the time and expense of cutting surgery. The phthisis rate with Nd:YAG cyclophotocoagulation of the ciliary body, my choice as the best and safest of the various techniques, is still 5%. (Note that this is an increase from last year, when I described our result as 1%; it may rise still further). Although the ocular morbidity with shunt procedures is formidable, the ocular mortality (phthisis) is approximately 1% in my hands. The disparity in disaster rates between the two techniques mandates the surgical creation of an outflow path before reducing inflow in patients with functional vision. This choice also maintains an appropriate supply of aqueous for those intraocular structures that depend on it for nutrition and oxygen, for example, the lens and central cornea.

In introducing to a patient the concept of reducing scarring postoperatively with a cancer drug, the vast difference in dosages needed must be pointed out. One course of treatment for cancer in a 70-kg man requires 4,800 mg versus 50 mg if 10 injections are given after filtration surgery. No systemic side effects have been recognized. The biggest stumbling block in selling the use of 5-FU to patients is the thought of periocular injections. In this, technique is important.

After proparacaine has been instilled in an eye, the tip of a wooden applicator stick is broken off, soaked in proparacaine, and placed under the lid over the location for the injection. This tip is allowed to remain there for 30 seconds to 1 minute. Care must be taken to warn the patient to avert his gaze from the applicator so the cornea is not injured. During this period, 0.5 cc of 5-FU, 10 mg/mL, is drawn up in a tuberculin syringe and the 27-gauge needle that comes with the syringe is exchanged for a 30-gauge needle. Bubbles are shaken to the top with the syringe held needle-up to insure consistent dosage and excess 5-FU is expressed until 0.1 cc remains. The applicator tip is removed, and the 5-FU injected subconjunctivally 180 degrees from the filtration site. Any reflux out the needle hole is caught on a dry cotton-tipped applicator or is irrigated out. Ointment is applied to protect the cornea from further leakage.

This technique allows no discomfort with the needle stick and only mild burning from the medicine. As the fistula heals and reflux into the eye is less likely, the 5-FU can be injected closer to the site of filtration. Complications are minimized by coating the cornea with a viscoelastic during surgery to prevent drying under the microscope light. No injections are given at the time of surgery. The cornea is allowed to recover overnight, and the bleb is inspected for leaks before 5-FU injections are started on the first day. My regimen is patterned after Weinreb (1) with four injections the first week and three the next 2 weeks if the corneal epithelium remains intact. Ointments are used instead of drops and application is spread out during the day to prevent exposure that can lead quickly to an erosion.

Superficial punctate keratitis is universal with the use of 5-FU. If such erosions become confluent and a corneal erosion threatens, the injections are held until the surface improves. Thus, 5-FU is titrated to an eye's ability to tolerate it. Avoiding erosions by this technique is not always successful, but the incidence is reduced to 25% to 33%.

Wound leaks have not been a problem in my series. Although I take pains to place my conjunctival incision as far posterior to the filtration site as I can, I use a standard 10-0 nylon suture and needle to close the conjunctiva. Attention to detail in the closure and 5-FU dose reduced from that of the regimen used in the national trial eliminates the necessity of a vascular needle.

Complete failure of filtration is unusual even in cases for which it would have been usual before 5-FU. Encysted blebs ("Tenon's cysts") are not prevented even with a full 10 injections. A factor contributing to filtration failure is the development of a choroidal detachment and secondary shallow chamber. Because of delayed fibrosis, aqueous filtration is greater than expected after surgery and, consequently, so is the incidence of choroidal detachments. This is the perfect place for a conservative closure with releasable sutures or the use of the Hoskins lens to laser flap sutures postoperatively. I usually would release a flap suture on the sixth or seventh day without the use of 5-FU, but with it I release the suture at 2 weeks for a similar result.

The early 5-FU injections are the most important. It may well be that three or four the first week are enough to effect a good result. Early in my experience with 5-FU, I stopped the injections if a shallow chamber occurred, restarting them only when the chamber started to reform. However, my failure rate for these cases was high. When I kept to the usual regimen right through the choroidal detachment and its medical or surgical treatment, the results were closer to those expected.

A unique complication of filtration surgery with adjunct 5-FU is hypotonia. Intraocular pressures of 2 to 4 are possible, especially in patients without previous surgery. Although the optic nerve may be more resistant to further glaucoma damage at this pressure, vision is impaired and quite variable. After working hard to get a low pressure, it may now be necessary to raise the pressure for some patients without losing control. The bleb can be limited with sutures or glacial acetic acid, cryotherapy, or argon laser treatment after painting with methylene blue.

I have spent so much time on 5-FU and its influence on filtration surgery because it is the state of the art. On the horizon is the creation of filtration fistulas ab interno. This technique has several advantages. The conjunctiva overlying the fistula that will form the bleb is not traumatized during creation of the filter, which should lead to less episcleral fibrosis, the most common cause of filtration failure. An additional advantage is access to the inferior and nasal conjunctiva, areas that are difficult to work in with conventional surgery. This access is important for patients with superior and temporal scarring that precludes raising a conjunctival flap. The procedure is short if a vitrectomy is not required. The conjunctiva is ballooned up with balanced saline solution through a distal wound. A small limbal incision is made 180 degrees from the proposed fistula. The chamber is filled with a viscoelastic, and the instrument is inserted across the anterior chamber to the opposite angle. A fistula is created there.

The options for creating the fistula include the Brown trabecuphine (2), a mechanized trephine, the Surgical Laser Technologies Nd:YAG laser that focuses its energy through a synthetic sapphire crystal (contact laser technology [3]), and a cauterizing needle developed by Thom Zimmerman. Which approach is the most effective remains to be seen. All share a common problem: each creates a full-thickness filter without a protective flap. In the diseased eyes that need this type of surgery, choroidal detachments are nearly universal when the intraocular pressure is abruptly lowered to the low single digits. So although the surgery is quick and straightforward, postoperative care is complicated and perilous, especially for an eye with a posterior chamber lens that can injure the cornea if a flat chamber occurs. With this complication in mind, it is hard to predict that these procedures will become favored outside the Boston area (with their penchant for full-thickness procedures) except for a circumscribed subset of patients. The combination of a trabeculectomy with releasable sutures and 5-FU provides such safe, excellent results that other methods pale by comparison.

References

1. Weinreb RN: Adjusting the dose of 5-fluorouracil after filtration surgery to minimize side effects. *Ophthalmology* 94:564, 1987.
2. Brown RH, Denham DB, Bruner WE, et al: Internal sclerectomy for glaucoma filtering surgery with an automated trephine. *Arch Ophthalmol* 105:133, 1987.
3. Javitt JC, O'Connor SS, Wilson RP, et al: Laser sclerostomy ab-interno using a continuous wave neodymium:YAG laser. *Ophthalmic Surg* 20:552, 1989.

Psychophysical Changes in Glaucoma
Stamper RL (Pacific Presbyterian Med Ctr, San Francisco)
Surv Ophthalmol 33 (suppl):309–318, February 1989   3–1

Observations with the relatively insensitive Snellen chart as well as kinetic and static perimetry have suggested that chronic glaucoma spares central vision until quite late in its course. More sensitive means of measuring central visual function recently have demonstrated defects early in the glaucomatous process, in some instances even before perimetry is abnormal. The functions tested are mediated largely by macular fibers.

Defects in color vision often are found early in the course of glaucoma, before visual field loss is apparent; however, different methods of measuring color perception vary widely in sensitivity. Because color vision is mediated largely by the fovea, impairment indicates that central vision is affected adversely by glaucoma. Most studies indicate a defect in spatial contrast sensitivity in glaucoma patients; this process presumably is mediated by the macula. Some evidence suggests that spatial contrast sensitivity loss may predate visual field loss. Temporal contrast sensitivity also may be defective early in the course of glaucoma. A few patients have been found to have decreased light sensitivity thresholds in the macula.

Diffuse and focal glaucomatous damage may occur together and may progress at different rates. Impaired central visual function is both more common and more profound than was previously thought.

► Evidence from increasingly sophisticated psychophysiologic tests is changing our concepts of how glaucoma loss occurs. However, the widespread of results from any of these tests in normal persons allows an overlap between that group and glaucomatous persons. This prevents present methodology from being helpful in diagnosing early glaucoma. It is hoped that in the not too distant future, new or improved testing modalities will enable us to winnow patients with ocular hypertension down to those subject to damage.—R.P. Wilson, M.D.

Risk Factors for the Development of Tenon's Capsule Cysts After Trabeculectomy
Feldman RM, Gross RL, Spaeth GL, Steinmann WC, Varma R, Katz LJ, Wilson RP, Moster MR, Spiegel D (Thomas Jefferson Univ; Univ of Pennsylvania; VA Hosp, Philadelphia)
Ophthalmology 96:336–341, March 1989   3–2

The Tenon's capsule cyst (TCC), or encapsulated bleb, is a complication of glaucoma filtering surgery. The cyst usually forms 2 to 8 weeks after surgery. Intraocular pressure is not always increased. Risk factors for development of TCC were studied in 438 trabeculectomies done on 434 eyes in a 4-year period. The mean age of the patients was 63 years, and the mean time since diagnosis of glaucoma was 8.5 years.

Tenon's capsule cyst occurred in 28% of patients having trabeculectomy. The risk of cyst development was increased by a history of previous TCC, argon laser trabeculoplasty, male sex, and the preoperative use of sympathomimetic agents. Use of a compression shell decreased the risk of TCC developing. All cysts were diagnosed within 2 months of trabeculectomy.

Advanced glaucoma was not associated with a higher risk of TCC in this study, but a relationship between TCC and glaucoma present for longer than 2 years may exist. Use of a Simmons compression shell was associated with a lower risk of TCC, but this technique was used only for patients with "low-tension" glaucoma.

▶ Encapsulated blebs (there is no endothelial or epithelial lining to justify the appellation *cyst*) are a frequent (28%) and frustrating complication of filtering surgery. The main risk factors revealed here are the previous use of epinephrine compounds, especially over a prolonged period, and previous laser trabeculoplasty. Any stimulus for chronic inflammation may encourage encapsulated bleb formation. Having responded in this manner before obviously predisposes patients to have encapsulation of the bleb again at any subsequent surgery. The risk factors for encapsulation may be becoming clearer, but the actual physiologic process still eludes us.— R.P. Wilson, M.D.

Long-Term Morphologic Effects of Antiglaucoma Drugs on the Conjunctiva and Tenon's Capsule in Glaucomatous Patients
Sherwood MB, Grierson I, Millar L, Hitchings RA (Univ of Florida, Gainesville; Inst of Ophthalmology; Moorfields Eye Hosp, London)
Ophthalmology 96:327–335, March 1989   3–3

Most patients coming to filtration surgery have taken different topical antiglaucoma drugs for several years, but the effects of such treatment on local tissues are uncertain. The effects of long-term treatment on the cell content of the conjunctiva and Tenon's capsule were examined in 20 patients having planned primary trabeculectomy within a few weeks of their diagnoses of glaucoma. Pilocarpine were given for a mean of 3 weeks before surgery. Twenty other patients had trabeculectomies after having received at least 2 different types of topical antiglaucoma drug for 1 year or longer.

The mean time of medical treatment for the multitreatment group was 7.5 years. The multitreatment patients had a significantly decreased number of goblet cells in the conjunctival epithelium and increased numbers of hyaline bodies and nonepithelial cells, chiefly lymphocytes. Macrophages, lymphocytes, fibroblasts, and mast cells were increased in both the substantia propria of the conjunctiva and the Tenon's capsule layer in patients given long-term antiglaucoma medication.

Long-term antiglaucoma drug therapy may increase tissue inflammatory cells, which may promote the risks of external bleb scarring and failure of filtration surgery. Further thought should be given to the best time for filtration surgery.

▶ Another basic science article also has serious implications for how we take care of our glaucoma patients. Doctor Sherwood and co-workers show that long-term use of topical medication increases inflammatory cells in the conjunctiva. Feldman and associates have shown an increased incidence of encapsulated blebs in those patients coming to surgery who have been taking medication for years. In both cases, long-term use of medicine is a risk factor for bleb failure. Perhaps the British are right that we wait far too long to operate on our patients with serious glaucoma.—R.P. Wilson, M.D.

Pathophysiology of Laser Trabeculoplasty
Van Buskirk EM (Oregon Health Sciences Univ, Portland)
Surv Ophthalmol 33:264–272, January–February 1989   3–4

Although argon laser trabeculoplasty lowers intraocular pressure by enhancing aqueous outflow, its exact effects on the trabecular meshwork are not understood completely. One explanation is primarily a mechanical one, based on heat-induced shrinkage of the superficial lamellar collagen of the corneoscleral meshwork. As a result, the entire inner part of the meshwork is pulled from the outer wall of Schlemm's canal toward the anterior chamber (Fig 3–1), preventing Schlemm's canal from collapsing. Alternatively, photocoagulation may initiate a chain of cellular and extracellular events that enhance aqueous outflow.

Clinical observations indicate that trabeculoplasty has nonspecific effects. Hypotensive effects are not specific to a particular wavelength or type of laser. High power actually leads to a postoperative rise in pressure. The hypotensive response usually is delayed. Although lasting months to years, the effect is transient in many instances. All these observations suggest that trabeculoplasty acts by enhancing aqueous outflow.

New information from histologic study of whole treated eyes suggests that laser photocoagulation of the meshwork is destructive locally but

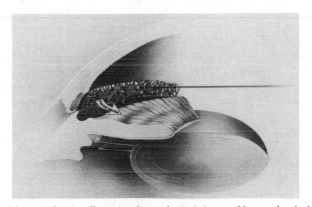

Fig 3–1.—Schematic drawing illustrating the mechanical theory of laser trabeculoplasty, whereby the laser burn contracts the inner trabecular meshwork, drawing it away from Schlemm's canal, preventing canalicular collapse. (Courtesy of Van Buskirk EM: *Surv Ophthalmol* 33:264–272, January–February 1989.

diffusely stimulates meshwork cells. Cellular stimulation probably activates molecular events, perhaps within the extracellular matrix, that improve the facility of aqueous outflow. Only at high levels of intraocular pressure may mechanical global stretching or tightening of the trabecular meshwork be important.

▶ Doctor Van Buskirk's research suggests that the trabecular tightening theory originated by Dr. Wise to explain why argon laser trabeculoplasties work is erroneous. Instead, the laser burns may stimulate trabecular cells in surrounding TM to divide and migrate into the injured area. These new cells may alter the biologic behavior of the area, for example, be more active in phagocytosing glycosaminoglycans blocking the PTM. Whether right or wrong, this work points out our ignorance concerning the most common glaucoma surgery in the United States, why it works, and its long-term consequences.—R.P. Wilson, M.D.

Therapeutic Ultrasound for Refractory Glaucoma: A Three-Center Study
Maskin SL, Mandell AI, Smith JA, Wood RC, Terry SA (Univ of Texas, San Antonio; Baylor College of Medicine; Mid South Glaucoma and Cataract Found, Memphis)
Ophthalmic Surg 20:186–192, March 1989   3–5

Therapeutic ultrasound lowers intraocular pressure by damaging the ciliary body, increasing uveoscleral outflow, or promoting scleral filtration. A total of 158 eyes with various types of glaucoma—most often open-angle glaucoma—were treated at 3 centers and followed up for a mean of 8 months afterward. The Sonocare CST-100 was used to apply varying numbers of 5-second exposures of high-intensity focused ultrasound. The "standard" number of applications during each session was 6.

Intraocular pressure fell 38%, on average. Success rates averaged about 70% and were highest in open-angle glaucoma. Six or more applications were most effective in lowering intraocular pressure to less than 25 mm Hg. Complications, occurring in 11% of cases, included phthisis bulbi in 0.6% and persistent hypotonia in 2.5%. The mean visual loss was less than 1 line of acuity. Forty patients had retreatment.

Ultrasound is effective and safe for refractory glaucoma of various types. Including retreated cases, success was achieved within 9 months in 85% of cases. External burns usually result from a patient's movement or a surgeon's inexperience. Future studies should include assessments of stability of the optic nerve and visual field after treatment.

▶ The use of therapeutic ultrasound to treat refractory glaucoma, a procedure promoted far more in the lay press than in scientific journals, is controversial at best. The machine was evaluated by Dr. Richard Simmons in Boston, Dr. Harry

Quigley in Baltimore, and me. It was returned promptly after a preliminary trial in all 3 instances. Doctor Simmons, in a large series, believed half of his treated patients were not helped. My experience was similar, but probably would have been better with practice. The biggest problem encountered was the postoperative pressure rises. Doctor Michael Yablonski, who probably has the greatest clinical experience, relates that intraocular pressure (IOP) often doubles after treatment. He has seen rises up to 118 mm Hg, and advises paracentesis if IOP is above 90. I don't know about you, but I promptly faint if a patient that I have just operated on gets an IOP above 80. This leads me to believe that, with precise ablation of the ciliary body ab externo using continuous-wave Nd:YAG laser energy already a proven modality, the time for therapeutic ultrasound has come . . . and gone.—R.P. Wilson, M.D.

Disc Hemorrhages in the Glaucomas
Drance SM (Univ of British Columbia, Vancouver)
Surv Ophthalmol 33:331–337, March–April 1989   3–6

A 20% prevalence of disk hemorrhages in patients with low tension glaucoma has been reported. Linear, flame- or splinter-shaped hemorrhages typically are found in the prelinar area of the disk and the adjacent superficial retinal nerve fiber layer (Fig 3–2). Most patients with low tension glaucoma who are followed up have recurrent hemorrhage. Most recurrent bleeds occur in the same disk site. Most hemorrhages last longer than 1 month; a majority are present for 2 months. A comparison of patients having open-angle glaucoma and disk hemorrhage with others lacking hemorrhage showed that only systemic hypertension differed significantly.

Disk hemorrhages are a sensitive marker of ensuing visual field defect in patients with glaucoma. Earlier signs of damage include notching of the disk and enlargement of the cup. Progression of field defects is more frequent in patients with disk hemorrhage. Isolated disk hemorrhage should be considered a sign of an active process that must be monitored closely. Other glaucomatous damage develops frequently. Possible causes of disk hemorrhages include microinfarction, mechanical rupture of capillaries, and a venous origin.

▶ Disk hemorrhages are seen more frequently when the disk is examined on each visit. That these small, nerve fiber layer hemorrhages often last 2 months increases the chance of their detection. Although their physiologic cause is not known, their significance as a marker for progressive glaucomatous damage is. Each occurrence mandates a review of the patient's intraocular pressure control (rule out diurnal spike), their compliance with the prescribed medical regimen, and, in most instances, an increase in therapy with the goal being a further 20% to 25% drop in intraocular pressure.—R.P. Wilson, M.D.

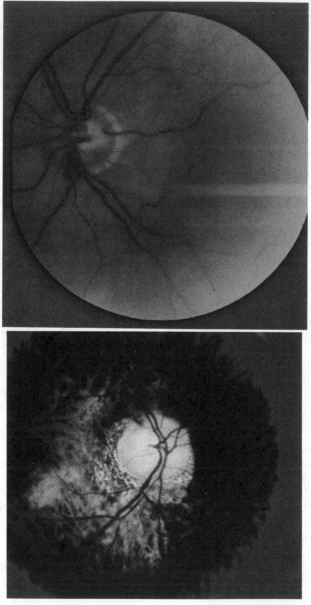

Fig 3–2.—Appearances of disk hemorrhages in glaucomatous disks. (Courtesy of Drance SM: *Surv Ophthalmol* 33:331–337, March –April 1989.)

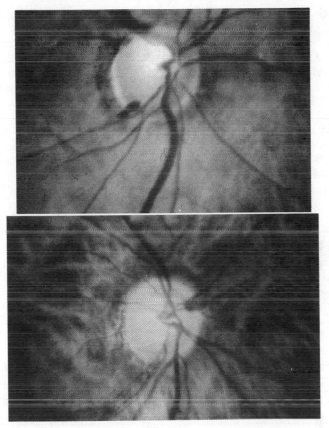

Fig 3–2, cont.

Angle-Closure Glaucoma Complicating Ciliochoroidal Detachment

Fourman S (Univ of Pittsburgh)
Ophthalmology 96:646–653, May 1989   3–7

Ciliochoroidal detachment usually is associated with low intraocular pressure and an open chamber angle, but rarely there may be anterior rotation of the ciliary body, angle closure, and elevated intraocular pressure. Six such patients were encountered, with acute angle closure glaucoma complicating ciliochoroidal detachment in 8 eyes.

Presenting findings included a shallow central anterior chamber, a flat peripheral anterior chamber, a closed angle, and elevated intraocular pressure. Three patients had uveal effusion syndrome, 2 had posterior scleritis, and 1 had arteriovenous malformation.

All of the eyes responded to intense cycloplegia with aqueous suppressant therapy. All patients received topical steroids, and 3 received high-dose oral prednisone as well. Resolution of glaucoma usually required 1 to 2 weeks. Withdrawal of antiglaucoma therapy and cycloplegia eventually was possible in all cases.

Angle-closure glaucoma complicating ciliochoroidal detachment can occur in a wide range of disorders and after surgery. It could be confused with primary angle-closure glaucoma or malignant glaucoma. Medical treatment with cycloplegia and aqueous suppressants is consistently effective.

▶ Choroidal detachment with anterior rotation of the iris around scleral spur causing angle closure is usually readily apparent by the difference in AC depth in the fellow eye. It is imperative that the etiology of the angle closure be recognized before treatment. This entity is one of several that pilocarpine makes worse. This list also includes aqueous misdirection, most pupillary blocks associated with an intraocular lens, and inflammatory angle closure secondary to either posterior synechiae or peripheral anterior synechiae.

The most common cause of angle closure secondary to iris rotation around scleral spur that I see is an overly tight scleral buckle causing choroidal congestion. An overly aggressive panretinal photocoagulation comes in second. Both may respond to argon laser peripheral iridoplasty (gonioplasty) if aggressive cycloplegics, corticosteroids, and aqueous suppressants are not successful. Drainage of the choroidal detachment is the last resort if a suprachoroidal effusion is present.—R.P. Wilson, M.D.

The Effect of Caffeine on Intraocular Pressure in Glaucoma Patients
Higginbotham EJ, Kilimanjaro HA, Wilensky JT, Batenhorst RL, Hermann D (Univ of Illinois, Chicago)
Ophthalmology 96:624–626, May 1989   3–8

Variable effects of caffeine on intraocular pressure (IOP) are reported. The effects of drinking regular coffee on IOP were compared with those of herbal tea in a single-blind crossover study of 13 patients with primary open-angle glaucoma or suspected glaucoma. The mean IOP was 1.04 mm Hg greater 90 minutes after ingestion of coffee, whereas the mean IOP was 0.42 mm Hg lower after drinking tea. At 30 and 60 minutes differences in pressure were not significant. Even the change at 90 minutes was not clinically significant.

These findings give no cause for discouraging glaucoma patients from drinking caffeinated coffee.

▶ "Should I not drink coffee?" is commonly asked by glaucoma patients. This paper provides reassurance that moderate amounts of coffee probably have no clinically significant effect on IOP. What it does not address and what is probably more significant, if difficult to determine, is the effect of a vasoconstrictor on posterior pole circulation. I ask patients with far-advanced disease or low-tension glaucoma to minimize the use of caffeine and nicotine. I also mention that doing this has no proven benefit, but theoretically it should help. Patients at this stage are grateful that one cares enough to look past pharmacology in their treatment and are happy to pursue any avenue open to them. —R.P. Wilson, M.D.

Assessing the Utility of Reliability Indices for Automated Visual Fields: Testing Ocular Hypertensives
Bickler-Bluth M, Trick GL, Kolker AE, Cooper DG (Washington Univ, St Louis)
Ophthalmology 96:616–619, May 1989   3–9

Automated perimetry increasingly is used to detect and follow up ophthalmic disease. The use of the reliability measures incorporated in the 30-2 Program and analysis program (STATPAC) of the Humphrey Visual Field Analyzer. Previous studies indicated that these programs yield unreliable data in more than one third of cases. Visual fields were recorded at baseline and after 6 and 12 months in 120 patients with elevated intraocular pressure who had normal Goldmann visual fields and were not taking antiglaucoma medication.

The indices of field reliability were fixation loss less than 20 with false positive and false negative errors less than 33%. Mean deviation and pattern standard deviation were also examined. Thirty-five percent of patients had low-reliability fields at baseline and about 25% after 6 and 12 months. More than half the patients produced at least 1 low-reliability field during this time, and 8% were unable to produce even 1 reliable field. Fixation errors declined 10% during the 1-year study period. Most patients had 20% to 32% fixation errors.

Increasing the fixation loss criterion for patient reliability to a cutoff level of 33% might raise the percentage of fields graded as reliable with minimal effects on the sensitivity and specificity of the test.

▶ Bickler-Bluth and colleagues again point out the difficulty of statistically analyzing a subjective test with visual thresholds that fluctuate both short-term (minutes) and long-term (months). They provide validation that the pattern standard deviation more accurately identifies significant defects than mean deviation. Their main point is that the acceptable fixation loss percentage on the Humphrey Visual Field Analyzer can be raised from 20% to 33% without seriously affecting the sensitivity and specificity of the test.—R.P. Wilson, M.D.

The Time Course of Intraocular Pressure in Timolol-Treated and Untreated Glaucoma Suspects
Chauhan BC, Drance SM, Douglas GR (Univ of British Columbia, Vancouver)
Am J Ophthalmol 107:471–475, May 1989   3–10

Timolol produces an immediate fall in intraocular pressure, but in some patients, its effect diminishes over the first few days and some treated patients have a gradual rise in pressure. The course of pressure response in patients randomly assigned to receive topical timolol or no treatment was examined. Twenty-four treated glaucoma suspects and 22 untreated patients were compared. The subjects had no localized field defect or disk changes after 6 years of follow-up, and their intraocular pressures were not increased dangerously.

Both groups had a rise in pressure, followed by a gradual leveling off and then a reduction toward the end of follow-up. The pressure-time curves paralleled one another and were separated by about 5 mm Hg.

The effect of treatment in this study was simply to lower the pressure-time curve by a fixed amount throughout the follow-up period. The behavior of intraocular pressure in individual patients was not dependent to a significant degree on treatment. Those who have a linear rise in intraocular pressure may be subjects in whom the linear part of the pressure-time curve is exaggerated, or they may be in an early stage of their time course. Those with a pressure peak relatively early in follow-up may be subjects with a short linear part of the curve, or they may be in a later stage of their time course of intraocular pressure.

▶ This report was chosen to counter the impression, mine included, that IOP gradually rises when the diurnal curve is averaged throughout life. Chauhan and his co-workers noted a flattening of the early rise, which at the end of 5 years appeared to have a slightly downward trend. It is interesting that the timolol group paralleled the control group but was lower by a fairly consistent amount. Because both curves were parallel, the long-term escape concept popularized at the end of the last decade probably was caused by progressive disease that increased outflow blockage rather than a lessening effect of the drug.—R.P. Wilson, M.D.

Retinal Ganglion Cell Atrophy Correlated With Automated Perimetry in Human Eyes With Glaucoma
Quigley HA, Dunkelberger GR, Green WR (Johns Hopkins Univ)
Am J Ophthalmol 107:453–464, May 1989   3–11

Loss of optic nerve fibers precedes the appearance of a typical glaucomatous field loss on Goldmann perimetry. The most sensitive measure of early glaucomatous damage would focus on the functional loss occasioned by the death of ganglion cells. The number and size of retinal ganglion cells in 6 human eyes with glaucoma were measured, and the findings were correlated with the results of visual field testing. Five age-matched normal eyes also were examined.

Large ganglion cells were fewer in retinal areas with atrophy. In the perifoveal region, however, no consistent pattern of cell loss by size was apparent. It seemed that visual field sensitivity on automated testing began declining shortly after the loss of ganglion cells began. In the central 30 degrees of the retina, 20% of cells were lost at sites with a 5-dB sensitivity loss, and a 40% cell loss was correlated with a 10-dB decrease in sensitivity. Some ganglion cells remained in areas with 0-dB sensitivity on field testing.

Some clinical evidence supports an early loss of larger ganglion cells in glaucoma. At a later stage of damage, testing of the physiologic responses of smaller ganglion cells would be useful. Different perimetric tests for early and late glaucoma would be helpful.

▶ Harry Quigley was the first to show how visual field loss was equated to axonal loss in the optic nerve. Now he and his colleagues move to a more basic level to quantify ganglion cell loss in relation to visual field loss. In addition, they find that large ganglion cells are the first to go in glaucoma, that damage more often is diffuse rather than localized, and that present psychophysiologic tests are not very sensitive in early disease and may be less so in advanced disease.—R.P. Wilson, M.D.

Lens Rim Artifact in Automated Threshold Perimetry

Zalta AH (Univ of Cincinnati)
Ophthalmology 96:1302–1311, September 1989   3–12

False positive rates as high as 20% are reported when automated perimeters are used for central threshold field testing. Lens rim artifact (LRA) is presumed to be among the more frequent errors in computerized perimetry. The visual fields of 445 eyes in 266 healthy subjects and patients with diagnoses of suspect or early glaucoma were reviewed. Central static threshold fields were examined with a corrective lens using the Humphrey 30-2 program.

Lens rim artifact was found in 10.4% of fields examined retrospectively and in 6.2% of those evaluated prospectively. It most often presented as a combination of absolute and relative defects involving the temporal quadrant alone or the temporal and 1 other quadrant. Several types of interpretational error were made; overdiagnosis was more prevalent than underdiagnosis. Risk factors for LRA included greater age and a high hyperopic correction. Defects involving only the 4 targets at 27 degrees eccentricity in the temporal quadrant were caused only by LRA.

Lens rim artifact is a significant cause of erroneous threshold values in automated threshold perimetry. The density criterion used to define abnormality is an important factor. Several of the associated interpretational errors have significant influence on the diagnosis and management of glaucoma. However, LRA can be minimized by properly educating the perimetrist and the patient, by correct setup of patient and corrective lenses at the perimeter, and by maintaining alignment of the eye and corrective lens during testing.

▶ Plotting central visual fields without refractive correction often results in relative scotomas. On the other hand, corrective lenses may introduce artifacts of their own. This phenomenon is seen most commonly if a patient's forehead is allowed to fall away from the headrest, or the head is allowed to tilt to 1 side during the test. The decreased interaction between technician and patient and rigid nature of the testing inherent in computerized perimetry have increased the incidence of LRA. Therefore, technicians must caution patients about the importance of positioning and must monitor patients vigilantly during examination.— R.P. Wilson, M.D.

Is It Worthwhile to Add Dipivefrin HCl 0.1% to Topical β_1-, β_2-Blocker Therapy?

Parrow KA, Hong YJ, Shin DH, Shi D-X, McCarty B (Wayne State Univ, Detroit)
Ophthalmology 96:1338–1342, September 1989   3–13

Whether adding an adrenergic agonist to a β_1-, β_2-blocker leads to a further reduction in intraocular pressure remains unclear. In this study the effects of dipivefrin were examined when used in combination with a β_1-, β_2-blocker in 32 patients having diagnoses of ocular hypertension or early primary open-angle glaucoma. The patients had received levobunolol or timolol for 6 months or longer at the time of the study. Dipivefrin 0.1% was instilled twice daily, 10 minutes after β-blocker application.

Addition of dipivefrin to the β-blockers significantly lowered mean intraocular pressure from 22.7 to 20.2 mm Hg at 1 week, and to 21.0 mm Hg at 12 weeks. No significant change occurred in the fellow, untreated eyes. Half the eyes had a pressure reduction of 2 mm Hg or more when dipivefrin was added, and one fifth of eyes had a reduction of 3 mm Hg or more.

An overall additive effect was noted in this study when dipivefrin was added to daily β-blocker therapy, but individual variation was considerable. It has been proposed that the additive effect reflects α-adrenergic–induced constriction of vessels supplying the ciliary processes. Alternatively, an increase in outflow facility and greater uveoscleral outflow may contribute to the effect. Whatever the mechanism, adding dipivefrin to nonselective β-blockers may prove helpful in the management of glaucoma.

▶ Fact: adding dipivefrin HCl to a nonselective β-blocker may add 1 to 3 mm Hg to IOP control. This effect is quite variable. Conclusion: if the patient needs an IOP more than 2 to 3 mm Hg lower, try the next step. If 2 or 3 mm Hg will help, add dipivefrin as a 1-eyed, therapeutic trial. This avoids long-term use of an ineffective drug with a high incidence of allergic reactions.

Fact: once-a-day use of dipivefrin is close to the top of the long-term dose response curve. Conclusion: once-a-day dipivefrin usually will give all the added effect possible when added to a nonselective β-blocker.— R.P. Wilson, M.D.

A Limited Comparison of Apraclonidine's Dose Response in Subjects With Normal or Increased Intraocular Pressure

Abrams DA, Robin AL, Crandall AS, Caldwell DR, Schnitzer DB, Pollack IP,

Rader JE, Reaves TA Jr (Johns Hopkins Univ; Univ of Utah, Salt Lake City; Tulane Univ, New Orelans; Alcon Labs, Fort Worth, Tex)
Am J Ophthalmol 108:230–237, October 1989   3–14

This multicenter randomized study compared the efficacy of 0.5% and 1.0% apraclonidine hydrochloride in 15 healthy persons and 17 patients with increased intraocular pressure. A double-masked crossover design with a vehicle placebo was used.

The 1% apraclonidine solution produced a maximum 30% reduction in mean intraocular pressure in healthy eyes and a 31% reduction in eyes with elevated pressure. The weaker solution produced a maximal 26% pressure reduction in healthy eyes and a 27% decrease in eyes with elevated pressure. The differences were not significant. Most subjects had a 20% or greater fall in intraocular pressure from baseline. Nine of the 15 healthy persons had pressures of 10 mm Hg or less 12 hours after instillation of apraclonidine. The degree of pressure reduction was unrelated to the initial pressure level.

Both 0.5% and 1% apraclonidine lowered intraocular pressure in this study, regardless of whether the irides were light or dark and whether the initial pressure was normal or increased. A 0.25% solution reportedly is as effective as 0.5% medication in glaucomatous eyes. The mechanism of action of apraclonidine remains to be clarified. The drug decreases aqueous flow in healthy eyes and may lower the episcleral venous pressure or increase uveoscleral outflow.

▶ Apraclonidine probably will beat a topical carbonic anhydrase inhibitor to market and surely will be approved for long-term use before the next new class of drug. This article does not reveal the mechanism of action or how additive apraclonidine is to other topical medications, but it does show a 31% reduction in IOP with its use. That an effective alternative to present medications soon will be ready justifies temporizing therapy in selected patients, for example, carbonic anhydrase inhibitors in those who will not tolerate long-term use or a second laser trabeculoplasty if the first was only effective for a year or 2.—R.P. Wilson, M.D.

An Autosomal Dominant Form of Low-Tension Glaucoma
Bennett SR, Alward WLM, Folberg R (Univ of Iowa)
Am J Ophthalmol 108:238–244, September 1989   3–15

Eight members of a family in consecutive generations had a distinct form of low-tension glaucoma transmitted in an autosomal dominant manner (Fig 3–3). Glaucomatous optic atrophy and field loss occurred at normal or borderline intraocular pressures. The disorder was manifest in early adult life and continued to progress slowly throughout life. Examination of 1 patient's eyes after death from myocardial infarction showed glaucomatous optic atrophy with loss of ganglion cells. The trabecular meshwork, retinal pigment epithelium, photoreceptors, and choroidal and optic nerve vessels all appeared normal.

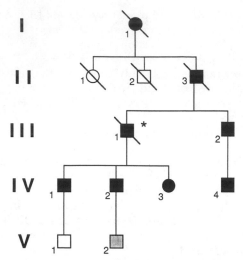

Fig 3–3.—Pedigree of family affected by autosomal dominant low-tension glaucoma. The eyes in case 1 (III-1) (*) were obtained post mortem for pathologic study. *Squares*, males; *circles*, females; *solid symbols*, affected; *shaded symbol*, uncertain diagnosis; *slash* through a symbol indicates deceased. (Courtesy of Bennett SR, Alward WLM, Folberg R: *Am J Ophthalmol* 108:238–244, September 1989.)

This family appears to have an inherited type of glaucomatous optic atrophy. Marked optic nerve head cupping is seen in childhood. The field loss is glaucomatous, with preservation of central vision until late in the course. Two successive generations have been affected, with male-to-male transmission documented. Intraocular pressures are not elevated substantially, and whether treatment of the pressure alters the course of visual loss is not clear. Some affected persons have received medical and laser treatments, which failed to dramatically alter either intraocular pressure or the visual field loss.

▶ The etiology of low-tension glaucoma remains an enigma. Some patients have obvious perfusion deficits because of pump or circulatory embarrassment. Others may have lamina cribrosa that in later life offers insufficient support in the face of normal IOPs. Many, if not most, have no apparent causative factors. The identification of a genetic line with autosomal inheritance may provide clues in the continuing investigation of this disorder. No abnormalities in the trabecular meshwork were found, supporting the view that outflow is normal and the fault lies posteriorly. The findings here of a normal choroidal and optic nerve vasculature may lead the hunt toward a more structural (mechanical) basis.—R.P. Wilson, M.D.

MK-927: A Topically Effective Carbonic Anhydrase Inhibitor in Patients
Bron AM, Lippa EA, Hofmann HM, Feicht BI, Royer JG, Brunner-Ferber FL, Panebianco DL, Von Denffer HA (Besançon Univ, Besançon, France; Merck

Sharp & Dohme Research Labs, West Point, Pa; Technical Univ of Munich, West Germany)
Arch Ophthalmol 107:1143–1146, August 1989   3–16

The water-soluble carbonic anhydrase inhibitor (CAI) MK-927 is new, potent, and available in ophthalmic preparations of 0.5% to 2.0%. Ocular tolerance is acceptable in healthy persons. MK-927 now has been evaluated in a patient population. Twenty-five patients with primary open-angle glaucoma or ocular hypertension participated in a double-masked placebo-controlled crossover study. Three drops of 2% MK-927 were instilled.

Treated eyes had a mean reduction of 7.7 mm Hg from a mean initial intraocular pressure of 27.8 mm Hg after 4.5 hours. Placebo was associated with a mean pressure fall of 3.9 mm Hg. At 6 hours mean peak changes in pressure were 26.7% in eyes given MK-927 and 13.7% in those given placebo. There was no contralateral effect of medication on IOP.

MK-927 had a clinically relevant pressure-lowering effect in patients with primary open-angle glaucoma and ocular hypertension. The drug most likely penetrates better than past compounds. Preliminary results of a further study in patients with elevated IOP confirm the efficacy of a single dose of 2% MK-927.

▶ The quest for an effective topically applied carbonic anhydrase inhibitor has been on for many years. The first real contender is MK-927. If approved, it would do away with most of the annoying and often dangerous side effects of the systemic CAIs. However, the development of aplastic anemia is not related to dose, and this frequently lethal complication still would be a serious concern.—R.P. Wilson, M.D.

Fluorouracil Filtering Surgery Study One-Year Follow-Up

The Fluorouracil Filtering Surgery Study Group (Schiffman J, Univ of Miami, Fla)
Am J Ophthalmol 108:625–635, December 1989   3–17

Reports of side effects related to the use of 5-fluorouracil have cautioned clinicians against employing 5-fluorouracil in all patients undergoing filtering surgery. To determine the long-term safety and efficacy of postoperative subconjunctivally injected 5-fluorouracil in eyes with uncontrolled glaucoma and poor prognoses for filtering surgery, 213 patients were studied; 27% of 105 eyes treated with 5-fluorouracil and 50% of 108 eyes treated by standard procedures were classified as failed (Fig 3–4). In the failed eyes, reoperation was needed for control of intraocular pressure during the first year or there was an intraocular pressure of more than 21 mm Hg 1 year after treatment. Corneal epithelial toxicity and transient visual acuity loss occurred more often in patients given 5-fluorouracil. However, visual acuities and the mean visual field sensitivities were comparable in both groups at 1 year.

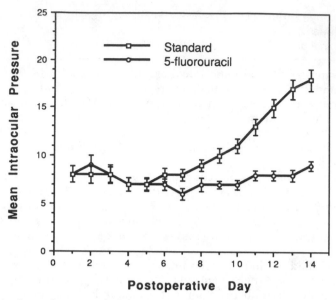

Fig 3–4.—Intraocular pressure during postoperative days 1–14 by treatment group. *Bars* indicate ± standard error. (Courtesy of The Fluorouracil Filtering Surgery Study Group: *Am J Ophthalmol* 108:625–635, December 1989.)

The use of subconjunctivally injected 5-fluorouracil was recommended after filtering surgery in eyes with uncontrolled glaucoma after cataract extraction and in phakic eyes after failed filtering surgery. The favorable effects of intraocular pressure control and the lack of a significant loss of visual acuity or field at 1 year outweigh the risks of corneal and conjunctival epithelial toxicity.

▶ 5-Fluorouracil (5-FU) has revolutionized my practice. Operating on aphakic eyes after multiple surgeries, especially when concomitant vitrectomy is required, is more difficult and hazardous. Until 5-FU, the success rate was depressing. Now, the success rate is in the 70% to 90% range depending on the case. I now resort to silicone tube shunts (Schocket or Molteno) with about one third the frequency I did before 5-FU. The adjunct use of 5-FU is applicable to any patient with a decreased prognosis for standard filtering surgery. This includes those patients with previously failed filters; those with aphakic, neovascular, or inflammatory glaucomas; those who heal too easily, for example, young or black patients; or those who need IOPs in the single digits. I have one 8-year-old boy and two 9-year-old girls who have submitted to postoperative injections and have excellent results to show for it. Vive la 5-FU.—R.P. Wilson, M.D.

A Long-Term Clinical Trial of Timolol Therapy Versus No Treatment in the Management of Glaucoma Suspects

Epstein DL, Krug JH Jr, Hertzmark E, Remis LL, Edelstein DJ (Massachusetts Eye & Ear Infirmary, Boston)
Ophthalmology 96:1460–1467, October 1989   3–18

Ophthalmologists disagree on whether it is appropriate to treat elevated intraocular pressure (IOP) in patients with neither glaucomatous optic nerve atrophy nor visual field defects. A randomized, prospective, clinical trial was done to compare timolol treatment with no treatment in patients with mildly increased IOP but without glaucomatous disk changes or anomalies in the visual field.

One hundred seven patients with IOPs between 22 and 28 mm Hg were assigned to timolol treatment or no treatment and were followed up for an average of 56 and 51 months, respectively. Failure was considered a confirmed IOP of more than 32 mm Hg, stereophotographically documented optic nerve progression, or development of glaucomatous visual field loss by perimetry. There were 9 failures in the treatment group and 17 in the no-treatment group. Six of the 9 treatment group failures had discontinued timolol before failing. Timolol was found to be significantly protective, with an adjusted risk ratio of 0.38. When only field and disk failure criteria were considered, timolol was significantly protective in an analysis where patients who stopped timolol treatment were considered lost to follow-up. There were seasonal fluctuations of IOP, with higher IOP occurring in the winter.

Earlier treatment of selected patients with mildly increased IOP was advocated. Timolol has a favorable influence on the clinical course of patients with mildly elevated IOP but no glaucomatous disk changes or anomalies in the visual field.

▶ Two caveats must be kept in mind when trying to apply this article clinically. One is the way studies like this are set up. To achieve any statistically reliable results, the number of patients in the control group that have conversion to definite glaucoma must be significant. Therefore, patients in both groups are skewed to the more suspect end of the glaucoma suspect spectrum. If you look at the glaucoma suspects in your practice, the conversion rate will be far less than the conversion rate reported here. The Academy home study course often has quoted a study that looked at patients who had elevated IOP but normal disks and fields. Glaucoma developed at a rate of 0.5%–1% per year over observation periods of 5 to 14 years. With present technology, earlier diagnosis is possible so the conversion rate would be slightly higher. Still, to expose unnecessarily even 90 patients for 5 years to the side effects of a powerful β-blocker to prevent the earliest changes of glaucoma in 10 people may not be in the interest of the common good or (the present buzzword) cost-effective.

This is my second caveat: systemic side effects of topical β blockers are widespread. As a brief example in just 1 area, a Canadian study looked at elderly patients placed in nursing homes for organic brain syndrome who were receiving timolol. This treatment was discontinued, with many patients showing improvement. Some had improvement to the extent that they could be discharged. Before treating a patient without demonstrable disease with long-term ocular antihypertensives, be sure the patient is suffering no side effects from your therapy. *Primum non nocere.*—R.P. Wilson, M.D.

The Effect of Chronic Miotic Therapy on the Results of Posterior Chamber Intraocular Lens Implantation and Trabeculectomy in Patients With Glaucoma
Chen HS-L, Steinmann WC, Spaeth GL (Wills Eye Hosp, Thomas Jefferson Univ, Philadelphia)
Ophthalmic Surg 20:784–788, November 1989   3–19

Preoperative pilocarpine treatment might affect the results of cataract–glaucoma surgery in glaucomatous eyes. Postoperative complications, intraocular pressure levels, required glaucoma medications, and visual acuity changes in patients who had used pilocarpine before surgery were compared with those in patients who had not.

The charts of 18 patients (20 affected eyes) having undergone trabeculectomy combined with or done after cataract extraction with posterior chamber lens implantation were reviewed. None of these patients used pilocarpine before treatment. Their results were compared with those of 35 patients, (40 eyes) who had used pilocarpine before these procedures. The groups were matched for age and sex. All patients were followed up for at least 6 months. No significant differences in postoperative intraocular pressure and required glaucoma medications were found between groups. Among pilocarpine-treated patients, however, there was a significantly higher incidence of complications, particularly intraocular lens capture, and of worse visual outcomes.

In this series, differences in preoperative and postoperative intraocular pressure levels or in required glaucoma medications were not significant between pilocarpine-treated and untreated patients. However, the incidence of intraocular lens capture was significantly greater in the treated eyes.

▶ Patients who have been treated long term with miotics have far different reactions to surgery than those who have not. There is more bleeding at the time of surgery, and after surgery the aqueous is turbid with serum proteins and cells. The iris, especially in a black patient, is sticky and adheres to cornea, lens, and especially intraocular lens if given an opportunity. It surprises me that the postoperative IOP was similar in the 2 groups. My experience is that fibrin and blood clots are more likely to block the filtering cleft in patients who were receiving miotics preoperatively than in those who were not. Phospholine iodide and carbachol should be discontinued 2 weeks before surgery and, if necessary, replaced with pilocarpine. A break from pilocarpine is also helpful if the health of the optic nerve permits. Preoperative steroid preparation to raise the blood-aqueous barrier is needed with the first 2 medications and sometimes is helpful with pilocarpine.—R.P. Wilson, M.D.

The Effect of Anterior Chamber Depth on Endothelial Cell Count After Filtration Surgery

Fiore PM, Richter CU, Arzeno G, Arrigg CA, Shingleton BJ, Bellows AR, Hutchinson BT (Massachusetts Eye and Ear Infirmary; Ophthalmic Consultants of Boston, Inc, Boston)
Arch Ophthalmol 107:1609–1611, November 1989   3–20

Glaucoma filtering surgery frequently is complicated by shallowing of the anterior chamber after surgery. The effect of shallowing of the anterior chamber with iridocorneal but not lenticular-corneal touch is not well documented. The effect of anterior chamber depth on endothelial cell count after filtration surgery was investigated.

Eighteen patients undergoing glaucoma filtration surgery were studied the day before and 4 to 6 months after surgery by specular microscopy. After surgery, patients were assessed for the presence of iridocorneal or lenticular-corneal touch, anterior chamber depth, and inflammation. Ten eyes that maintained their anterior chamber after glaucoma filtration surgery had no significant reduction in corneal endothelial cell density. However, 8 eyes in which shallow anterior chambers with iridocorneal touch were developing and a mean reduction of 265 cells peripherally and 250 cells centrally in corneal endothelial cell count. These represented reductions of 12.4% and 11.6%, respectively. After a mean follow-up of 44.4 months, no patient with iridocorneal touch had corneal edema.

In this series, the eyes maintaining deep anterior chambers after filtration surgery had a mean reduction of 1.7% to 3% in corneal cell density. The eyes with iridocorneal touch, however, had an 11.6% reduction centrally and a 12.4% reduction peripherally. After glaucoma filtration surgery, iridocorneal touch is associated with loss of endothelial cells, but it is apparently well tolerated by the cornea.

▶ The lesson from this article is that a flat chamber, even if it does not result in lens-corneal touch, is not benign. The authors conclude that their patients' corneas survived a sudden 12% loss of endothelial cells for the ensuing 4 to 5 years, and point out that both groups had patients that underwent subsequent cataract surgery without corneal decompensation, but I again have 2 caveats. The authors are excellent surgeons, and patients of other surgeons might not fare as well. Also, the longest follow-up in this study was 62 months, and the average, 44.4. My perspective during my first 5 years in practice has changed during the next 6. Corneas in patients that appeared to be doing fine have decompensated, often leaving me to wonder whether it was them or me.

The usual objective for patients with flat chambers after filtering surgery is to maintain fistulas. If there is a moderate bleb, enough aqueous formation to maintain the fistula is likely. If the bleb is flat, then reformation and probably drainage of the choroidal detachment and reformation are indicated. The optimal period for this is postoperative day 4 or 5. This article will influence me to be less tolerant of prolonged iris-corneal apposition.—R.P. Wilson, M.D.

Investigations Into a Vascular Etiology for Low-Tension Glaucoma

Carter CJ, Brooks DE, Boyle DL, Drance SM (Univ of British Columbia, Vancouver)
Ophthalmology 97:49–55, January 1990   3–21

Elevated intraocular pressure is an accepted primary cause of atrophy of the optic nerve head and visual field defects in high-tension glaucoma. Other etiologic factors must be present to produce this finding in low-tension glaucoma. Low-tension glaucoma may result from reduced optic nerve perfusion because of vascular disease or other factors, such as changed blood viscosity. The noninvasive vascular profiles, coagulation test results, and rheologic profiles of patients with low-tension glaucoma were compared with those of patients with high-tension glaucoma and controls.

Forty-six consecutive cases of low-tension glaucoma, 69 similarly unselected cases of high-tension glaucoma, and 47 age-matched controls were studied (Table 1). A multifactorial design and previously validated objective tests were used. However, there were no significant group differences in markers of atherosclerotic vascular disease. No rheologic differences could be found.

These findings do not support the hypothesis that an organic vascular pathologic condition underlies low-tension glaucoma. If vascular disease is important in this condition, it must be localized or vasospastic.

▶ This study points out the problems with retrospective studies. Doctor Drance previously has pointed out the unexpectedly high incidence of hypovolemic shock in patients with low-tension glaucoma. Yet another study looking at cohort of patients after hypovolemic shock found no cases of low-tension glaucoma. This article in essence retracts previous publications espousing a vascular cause for this entity. Richard Lewis, on the other hand, demonstrated a 48% incidence of migraines in low-tension glaucoma patients, whereas 25% of the general population has them. A vasospastic cause is possible, as is an age-induced flaccid lamina cribrosa that crimps the axons stopping axoplasmic flow. In all likelihood there are a variety of causes. Age will be a factor as both

TABLE 1.—Patient Characteristics	HTG	LTG	CONTROLS
Age (yrs)	66	64	66
Range	37–86	42–84	66–85
Male to female ratio	42:27	16:30	20:27
Percentage of smokers	33	25	35

Abbreviations: HTG, high-tension glaucoma; *LTG,* low-tension glaucoma.
(Courtesy of Carter CJ, Brooks DE, Coyle DL, et al: *Ophthalmology* 97:49–55, January 1990.)

TABLE 2.—Glaucoma Survey of General
Population by Age

Age, yr	Incidence
40–49	0.22%
50–59	0.10%
60–69	0.57%
70–79	2.81%
80+	14.29%

the incidence of glaucoma and the proportion of the glaucoma population with the low-tension variety increase with age (Table 2).—R.P. Wilson, M.D.

Management of Encapsulated Filtration Blebs

Shingleton BJ, Richter CU, Bellows AR, Hutchinson BT (Ophthalmic Consultants of Boston, Inc; Massachusetts Eye and Ear Infirmary, Boston; Harvard Med School)
Ophthalmology 97:63–68, January 1990   3–22

Encapsulation of filtering blebs after surgery can lead to increased intraocular pressure (IOP), necessitating antiglaucoma medical or operative treatment (Fig 3–5). To establish the efficacy of medical treatment for increased IOP in encapsulated filtering blebs and to determine the frequency and results of surgical revision, 49 patients with 49 affected eyes were followed up for 6 to 48 months.

Intraocular pressures rose from 10.2 mm Hg at 1 week after filtration surgery to a maximum of 26.1 mm Hg at 3 weeks after surgery. Pressures then decreased to 16.2 mm Hg at 16 weeks and remained stable for the rest of the follow up period. Thirty-nine eyes had a final IOP of 19 mm Hg or less. Thirty-five needed medical treatment alone and had a final IOP of 14.1 mm Hg. Medical treatment consisted of antiglaucoma drops, oral carbonic anhydrase inhibitors, or digital massage, or a combination of these. Fourteen eyes needed reoperation for IOP elevation uncontrolled by medical treatment. Five of these eyes needed 2 or more reoperations.

Clinicians should maintain a high index of suspicion in the early postoperative period for the development of encapsulated blebs. Detecting such formations often is heralded by an early increase in IOP. Aggressive medical treatment, including glaucoma medications and digital massage, is indicated, especially in the first 2 postoperative months, when IOP elevation tends to be at its highest.

▶ When first presented with an encapsulated bleb, I regarded it as a severe

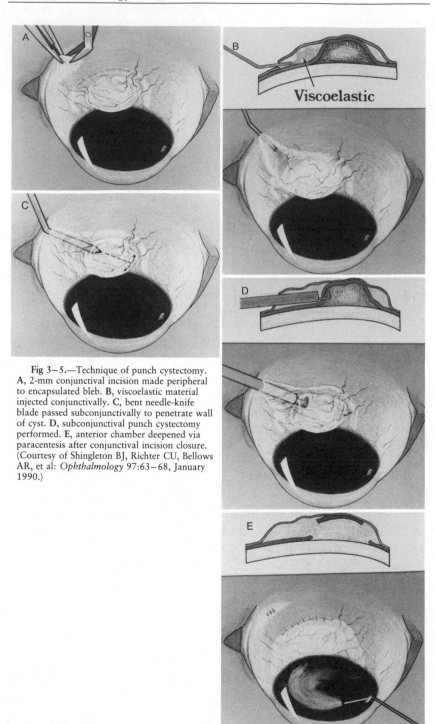

Fig 3–5.—Technique of punch cystectomy.
A, 2-mm conjunctival incision made peripheral
to encapsulated bleb. **B,** viscoelastic material
injected conjunctivally. **C,** bent needle-knife
blade passed subconjunctivally to penetrate wall
of cyst. **D,** subconjunctival punch cystectomy
performed. **E,** anterior chamber deepened via
paracentesis after conjunctival incision closure.
(Courtesy of Shingleton BJ, Richter CU, Bellows
AR, et al: *Ophthalmology* 97:63–68, January
1990.)

complication. Now I know that the IOP at 6 months almost always will be controlled. In fact, the only danger in a typical encapsulated bleb is for a patient with far advanced disease. If the optic nerve cannot tolerate a mildly elevated IOP (few encapsulated blebs result in high IOP or maximal medication), then needling with postoperative 5-FU is my treatment of choice.—R.P. Wilson, M.D.

Risk Factors for the Development and Severity of Glaucoma in the Pigment Dispersion Syndrome
Farrar SM, Shields MB, Miller KN, Stoup CM (Duke Univ Eye Ctr, Durham, NC)
Am J Ophthalmol 108:223–229, September 1989   3–23

Both pigment dispersion syndrome and pigmentary glaucoma typically affect young adults, and early detection is especially important in preventing a lifetime of blindness. If miotic treatment can arrest pigment dispersion and prevent or reverse glaucoma, knowing which patients are at particular risk of glaucoma would be most helpful. The records of 93 patients with pigmentary glaucoma and 18 with pigment dispersion syndrome were retrospectively reviewed.

Possible risk factors included maleness, black race, severe myopia, and the presence of Krukenberg spindles: pigment granules deposited on anterior segment structures. Two thirds of all patients were men, and men had diagnoses at an earlier age than women had. In addition, men required more aggressive treatment for glaucoma. All 4 black patients needed surgery. Patients with glaucoma had more severe myopia and more frequently had Krukenberg spindles.

A preponderance of men was noted in this study, as in past series. Black race also may indicate a high risk of pigmentary glaucoma developing, as may a family history of glaucoma. Refractive error has apparent prognostic significance. Follow-up of about half the present study group suggests that more than half of patients with pigment dispersion syndrome will develop pigmentary glaucoma, and that about half of these eventually will need surgery.

▶ The major aim of this study was to discover the risk factors that would predict which patients with pigmentary dispersion syndrome would go on to have glaucoma. Under optimal conditions, accurate selection would allow prophylactic treatment. However, in a civilized country where the legal system has run amuck, treating myopes without definite disease with a miotic that has been linked to retinal detachment formation is asking for a liability suit. Thymoxamine, an α-adrenergic blocking agent that causes miosis by blocking the dilator muscle of the iris, would be a perfect solution. Although available in Europe for years, the market for this drug unfortunately is small and has not yet justified the product liability costs to produce it here. Early detection remains the cornerstone of pigmentary glaucoma treatment. The risk factors presented here—male sex, black race, myopia greater than 3 D, and presence of Krukenberg spindles—will help in this assessment.—R.P. Wilson, M.D.

4 Neuro-Ophthalmology

CT and Magnetic Resonance Imaging "Negative" Neuro-Ophthalmology: The Medical and Economic Impact

ROBERT C. SERGOTT, M.D.

Neuro-Ophthalmology Service, Wills Eye Hospital, Philadelphia, Pennsylvania

Neuro-ophthalmology in 1989 is best described as a subspecialty in transition. This evolutionary phase is illustrated dramatically by the articles chosen for the 1989 YEAR BOOK. All the articles except one (1) explore new developments about diseases and symptomatology in which the CT and magnetic resonance imaging (MRI) scans are negative for significant structural abnormalities. We therefore have entered the era of CT and MRI "negative" diseases as the primary research thrust of clinical neuro-ophthalmology.

From 1971 to 1988, advances in neuroimaging techniques dominated neuro-ophthalmology. Computed tomographic and MRI scans converted the basic neuropathologic processes of ischemia, demyelination, neoplasia, and degeneration from abstract ideas into dynamic concepts. New developments in imaging such as MRI angiography and the three-dimensional reconstruction will fuel some future progress in neuro-ophthalmology, but the current focus centers on CT and MRI negative disease. Because of the dissemination of imaging technology from tertiary care academic centers to community-based institutions, patients with structural problems such as mass lesions compressing the chiasm are diagnosed and treated at local hospitals. Therefore, neuro-ophthalmologists, the majority of whom practice in large urban university medical centers, now evaluate young and old patients who arrive with several pounds of negative imaging studies. This changing referral pattern, initiated by the improved diagnostic ability of CT and MRI, has stimulated investigations of amaurosis fugax and migraine for younger patients (2–5), and of nonarteritic ischemic optic neuropathy (NAION), Graves' ophthalmopathy, and Alzheimer's disease for older patients (6–9). The recognition of the antiphospholipid antibody syndromes should prevent blindness and neurologic morbidity for many younger patients.

Surgical intervention for NAION is highly controversial but appears to have much more rationale than the previous, rather indiscriminate administration of corticosteroids and anticoagulants (6). The visual system in Alzheimer's disease may provide a precise window into this enigmatic condition through which we may view and assess various therapeutic strategies (9). All these developments have been positive because of the neuro-imaging revolution.

Nevertheless, these techniques have had a negative impact on the economics of medicine. Now, almost any patient with a headache, blurred vision, or ocular pain undergoes a neuroimaging procedure before receiving a thorough neuro-ophthalmic evaluation. Although some patients clearly have benefited from the spread of imaging technology, many others have undergone needless studies because of poor history taking and physical examination by physicians or because of the fear of malpractice suits.

The burden of the negative economic impact of CT and MRI scanning rests with both the medical community and the government. First, family practitioners, internists, ophthalmologists, neurologists, neurosurgeons, and even optometrists who are not trained in the neurology of the visual system are allowed to order CT and MRI scans. America is almost certainly headed in the direction of "rationing" health care, and because no one is comfortable with rationing access based on personal economic means, an alternative method of rationing is to limit which practitioners may request certain expensive, high-technology investigations. In this scenario, many needless studies would be avoided. Such a system now exists in Scotland, where any ophthalmologist who believes an MRI scan is necessary for a visual problem must consult with a neuro-ophthalmologist (McFadzean R: Personal communication, 1990).

Physicians' culpability in this overabundance of imaging studies is compounded by doctor ownership of imaging centers. Referring physicians who are shareholders in any center for imaging or diagnosis and treatment have with the best interpretation the appearance of a conflict of interests, and, under a more rigorous and probably more accurate interpretation, have the reality of financial interests superseding patient care decisions. Yet, challenge of these "centers" is an intricate legal maze in which restraint-of-trade laws provide convenient and effective protective armor for the physician–entrepreneur.

The government's role in the negative economic impact of advanced CT and MRI scanning arises from the bureaucracy of the United States' health care system. Ever since federal and state governments insinuated themselves into the previously free market system of health care, these organizations have paid indiscriminately for service—any service. The bureaucracy has requested only that service be provided and has never considered the quality of the health care provided. Therefore, Medicare and Medicaid pay the same fee for a CT or MRI scan regardless of the quality of the scan or the quality of the physician reading the scan. A scan on a "first generation" machine, which is invariably useless, receives the same reimbursement as a study performed on the best available apparatus. Likewise, an interpretation of a CT or MRI scan of the brain or orbits rendered by a general radiologist merits the same compensation as a report from a neuroradiologist with at least 2 years of subspecialty training. Whether the subject is law, medicine, neuroradiology, or neuro-ophthalmology, all practitioners and machines are not created equal. Until the government recognizes inherent differences in practitioners and imaging technology, unnecessary and inadequate CT and MRI scanning will continue to be a large financial drain on the United States health care system.

References

1. Vrabec TR, Sergott RC, Savino PJ, et al: Intermittent obstructive hydrocephalus in the Arnold-Chiari malformation. *Ann Neurol* 26:401–404, 1989.
2. Briley DP, Coull BM, Goodnight SH Jr: Neurologic disease associated with antiphospholipid antibodies. *Ann Neurol* 25:221–227, 1989.
3. Digre KB, Durcan FJ, Branch DW, et al: Amaurosis fugax associated with antiphospholipid antibodies. *Ann Neurol* 25:228–232, 1989.
4. Tippin J, Corbett JJ, Kerber RE, et al: Amaurosis fugax and ocular infarction in adolescents and young adults. *Ann Neurol* 26:69–77, 1989.
5. Lewes RA, Vijayan N, Watson C, et al: Visual field loss in migraine. *Ophthalmology* 96:321–326, 1989.
6. Sergott RC, Cohen MS, Bosley TM, et al: Optic nerve decompression may improve the progressive form of nonarteritic ischemic optic neuropathy. *Arch Ophthalmol* 107:1743–1754, 1989.
7. Bartelena L, Marcocci C, Bogazzi F, et al: Use of corticosteroids to prevent progression of Graves' ophthalmopathy after radioiodine therapy for hyperthyroidism. *N Engl J Med* 321:1349–1352, 1989.
8. Prummel MF, Mourits MPL, Berhout A, et al: Prednisone and cyclosporine in the treatment of severe Graves' ophthalmopathy. *N Engl J Med* 321:1353–1359, 1989.
9. Kiyosawa M, Bosley TM, Chawluk J, et al: Alzheimer's disease with prominent visual symptoms: Clinical and metabolic evaluation. *Ophthalmology* 96:1077–1086, 1989.

Amaurosis Fugax Associated With Antiphospholipid Antibodies
Digre KB, Durcan FJ, Branch DW, Jacobson DM, Varner MW, Baringer JR (Univ of Utah; Marshfield Clinic, Marshfield, Wis)
Ann Neurol 25:228–232, March 1989   4–1

Amaurosis fugax in older persons often is caused by embolization of carotid atherosclerosis, but no cause is identified in a high proportion of young persons. Of 6 patients aged 21 to 33 years in whom amaurosis fugax was associated with increased antiphospholipid antibodies (table), most had splinter hemorrhages of the nail beds (Fig 4–1), which have not previously been related to antiphospholipid antibodies. Treatment with antiplatelet agents or anticoagulants, or both, led to a significant reduction in episodic visual loss in 5 of the 6 patients.

The 2 clinically important antiphospholipid antibodies, lupus anticoagulant (LA) and anticardiolipin antibodies (ACLA), probably belong to the same family of autoantibodies. They have been related to several disorders including thromboembolism, myocardial infarction, peripheral arterial occlusion, stroke, and central retinal artery or vein occlusion. The splinter hemorrhages may represent microemboli caused by intravascular platelet aggregation.

Work-up of young patients with amaurosis fugax should include ocu-

Summary of Clinical Features of Patients*

Patient No.	Age (yr)	Sex	Visual Symptoms	Other Neurological Symptoms	Splinter Hemorrhages (Fingernail)	Other Neurological Findings	Echocardiography	CT/MRI Findings
1	23	F	Unilateral total visual loss—2 min	R hand clumsiness; headaches; severe pre-eclampsia	Present	R upper extremity weakness	Thickened mitral valve without vegetation	Multiple infarctions on CT and MRI
2	31	F	Unilateral altitudinal visual loss—1–5 min	Vertigo; diplopia; headaches	Present	None	Mitral valve prolapse	Normal MRI
3	25	F	Constriction of visual field 20 times/day; central scotoma	None	Present	None	Normal	Normal CT
4	21	F	Unilateral total visual loss—5 min	Two episodes of transient amnesia; vertigo	Not examined	None	Normal	Normal CT
5	26	M	Altitudinal visual loss—30 sec –20 min	Vertical diplopia; classic migraines	Present	None	Mild aortic regurgitation	Normal MRI
6	33	M	Central scotoma—5 min; oblique curtain to total visual loss	Diplopia; vertigo	Not examined	None	Mildly thickened mitral valve	Normal CT

*R, right; CT, computed tomography; MRI, magnetic resonance imaging.
(Courtesy of Digre KB, Durcan FJ, Branch DW, et al: Ann Neurol 25:228–232, March 1989.)

lar examination, echocardiography, a platelet count, estimation of activated partial thromboplastin time, and an ACLA test. If the findings suggest cerebral ischemia, MR imaging or CT should be done.

▶ Amaurosis fugax in young patients previously has been attributed most frequently to migraine phenomenon and much more rarely to atrial myxoma and

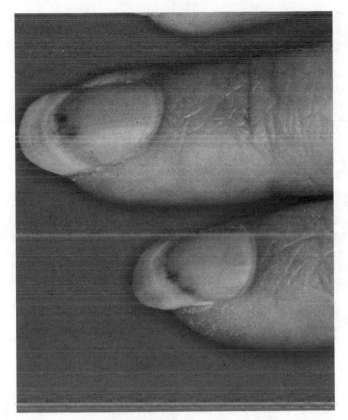

Fig 4–1.—Splinter hemorrhages were present on general physical examination. (Courtesy of Digre KB, Durcan FJ, Branch DW, et al: *Ann Neurol* 25:228–232, March 1989.)

carotid atresia. This study now presents an important new syndrome compelling clinicians to search for splinter hemorrhages of the nasal beds and to estimate an activated partial thromboplastin time, screen for lupus anticoagulant, and test for ACLA. Unless noninvasive carotid imaging suggests a stenotic carotid lesion, these patients *never* should be subjected to carotid angiography. This syndrome is an important step in decreasing the size of the "wastebasket" diagnosis of "atypical migraine."—R.C. Sergott, M.D.

Neurological Disease Associated With Antiphospholipid Antibodies
Briley DP, Coull BM, Goodnight SH Jr (Oregon Health Sciences Univ, Portland; VA Med Ctr, White City, Ore)
Ann Neurol 25:221–227, March 1989   4–2

Antiphospholipid antibody in general and anticardiolipid antibody (ACLA) in particular are closely associated with pathologic thrombotic events. Data were studied on 80 patients who had significantly elevated

ACLA levels according to a sandwich-type enzyme-linked immunosorbent assay that identified both immunoglobulin M (IgM) and IgG anticardiolipin antibodies.

Twenty-five patients had neurologic disorders, including 15 with systemic lupus or a lupus-like syndrome. Sixteen patients had brain infarction, and 4 had acute ischemic encephalopathy. Six patients each had migraine-like headaches and ophthalmologic complications. Six of the patients with brain infarction had multi-infarct dementia. The ophthalmic disorders included amaurosis fugax, retinal infarction, and acute ischemic optic neuropathy. One patient had recurrent episodes of optic neuropathy over 6 years.

This experience supports a relationship between antiphospholipid antibodies and cerebrovascular thrombosis. Most of the neurologic symptoms indicate ischemic involvement of medium-sized vessels. Migraine-type headaches often were accompanied by cognitive dysfunction. The only evident treatment effect was a response in 3 patients given plasmapheresis and immunosuppressive therapy. The latter may be helpful in cases of acute ischemic encephalopathy. Screening should utilize both an ACLA assay and a test for lupus anticoagulant.

▶ In general, we achieve major therapeutic success when we can detect and treat important refactors for ischemic neurologic and ophthalmic diseases before the development of permanent defects. The high occupancy rates in rehabilitation units is testimony to how poorly we reverse these problems once an ischemic event has been completed. This article corroborates some of the findings in the preceding article. Because ophthalmologists see a large number of patients who report amaurosis fugax and even symptoms of cerebral transient ischemic attack, they must remember to screen patients for antiphospholipid antibodies. Detecting just 1 patient with elevated ACLA or lupus anticoagulant and preventing a stroke is more cost-effective than a long-term rehabilitation medicine admission (so do not let the managed health care providers tell you these tests are not indicated; they represent medical progress).—R.C. Sergott, M.D.

Pseudotumor Cerebri Induced by Danazol
Hamed LM, Glaser JS, Schatz NJ, Perez TH (Univ of Miami; FDA, Rockville, Md)
Am J Ophthalmol 107:105–110, February 1989   4–3

Two patients given danazol for cyclic neutropenia or immune hemolytic anemia had intracranial hypertension. Danazol is used effectively to treat a variety of disorders. No apparent cause was found for one patient, in whom papilledema was resolved a month after danazol was withdrawn. The other patient (Fig 4–2) had cerebral venous sinus thrombosis. Papilledema also improved in this case after the cessation of danazol therapy. Seven other cases of pseudotumor cerebri associated

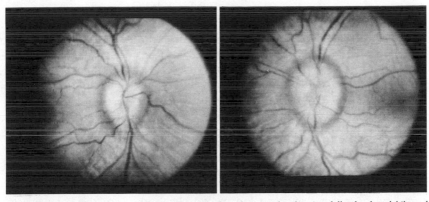

Fig 4–2.—**Left,** right eye. **Right,** left eye. Fundus photographs showing fully developed bilateral papilledema. (Courtesy of Hamed LM, Glaser JS, Schatz NJ, et al: *Am J Ophthalmol* 107:105–110, February 1989.)

with danazol therapy have been reported to the FDA. In all cases the papilledema was resolved shortly after the end of danazol administration.

Intracranial hypertension induced by danazol responds favorably to withdrawal of the drug or to diuretic therapy. Alternate treatment should be used if feasible when this complication develops.

▶ This medication (danazol) is another to be added to the list of drugs associated with pseudotumor cerebri syndromes. Remember that pseudotumor cerebri may produce optic atrophy and blindness. Neglecting to discontinue a medication like danazol, which is known somehow to be associated with this disease, could have disastrous results. Other medications to be wary of are corticosteroids, nalidixic acid, hypervitaminosis A or hypovitamenosis A, nitrofurantoin, tetracycline, oral contraceptives, psychotherapeutic agents, antiinflammatory compounds, and amiodarone.—R.C. Sergott, M.D.

Transient Ocular Motor Paresis Associated With Acute Internal Carotid Artery Occlusion

Wilson WB, Leavengood JM, Ringel SP, Bott AD (Univ of Colorado)
Ann Neurol 25:286–290, March 1989   4–4

Sudden monocular blindness and central artery occlusion are associated with acute internal carotid thrombosis, but unilateral ophthalmoparesis is not a recognized association. Three patients, all adult men, who had the complete syndrome but lacked other major signs of vascular disease were encountered. Paresis of the oculomotor, trochlear, and abducens nerves was variable and resolved slowly over days to weeks. However, vision did not return in any of the patients. Mild to moderate signs of hemispheric dysfunction were constantly noted. Thrombus extended from the internal carotid origin to its intracranial bifurcation and occluded the proximal half to two thirds of the ophthalmic artery. No patient had evidence of vasculitis.

The occurrence of transient partial oculomotor paresis ipsilateral to acute internal carotid occlusion suggests that transient ischemia occurred in the nutrient circulation of the ocular motor nerves. Ischemia likely occurred in the cavernous sinus or the posterior orbit, or both. The partial involvement and transiency of the ophthalmoparesis suggest that some collateral supply persists.

▶ This is a new variation of the syndrome of central retinal artery occlusion with acute internal carotid thrombosis. Be careful of the insulin-dependent diabetic patient who may present in an identical manner with a central retinal occlusion and ophthalmoplegia. In a diabetic patient, this syndrome still represents mucor mycosis invading the carotid circulation from the paranasal sinuses until proven otherwise. All patients in this series were surprisingly young (aged 42, 44, and 57 years) nondiabetic persons. It is interesting that, in light of the 2 previous articles, these patients apparently were not screened for lupus anticoagulant and anticardiolysis antibodies.— R.C. Sergott, M.D.

Visual Field Loss in Migraine
Lewis RA, Vijayan N, Watson C, Keltner J, Johnson CA (Univ of California, Davis)
Ophthalmology 96:321–326, March 1989   4–5

Permanent visual loss is reported in a limited number of patients with migraine, but detailed visual field studies are lacking. Visual fields were examined with an automated static perimeter in 60 patients with at least a 2-year history of migraine diagnosed by a neurologist and no history of ocular problems. A visual screening study was negative in all cases. The 48 women and 12 men in the study had an average age of 49 years and had had migraine for a mean of 24 years.

All patients had acuity of 20/30 or better. The average intraocular pressure was 15 mm Hg. One third of the patients had visual field sensitivity loss beyond the 95% normal confidence limits. Seven patients had field loss in both eyes, whereas 3 had a left homonymous deficit. Generalized depression of the visual field was the most frequent abnormality. Field loss was more frequent in older patients and those with a longer history of migraine.

Studies of visual fields in migraine patients are confounded by the criteria used to diagnose migraine and by the selection of patients with associated disorders. Whether the visual field defects are transient or permanent remains unclear.

▶ This interesting finding has potential great importance given the tremendously high incidence of migraine headaches within the general population. Because of the high incidence, this article is both fascinating and potentially treacherous for the unsuspecting clinician. Just as the diagnosis of migraine headaches is made after other causes of headache have been excluded, migraine as a cause of visual field loss also must be an exclusionary diagnosis. Glaucoma still must be the first consideration for patients with nerve fiber layer defects, and strokes and tumors must be the initial diagnosis for homonymous hemianopias, even for the patients with the worst migraine headaches.—R.C. Sergott, M.D.

Orbital Inflammation and Optic Neuropathies Associated With Chronic Sinusitis of Intranasal Cocaine Abuse: Possible Role of Contiguous Inflammation

Goldberg RA, Weisman JS, McFarland JE, Krauss HR, Hepler RS, Shorr N (Univ of California, Los Angeles)
Arch Ophthalmol 107:831–835, June 1989   4–6

Ophthalmic effects of cocaine abuse are unusual, but 3 long-term abusers of intranasal cocaine who had orbitopathy or optic neuropathy were encountered. All of them had chronic sinusitis with histologic evidence of acute and chronic inflammation in the sinus and orbital tissues. Two of the patients had radiographic evidence of sinusitis with contiguous orbital inflammation. These patients responded to steroid therapy, but 1 had recurrent inflammation during tapering. One patient had complete loss of vision in the involved eye secondary to fulminant orbital inflammation and optic nerve dysfunction.

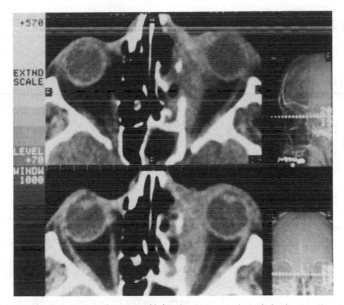

Fig 4–3.—Axial CT scan reveals extent of left orbital mass. Left medial orbital wall and ethmoidal sinus are partially surgically absent. (Courtesy of Goldberg RA, Weisman JS, McFarland JE, et al: *Arch Ophthalmol* 107:831–835, June 1989.)

Optic neuritis was the only ophthalmic abnormality in 1 of these patients. The other 2 had direct evidence of orbital involvement with an inflammatory medial orbital mass (Fig 4–3). The patients went to ophthalmologists early in their clinical course. It is important that drug abuse be considered when patients have unusual orbital and optic nerve findings.

▶ Much of Sigmund Freud's early research investigated the ocular anesthetic effects of cocaine. Now the current generation of cocaine "researchers" has rediscovered the anatomical connections of the nostrils, paranasal sinuses, orbits, and optic nerves.

When confronted with an unusual optic neuropathy or "orbital pseudotumor" in association with sinusitis, a clinician must suspect cocaine use as a possible cause. One patient in this report actually preferred to continue cocaine use and risk blindness. It is possible to imagine a plaintiff's attorney constructing a theory of liability against an ophthalmologist who failed to warn a patient about potential blindness secondary to cocaine use, even though the drug is illegal. The physician would be found guilty of negligence, and the malpractice monetary award would pay for the cocaine user's legal fees and recreational drug expenses.—R.C. Sergott, M.D.

Hyperdeviation Associated With Isolated Unilateral Abducens Palsy

Slavin ML (Long Island Jewish Med Ctr, New Hyde Park, NY)
Ophthalmology 96:512–516, April 1989   4–7

A recently seen patient with presumed isolated abducens palsy caused by ischemia was found to have significant associated hyperdeviation (HD). Fifteen further patients with isolated abducens palsy were evaluated prospectively for HD. Hyperdeviation was found in each instance. A small HD in primary gaze, detected with the alternate cover test, may be masked by a much larger esodeviation that is invariably present. A recent study showed that three fourths of a large group of adults had HD, which followed the pattern of primary overaction of the inferior oblique muscle.

For 4 of the 16 study patients the chief complaint was vertical as well as horizontal diplopia. Vertical ductions were consistently normal. For 10 patients the maximal HD ranged from 8 to 16 prism D, and for 6 patients it ranged from 4 to 7 prism D. Ten patients had a HD in primary as well as peripheral gaze. The magnitude of HD was not correlated with the degree of abduction defect. It usually was maximal to the side of the paretic lateral rectus muscle. The double Maddox rod test showed no cyclodeviation in 10 of 12 patients.

Hyperdeviation caused by childhood vertical strabismus or dissociated vertical divergence should be considered in these cases. Ocular electromyography may help clarify the mechanism in patients with variable HD and an abduction defect.

▶ Finding a vertical deviation in association with an otherwise isolated lateral rectus palsy does not preclude the diagnosis of a microvascular sixth nerve palsy. Ophthalmologists must be certain that the HDs are not manifestations of thyroid eye disease, ocular myasthenia, metastatic orbital disease, or a cavernous sinus syndrome. These differential diagnostic possibilities mandate a careful neuro-ophthalmic examination for the following findings: (1) ptosis and lid retraction, (2) proptosis and enophthalmos, and (3) ductional deficits of the involved eye.

A key clinical observation in this study is that only 3 of the 16 patients with HDs had symptoms of oblique diplopia. Therefore, if patients have HD and describe only horizontal double vision, clinical observation is reasonable. But if they describe oblique diplopia, a search for disorders other than an isolated sixth nerve palsy becomes important.—R.C. Sergott, M.D.

The Spectrum of Optic Nerve Disease in Human Immunodeficiency Virus Infection
Winward KE, Hamed LM, Glaser JS (Univ of Miami, Fla)
Am J Ophthalmol 107:373–380, April 1989   4–8

Four patients with HIV-associated optic neuropathies were encountered. Optic neuropathy was among the initial clinical features of HIV infection in 2 patients. One patient had syphilitic optic perineuritis that responded well to penicillin therapy. One had cytomegalovirus papillitis and a severe decline in acuity. The third patient had varicella zoster optic neuritis, which improved on intravenous acyclovir therapy. The fourth patient had cryptococcal retrobulbar neuritis and died shortly afterward.

Human immunodeficiency virus infection may be associated with optic perineuritis, papillitis, retrobulbar neuritis, or papilledema secondary to intracranial hypertension. The ophthalmologist may be the first to diagnose HIV infection. Affected patients may well have multiple infections at the same time. Some of the causes of optic neuropathy, such as syphilis, are responsive to treatment. Systemic corticosteroids should not be used in patients with known or suspected HIV infection until a thorough infectious work-up is negative. Human immunodeficiency virus–associated disorder should be included in the differential diagnosis of optic neuropathy, especially in persons at risk for AIDS.

▶ All optic neuritis is not "idiopathic" or associated with multiple sclerosis. Certainly every patient with inflammatory optic neuropathy does not merit HIV testing. However, the astute clinician must be cautious that virtually any optic neuropathy or uveitis syndrome may represent an infection such as syphilis and ultimately herald HIV infection. Then the ophthalmologist must refer the patient for appropriate care.—R.C. Sergott, M.D.

Alzheimer's Disease With Prominent Visual Symptoms: Clinical and Metabolic Evaluation

Kiyosawa M, Bosley TM, Chawluk J, Jamieson D, Schatz NJ, Savino PJ, Sergott RC, Reivich M, Alavai A (Univ of Pennsylvania; Wills Eye Hosp, Philadelphia)

Ophthalmology 96:1077–1086, July 1989

4–9

Five of 8 patients with Alzheimer's dementia had prominent visual symptoms early in the course of illness. Neuro-ophthalmologic work-up showed relatively consistent abnormalities in figure copying, color vision testing with isochromatic plates, and stereopsis. Cerebral glucose metabolism, determined with positron emission tomography with ^{18}F-fluoro-2-deoxyglucose, was unchanged in the primary visual cortex in both visually and not visually symptomatic groups of subjects. Glucose metabolism, however, was reduced in the visual association cortex and the inferior parietal cortex in patients with early visual symptoms.

Some patients with progressive dementia have prominent visual symptoms early in the course of disease. Minor visual field abnormalities were frequent in the present patients, and stereopsis was poor in those with early visual symptoms. Patients with Alzheimer's dementia and visual symptoms form a distinct subgroup. They tend to seek ophthalmic aid before cognitive deficit is manifest. The visual symptoms probably are attributable to malfunction of association cortices in the parietal and occipital lobes. Atrophy is evident in these areas, as is hypometabolism.

▶ For those ophthalmologists who choose their subspecialty as an escape from "real medicine," this paper and the preceding one (4–8) are harsh reminders that patients are not always interested in posterior chamber lenses, keratorefractive surgery, and blepharopigmentation. Moreover, these 2 papers illustrate why eye care providers must be educated in all aspects of medicine and not just the eye (poor education and training are never cost-effective despite what some congressmen and senators think).

This interesting group of patients shows that Alzheimer's disease may have a special predilection for the afferent visual system. More patients with this syndrome must be identified and studied with detailed clinical, electrophysiologic, metabolic, and neuropathologic analyses in an effort to understand the pathophysiology of Alzheimer's disease.—R.C. Sergott, M.D.

Superior Segmental Optic Hypoplasia: A Sign of Maternal Diabetes

Kim RY, Hoyt WF, Lessell S, Narahara MH (Univ of California, San Francisco; Massachusetts Eye and Ear Infirmary, Boston)

Arch Ophthalmol 107:1312–1315, September 1989

4–10

Researchers in the mid-1970s described a syndrome in children of diabetic mothers characterized by segmental optic nerve hypoplasia, altitudinal or sector visual field defects, and normal visual acuity. The appearance of optic disks in the eyes of patients with maternal diabetes—segmental optic nerve hypoplasia syndrome was described.

Ten patients with superior segmental optic nerve hypoplasia, all of whom were born to diabetic mothers, were studied. Seventeen eyes had at least 1 of 4 characteristic findings in the optic disk: relative superior entrance of the central retinal artery, pallor of the superior disk, superior peripapillary halo, and thinning of the superior peripapillary nerve fiber layer. In 15 disks, the central artery entered relatively superiorly. Thirteen disks showed superior segmental hypoplasia with pallor and an adjacent pale scleral "halo." Seven disks had generalized hypoplasia. All 17 fundi had thinned superior peripapillary nerve fiber layers. Generalized arteriolar tortuosity was noted in 2 cases. Eleven optic disks were flat, and 6 had small but identifiable cups.

The presence of these 4 signs of superior segmental optic nerve hypoplasia is strongly suggestive of maternal diabetes. The characteristic findings usually occur bilaterally and affect women more often than men. The visual acuity of these patients is generally normal.

▶ Recognition of this unusual syndrome is important for several reasons: (1) these patients do not require extensive and expensive neuroimaging studies; (2) visual field defects should not be diagnosed as glaucomatous in nature; and (3) visual acuity is normal in this syndrome, and an alternative explanation must be found for any decrease in central vision.—R.C. Sergott, M.D.

Intermittent Obstructive Hydrocephalus in the Arnold-Chiari Malformation

Vrabec TR, Sergott RC, Savino PJ, Bosley TM (Wills Eye Hosp, Philadelphia)
Ann Neurol 26:401–404, September 1989   4–11

The Arnold-Chiari malformation consists of a spectrum of congenital hindbrain abnormalities. It often is associated with cerebellar tonsil and medulla herniation, hydrocephalus, and increased intracranial pressure. A case of Chiari-I malformation was presented.

Woman, 26, had intermittent symptoms of headache, arm pain, and scotomatous visual loss. Papilledema was associated clinically with midperipheral retinal hemorrhages. Computed tomographic scans and lumbar punctures done repeatedly yielded normal results. The Chiari-I malformation was demonstrated with posterior fossa-directed magnetic resonance imaging. Intraventricular monitoring was done to assess the marked but unsustained increase in intracranial pressure.

This woman's unusual clinical course demonstrates that transient neuro-ophthalmologic signs and symptoms of the Arnold-Chiari malformation can be related directly to intermittently obstructive hydrocephalus and increased intracranial pressure. The patient's transient symptoms and simultaneous extreme but unsustained intracranial pressure increases presumptively were produced by a process of intermittent obstruction.

▶ Arnold-Chiari malformations frequently are considered an "incidental" finding detected with MRI studies. The most common neuro-ophthalmic disorder associated with these abnormalities is downbeat nystagmus. However, this case demonstrates how an Arnold-Chiari malformation may produce papilledema and increased intracranial pressure without downbeat nystagmus.—R.C. Sergott, M.D.

Amaurosis Fugax and Ocular Infarction in Adolescents and Young Adults
Tippin J, Corbett JJ, Kerber RE, Schroeder E, Thompson HS (Univ of Iowa Hosps and Clinics, Iowa City)
Ann Neurol 26:69–77, 1989   4–12

The cause and natural history of amaurosis fugax (AF) and ocular infarction (OI) in younger patients are not known. To identify possible causes, records of 83 patients whose symptoms began before the age of 45 years were reviewed. Forty-one percent of these patients had headache or orbital pain accompanying ameurotic spells. Another 25.3% had severe headaches independent of loss of vision. Laboratory test results rarely were abnormal. Echocardiography showed that only 1 patient had previously undiagnosed heart disease. Mitral valve prolapse was found in 6.5% of patients, which is comparable to the incidence expected in the general population.

Forty-two patients were followed up for a mean of 5.8 years. None had a stroke. Clinical status at follow-up was not correlated with the duration of visual loss, frequency of visual loss, sex, presence of headache or heart disease, cigarette smoking, use of oral contraceptives, or abnormal echocardiography or laboratory test results.

A high frequency of headache is temporally associated with episodic visual loss. In younger patients, AF and OI probably are associated with a more benign clinical course than that in older patients. Migraine is a likely cause for visual loss episodes in most of these younger patients. Therefore, a conservative approach to the assessment of such patients is warranted.

▶ Transient visual loss in young patients is always a perplexing management problem. When symptoms are classic for migraine, diagnosis and treatment are straightforward. However, once a fixed ischemic defect occurs, we still would recommend an aggressive search for an underlying cardiac, vascular, hematologic, or autoimmune abnormality. Even if the yield is low, a delay in diagnosis could result in additional permanent visual or neurologic defects in young patients.—R.C. Sergott, M.D.

Use of Corticosteroids to Prevent Progression of Graves' Ophthalmopathy After Radioiodine Therapy for Hyperthyroidism

Bartalena L, Marcocci C, Bogazzi F, Panicucci M, Lepri A, Pinchera A (Univ of Pisa, Italy)
N Engl J Med 321:1349–1352, Nov 16, 1989   4–13

Because Graves' ophthalmopathy has autoimmune origins, it may be treated with corticosteroids, which have immunosuppressive and anti-inflammatory properties. The effect of radioiodine treatment for hyperthyroidism caused by Graves' disease on Graves' ophthalmopathy and the protective role of corticosteroids were studied.

Fifty-two patients were assigned randomly in equal numbers to treatment with radioiodine alone or radioiodine plus systemic prednisone for 4 months. Prednisone was given initially in a dose of 0.4 to 0.5 mg per kilogram of body weight for 1 month. The drug then was withdrawn gradually during the next 3 months. All patients were examined every 3 months for 18 months after treatment. Before therapy, 10 patients in the first treatment group (radioiodine alone) and 5 in the second treatment group (radioiodine and prednisone) showed no evidence of ophthalmopathy. No ocular symptoms appeared in any patient after radioiodine treatment. Of group 1 patients with an initial ophthalmopathy index of 1 or more, ocular disease worsened in 56% and was unchanged in 44%. The worsening mostly involved soft tissue changes and extraocular-muscle function. By contrast, ophthalmopathy improved in 52% and did not change in 48% of the patients in group 2. The mean ophthalmopathy index in group 1 rose from 1.5 to 3 and in group 2 dropped from 2.2 to 1.3.

Systemic corticosteroid therapy appears to prevent the exacerbations of Graves' ophthalmopathy that occur after radioiodine treatment in many patients with hyperthyroidism and some degree of ocular involvement before treatment. However, it is possible that, in view of the close temporal relationship between the onset of Graves' hyperthyroidism and ophthalmopathy, the progression of ophthalmopathy after radioidine treatment might have been coincidental.

▶ A far from perfect study about an exceedingly complex disease. The use of systemic prednisone, a potentially dangerous medication, prevented only more advanced soft tissue and extraocular muscle problems, 2 indices that are somewhat subjective. No patient in either group had dysthyroid optic neuropathy. The practitioner must decide whether the risks of systemic corticosteroid therapy are warranted to "maybe" prevent lid edema and extraocular muscle imbalance, 2 problems that many times do not require intervention. We believe that this study is not a "New England Journal gold standard manuscript" because of the variability of the end points used and the reasonable possibility that the result could be coincidental.— R.C. Sergott, M.D.

Prednisone and Cyclosporine in the Treatment of Severe Graves' Ophthalmopathy

Prummel MF, Mourits MP, Berghout A, Krenning EP, van der Gaag R, Koornneef L, Wiersinga WM (Univ of Amsterdam; Netherlands Ophthalmic Research Inst, Amsterdam; Dijkzigt Hosp; Erasmus Univ, Rotterdam, The Netherlands)
N Engl J Med 321:1353–1359, Nov 16, 1989   4–14

The best medical therapy for patients with severe Graves' ophthalmopathy has not been established. A prospective, single-blind, randomized clinical trial was done to compare the efficacy, safety, and tolerability of prednisone and cyclosporine in untreated patients with severe Graves' ophthalmopathy and stable thyroid function.

Thirty-six patients were given either cyclosporine, 7.5 mg/kg/day, or prednisone, 60 mg/day. The prednisone dose was tapered to 20 mg/day. Treatment lasted for 12 weeks. Sixty-one percent of the prednisone-treated patients and only 22% of the cyclosporine-treated patients responded to treatment. Response consisted of reductions in eye-muscle enlargement and proptosis and improved visual acuity and total and subjective eye scores. Patients did not tolerate prednisone as well as cyclosporine. Patients who did not respond to treatment in the first 12 weeks were treated for another 12 weeks with combined prednisone and cyclosporine. Of the 9 patients who initially received prednisone, 5 (56%) had improvement after cyclosporine was added. Sixty-two percent of the 13 patients who were given cyclosporine initially had improvement with the addition of prednisone.

Single-drug treatment with prednisone is more effective than cyclosporine in patients with severe Graves' ophthalmopathy. For patients who do not respond to either drug alone, the 2 combined may be effective.

▶ This study had a much better design than the previous one, but it is still not a classic. Several valuable facts are established: (1) cyclosporine alone should not be used for severe Graves' ophthalmopathy; and (2) the combination of prednisone and cyclosporine may help desperation cases after prednisone has failed. However, we believe that ophthalmologists should recommend transantral orbital decompression surgery or orbital irradiation before risking the complications of prednisone and cyclosporine together. Properly performed surgery to decompress the orbital apex is the most effective and usually the safest method to treat Graves' optic neuropathy.—R.C. Sergott, M.D.

Optic Nerve Decompression May Improve the Progressive Form of Nonarteritic Ischemic Optic Neuropathy

Sergott RC, Cohen MS, Bosley TM, Savino PJ (Wills Eye Hosp, Philadelphia)
Arch Ophthalmol 107:1743–1754, December 1989   4–15

Nonarteritic ischemic optic neuropathy (NAION) is considered an untreatable cause of visual acuity and field loss in adults. Twenty-five percent of patients have progressive deterioration of visual function 1 to 4

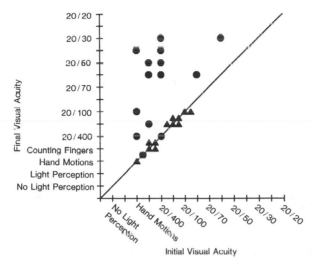

Fig 4–4.—*Circles* indicate preoperative and postoperative visual acuities in 14 patients with progressive nonarteritic ischemic optic neuropathy treated by optic nerve sheath decompression; *triangles*, initial and final visual acuities for 12 control patients who did not undergo surgery. (Courtesy of Sergott RC, Cohen MS, Bosley TM, et al: *Arch Ophthalmol* 107:1743–1754, December 1989.)

weeks after symptom onset. Experimental ischemia and NAION may be associated with blocked axoplasmic transport. Modified optic nerve sheath decompressions with lysis of subdural adhesions was done in a group of patients with severe visual loss caused by NAION.

Visual function in 12 of 14 patients with NAION was improved after optic nerve sheath decompression (Fig 4–4). Visual recovery was maintained in all patients 6 to 18 months after the procedure. Seven patients previously had had a NAION in the eye that was not treated surgically; it did not improve spontaneously. Two of these eyes with long-standing reduced vision had some improvement in vision after surgery on the contralateral, acutely affected eye. Spontaneous visual improvement did not occur in 12 controls matched for age and sex with similar baseline visual acuity and field loss. Of 3 patients with sudden, nonprogressive visual loss caused by NAION, only 1 had improvement after surgery. In a matched control group, 2 of 15 eyes in 14 patients improved spontaneously.

Optic nerve sheath decompression reversed visual deficits in 12 of 14 patients with progressive NAION. Surgery for a presumed ischemic optic neuropathy is a radical departure from previously accepted beliefs. Although this study had some methodologic flaws, it showed that such treatment can produce striking improvement. This surgical procedure should be considered when NAION results in progressive, profound loss of visual function.

▶ This is a candidate for most controversial publication of the year. At present, the procedure should be limited to that small group of patients with progressive visual loss and NAION. The results of other independent investigations now are required to determine the applicability of this approach.— R.C. Sergott, M.D.

Retinal Hemorrhage Predicts Neurologic Injury in the Shaken Baby Syndrome
Wilkinson WS, Han DP, Rappley MD, Owings CL (Univ of Michigan, Ann Arbor; Med College of Wisconsin, Milwaukee)
Arch Ophthalmol 107:1472–1474, October 1989   4–16

The shaken baby syndrome is a type of child abuse in which intracranial injury and intraocular hemorrhage can exist without external signs of direct head trauma. Babies with this syndrome often have a vague clinical presentation with minimal history of trauma. However, there may be substantial intracranial bleeding or other cerebral injury. Ophthalmologists may be asked to assess an early manifestation of this condition, before its neurologic complications evolve completely. To determine whether a relationship between the severity of intracranial injury and severity of retinal hemorrhage exists, 14 consecutive cases of presumed shaken baby syndrome were evaluated.

The severity of retinal hemorrhage was based on hemorrhage type, and size, and on the extent of fundus involvement. Retinal hemorrhage severity was significantly correlated with acute neurologic results. More severe acute neurologic injury was associated with diffuse fundus involvement, vitreous hemorrhage, or large subhyaloid hemorrhages.

The severity of retinal hemorrhage is predictive of the severity of acute neurologic injury in children with the shaken baby syndrome. The presence of large subhyaloid hemorrhages, vitreous hemorrhage, or diffuse involvement of the fundus can be used to identify battered or shaken babies who are likely to have severe neurologic injury.

▶ In such a clinical situation, an ophthalmologist may make a life-saving diagnosis. Retinal hemorrhages in infants are never an incidental finding and always demand an explanation.— R.C. Sergott, M.D.

Bilateral Anterior Ischaemic Optic Neuropathy Associated With Optic Disc Drusen and Systemic Hypotension
Michaelson C, Behrens M, Odel J (Boston Univ Med Ctr; Columbia Presbyterian Med Ctr, New York)
Br J Ophthalmol 73:762–764, 1989   4–17

Nonarteritic anterior ischemic optic neuropathy (AION) seems to be caused by obstruction of axoplasmic flow because of ischemia, resulting in a cascading effect through further small vessel compromise in underlying disk crowding. A young woman with systemic hypotension and optic disk drusen who had bilateral AION while undergoing home peritoneal dialysis was described.

Woman, 23, noticed a painful loss of inferotemporal vision in the left eye when she awoke one morning. Her visual acuity was found to be 20/20 on the right and 20/25 +3 with marked relative afferent pupillary defect and constriction of visual field on the left. There were drusen of both optic disks. The left was swollen. Findings on a CT scan of the head and orbits were normal. Two months later, her visual acuity was 20/20 in each eye. There was no relative afferent pupillary defect. A few weeks later, she awoke with marked diminution of vision in her right eye. At this time, her visual acuity was finger counting at 2 to 3 feet, with hand motion only superotemporally in the right eye, and 20/20 +3 in the left eye with the field concentrically constricted on tangent screen. Findings were normal on external, motility, and slit lamp examinations. In each eye tension by applanation was 16. The pupils were sluggish and had a marked right relative afferent defect. There were bilateral disk drusen and diffuse thinning of the nerve fiber layer. She had calcification in both optic nerve heads as demonstrated with orbital CT scan.

Through mass effect, drusen might have increased the intraneural tissue pressure, resulting in greater susceptibility to ischemia.

▶ Any patient with chronically swollen optic disks—either from chronic papilledema or, as described here, from drusen—is at risk for visual loss during dialysis procedures because of hypotension. Ophthalmologists and nephrologists must screen all potential dialysis patients for chronic optic nerve elevation. Failure to detect this problem can result in severe, irreversible visual loss.—R.C. Sergott, M.D.

5 Oculoplastics

A New Orbital Implant to Increase Enucleation Prosthesis Motility

JOSEPH C. FLANAGAN, M.D., F.A.C.S.
Oculoplastic Service, Wills Eye Hospital, Philadelphia, Pennsylvania

Orbital implants have been used after enucleation for the past 100 years. A variety of orbital implants has been designed and used in attempts to increase motility so that patients can have natural movement of enucleation prostheses. Most of these implants were designed so that the recti muscles could be sutured and fixated to the implant, thereby imparting motion to the prosthesis. The implants that provided the greatest motility had portions that were exteriorized to conjunctiva surfaces so that the external prostheses could be coupled to the orbital implant to give optimal motility. These old, integrated types of implants did provide excellent motility; however, most became infected because of that portion of the implant that was exposed to the external environment. The incidence of infection was quite high and necessitated the subsequent removal of the implant.

Arthur C. Perry, M.D., of La Jolla, California, has designed a new, integrated orbital implant, which was approved by the FDA in August 1989. This implant can be used after enucleation or evisceration, or as a secondary implant if the original implant must be removed because of extrusion or migration or if improvement in motility is desired for cosmetic reasons. The concept of this implant is different in that integration in this instance means that the implant becomes integrated as a living portion of the recipient's orbital tissues; therefore, extrusion and migration should not occur. It is made of a natural component of coral reefs known as porous hydroxyapatite. The natural material is modified chemically so that it is similar to the mineral portion of human cancellous bone. Therefore, it is porous, which allows a recipient's blood vessels and fibrous tissues to grow into the implant, and in this manner it does become a "living" portion of the orbital tissues. When the fibrovascular infiltration is complete, migration or extrusion should not occur.

Some months after an implant has been inserted into an orbit and has become a fully integrated part of the recipient's body, a 10-mm cylindrical portion of the implant is drilled out so that a peg can be placed to maintain patency. Conjunctiva and fibrovascular tissue line the cylindrical space, which seals the area from the external environment. The ocularist then can design a cylindrical peg on the posterior surface of the prosthesis, which fits into the implant and gives excellent motility to the external prosthesis. An alternate method involves placement of a cylindrical peg into the implant space, with a 3-mm ball on the external end of the peg. The ocularist designs a corresponding socket into the posterior surface of the prosthesis, creating a ball-and-socket junction to provide motility.

If the hydroxyapatite implant is used for enucleation, enucleation is done in a routine fashion; however, the four recti muscles and superior and inferior oblique are isolated and secured with 5-0 Vicryl sutures in a manner similar to that used for extraocular muscle surgery. When enucleation is completed, the hydroxyapatite implant is used for the orbital implant. It may be encased in a covering of donor sclera or donor or autologous fascia lata. Sclera or fascia lata is believed to impart more motility than the implant being placed uncovered into the muscle cone. If a covering of sclera or fascia lata is not used, drill holes can be made into the implant at the time of surgery so the extraocular muscles can be sutured to the implant surface. In either case, attachment of the muscles is important to allow for the ingrowth of fibrovascular tissues into the hydroxyapatite substance.

The patient receives the usual postoperative treatment and may be fitted for a prosthesis in approximately 4 weeks. Four to 6 months should elapse before the drill hole is made to receive the cylindrical peg. A bone scan can be done to determine the extent of the fibrovascularization of the implant. At the time of the drilling, a temporary peg is placed in the cylindrical receptacle and is left in place for approximately 3 weeks so that the area is completely covered by fibrovascular tissue and conjunctival epithelium. The patient returns to the ocularist for modification of the prosthesis by one of the two methods previously described.

Time and widespread use of hydroxyapatite implants will tell the final story, but at present their use appears to provide a great advance to ophthalmic surgery. To date, this implant has been used successfully for enucleation and evisceration and as a secondary implant. Its advantages include decreased incidence of migration and extrusion and a significant increase in motility of the enucleation prosthesis, as well as support for the prosthesis, which should reduce lower lid sagging, often seen in patients who have worn enucleation prostheses for several years. Vastly improved motility appears to be the primary advantage, however. Use of the prosthesis is contraindicated when orbital infection or severe orbital trauma with retained foreign bodies is present and when poor vascularization might be expected, that is, in cases of irradiation.

Treatment of Congenital Unilateral Upper Eyelid Retraction With a Marginal Myotomy Procedure
Rovit AJ, Deupree DM, Zang Y-F, Biglan AW (Univ of Pittsburgh; First Teaching Hosp, Beijing)
Ophthalmic Surg 19:872–875, December 1988   5–1

Two children with congenital unilateral upper lid retraction were successfully operated on at age 2 years, using a modification of Grove's mar-

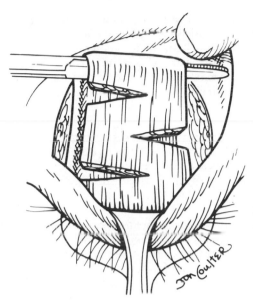

Fig 5–1.—Vertical levator lengthening after 3-incision marginal myotomy. Note each horizontal cut extends greater than 50% of muscle width. (Courtesy of Rovit AJ, Deupree DM, Zang Y-P, et al. *Ophthalmic Surg* 19:872–875, December 1988.)

ginal myotomy procedure for lengthening the levator palpebrae superiorus muscle.

Technique.—Under general anesthesia a 12- to 14-mm horizontal incision is made through the orbicularis muscle, and the latter is dissected from the tarsal plate to expose the levator insertion. The septum is incised, and 25 mm of levator muscle and aponeurosis are exposed by blunt dissection. Small cuts are made through the levator to obtain the desired lengthening (Fig 5–1) after blanching with wet-field cautery applications. The skin is closed, taking deep bites through the levator aponeurosis to recreate the lid crease.

The timing of surgery is dependent on symptoms of exposure keratitis. The possibility of upper lid retraction caused by overaction of the superior rectus-levator complex acting on a restricted inferior rectus is excluded by normal versions and unrestricted forced ductions.

► This condition simulates closely the eyelid retraction that occurs in patients with thyroid ophthalmopathy. The technique described here is useful, or one may choose any other technique that is used to correct eyelid retraction such as levator recession with or without fascia lata graft or other spacers.—J.C. Flanagan, M.D.

Orbital Decompression for Decreased Visual Acuity or for Cosmetic Reasons
Koornneef L, Mourits M (Academic Med Ctr, Amsterdam)
Orbit 7:225–238, August 1988

Excellent results with orbital decompression in patients with reduced visual acuity have encouraged decompression on cosmetic indications alone. Ninety-nine orbits were decompressed, 58 for malignant Graves' ophthalmopathy. Fifty-one of these procedures were for cosmetic reasons: 22 involved the anterior approach, and 29 were decompressed coronally. The mean reduction in Hertel readings was 4 mm; it was greater in patients treated coronally. Diplopia occurred in 11% of patients, but was managed successfully with conventional squint surgery.

These patients were quite satisfied with the surgical outcome, and discomfort was comparatively minimal. One fifth of patients had less diplopia after surgery. The coronal approach allows the surgeon to sever adhesions between the orbital septa, extraocular muscle sheaths, and periorbital fascia.

▶ Orbital decompression in cases of severe thyroid ophthalmopathy should be considered for cosmetic reasons. In this instance I prefer to decompress the orbit through an inferior cul-de-sac approach. If vision is compromised, I prefer the Caldwell Luc approach, which provides better exposure of the posterior and medial aspect of the orbital walls.—J.C. Flanagan, M.D.

Balloon Catheter Dilatation in Lacrimal Surgery
Becker BB, Berry FD (Univ of California, Los Angeles; Vision Care Ctr, Fresno, Calif)
Ophthalmic Surg 20:193–198, March 1989   5–3

Balloon catheter dilation was performed in 4 patients for whom dacryocystorhinostomy had failed because of obstructed nasal ostia.

Technique.—Under topical anesthesia a Bowman probe is advanced through the canaliculus through the nasal ostium into the nose. A guide wire then is placed through the inferior and common canaliculus into the lacrimal sac and pushed through the obstructed ostium. A balloon catheter is guided over the wire until it is just distal to the common canaliculus in the lacrimal sac (Fig 5–2), and the balloon is inflated. Dilation is done twice for 10 minutes at 10 bars, and patency then is confirmed by irrigating the lacrimal system with fluorescein dye. Topical antibiotic-steroid drops are used for a week.

In 3 cases epiphora was relieved, and a patent lacrimal drainage system achieved. The fourth patient had a transient partial response. In 1 case epiphora recurred after 3.5 months and responded to a second dilation.

This method is a simple nonoperative approach to the failed dacryocystorhinostomy where the ostium is blocked. Topical anesthesia usually is adequate, and the procedure can be done in the office. Smaller balloons may prove useful in treating canalicular stenosis.

▶ This technique may be an excellent way to salvage failed DCRs if the stricture is picked up early postoperatively. We attempted this several years ago,

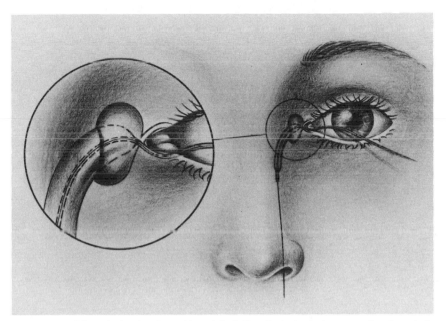

Fig 5–2.—Schematic showing the position of the balloon in the lacrimal sac extending through the ostium into the nose. The guide wire extends from the external nare. The catheter shaft fits over the guide wire and a short tip extends beyond the balloon over the wire. (Courtesy of Becker BB, Berry FD: *Ophthalmic Surg* 20:193–198, March 1989.)

found it technically difficult, and abandoned the effort. However, with these new findings, my interest has been renewed.   J. G. Flanagan, M.D.

Primary Liposarcoma of the Orbit: Problems in the Diagnosis and Management of Five Cases
Jakobiec FA, Rini F, Char D, Orcutt J, Rootman J, Baylis H, Flanagan J (Manhattan Eye, Ear & Throat Hosp, New York; Univ of California, San Francisco; Univ of Washington, Seattle; Univ of British Columbia, Vancouver; Univ of California, Los Angeles; et al)
Ophthalmology 96:180–191, February 1989   5–1

Malignancies of fat tissue are surprisingly rare considering the large volume or orbital fat. In 5 patients with primary orbital liposarcoma the chief features were diplopia and proptosis. Vision generally was maintained well. Three CT studies showed a central fat density surrounded by a variably dense pseudocapsule. Ultrasonography excluded a truly cystic tumor by showing internal acoustic interfaces. Magnetic resonance imaging suggested fat within the lesion in 1 instance. Bowing of an involved extraocular muscle was a useful feature.

There were 2 well-differentiated liposarcomas and 3 myxoid liposarcomas, all with univacuolar signet ring lipoblasts. Bizarre hyperchromatic mesenchymal cells also were found in the lesions. The patients were free of metastasis on follow-up for a mean of 5 years. Three patients, however, needed orbital exenteration after local recurrence. Two patients who refused exenteration received orbital radiotherapy.

The light microscopic differential diagnosis of myxoid liposarcoma in the orbit includes a number of lesions with loose stroma. Most of these lesions cannot be widely excised without causing irreversible damage to infiltrated structures, especially the extraocular muscles. Myxoid liposarcomas are considered somewhat radiosensitive, but well-differentiated tumors are less responsive to irradiation. The chief threat is direct spread outside the orbit. Chemotherapy may have a limited role. Orbital exenteration is best reserved for postsurgical failures or progressive cases for which spread beyond the orbit is a concern.

▶ Clinically, liposarcoma of the orbit is extremely difficult to diagnose, and complete surgical excision is the treatment of choice. These tumors are not encapsulated, and therefore it is difficult to determine complete removal. Once surgery has been done and the diagnosis is established, the patient should be followed up carefully clinically and by periodic CT scan to rule out recurrence. If there is recurrence, orbital exenteration should be considered.—J.C. Flanagan, M.D.

Eyelid Depigmentation Following Corticosteroid Injection for Infantile Ocular Adnexal Hemangioma
Cogen MS, Elsas FJ (Univ of Alabama, Birmingham)
J Pediatr Ophthalmol Strabismus 26:35–38, January–February 1989   5–5

Infantile hemangioma in or about the orbit is associated with amblyopia and strabismus in many instances.

Young infant had delayed, progressive upper eyelid depigmentation 4 to 6 months after steroid injection of a capillary hemangioma of the lid. The lesion had an appearance typical of a capillary hemangioma. The mass decreased markedly in size after injection with a mixture of triamcinolone and betamethasone. The lid skin was stark white 6 months after treatment, but pigmentation began returning a year after steroid injection. The hemangioma involuted.

Capillary hemangioma, or strawberry nevus, is the most common orbital tumor of childhood. Amblyopia occurs in as many as half of patients, and strabismus, in up to a third. Significant astigmatism and asymmetric refractive errors also are frequent. Injection with repository steroids is a treatment of choice. The case described is the first known instance of loss of skin pigmentation after steroid injection of an infantile ocular adnexal hemangioma.

Steroids may reduce melanosomes in basal keratinocytes. Removal of the steroid effect is followed by rapid restitution of functional melanocytes in normal skin and rebound hyperpigmentation.

▶ Infantile capillary hemangiomas are best treated conservatively, unless vision is threatened. Injection of steroids, if necessary, should be done with caution and should be given into the tumor itself and not subcutaneously. I dilate the pupils and examine the fundus immediately after the injections to evaluate retinal perfusion because of the remote possibility of occlusion of the retinal circulation caused by the rich anastomosis in this area.—J.C. Flanagan, M.D.

Conservative Management of Congenital Nasolacrimal Duct Obstruction
Nucci P, Capoferri C, Alfarano R, Brancato R (Univ of Milan; San Raffaele Hosp, Milan)
J Pediatr Ophthalmol Strabismus 26:39–43, January–February 1989   5–6

The best way to treat congenital nasolacrimal duct obstruction (CNDO) always has been controversial. The value of conservative treatment by hydrostatic massage and antibiotic eyedrops was assessed in 59 children aged 1 month to 2 years with CNDO. The patients had had epiphora and recurrent mucopurulent discharge since the first month but was in good general health.

Children aged 1 to 12 months had a cure rate of 93%, and only 2 underwent nasolacrimal probing. Children aged 1 to 2 years had a cure rate of 79% with conservative management; 6 had probing. Initial probings were successful in both age groups. In all, 86% of patients in this series were spared nasolacrimal probing. All cases that had probing were unilateral.

The authors' policy has been to advise probing when conservative management fails for 3 months. Such treatment can, however, be effective even in children aged 1 to 2 years. A prospective study is needed to determine the true efficacy of conservative management in children aged more than 1 year, and the optimal time for probing.

▶ I believe that CNDO should be treated conservatively in the manner described here, for 9 months. If one waits longer, the incidence of spontaneous recovery is low and the incidence of failed probing is increased. Therefore, after 9 months, probing and irrigation of the nasolacrimal duct combined with infracturing of the inferior turbinate is suggested. If this fails, or there is a severe obstruction, the above should be repeated in combination with silicone intubation.—J.C. Flanagan, M.D.

Strategies for the Initial Management of Acute Preseptal and Orbital Cellulitis
Jones DB, Steinkuller PG (Baylor College of Medicine, Houston)
Trans Am Ophthalmol Soc 86:94–107, 1988   5–7

Preseptal and orbital cellulitis are potentially life-threatening infections. The former is an infection of the soft tissue of the eyelids and periocular region anterior to the orbital septum, whereas the latter involves the orbital soft tissues posterior to the septum. Preseptal cellulitis is characterized by hyperemia of the skin and lid distention without apparent orbital congestion. In orbital cellulitis there are orbital pain, proptosis, and limited ocular motility. High-resolution CT is important in assessing and managing all forms of suspected orbital cellulitis. Both axial and coronal views are useful; intravenous contrast generally is not necessary.

A distinction between preseptal and orbital cellulitis is basic to planning treatment. Exogenous infections are caused chiefly by *Staphylococcus aureus* and *Streptococcus pyogenes*. Initially a β-lactam antibiotic resistant to β-lactamase activity is selected. Intravenous nafcillin is preferred for serious infections, and oral cloxacillin is preferred for mild posttraumatic preseptal cellulitis. Exogenous orbital cellulitis is treated with intravenous nafcillin and tobramycin. Nafcillin and chloramphenicol are preferred for children with orbital cellulitis secondary to sinusitis. The role of the newer β-lactam and fluoroquinolone antibiotics remains to be defined.

▶ This article outlines an excellent algorithm in the management of preseptal and orbital cellulitis. It presents a logical approach to the treatment of most cases of orbital cellulitis. If a patient does not respond, an infectious disease consult is imperative to monitor high doses of antibiotics and the systemic side effects of same.—J.C. Flanagan, M.D.

Mascara and Eyelining Tattoos: MRI Artifacts
Weiss RA, Saint-Louis LA, Haik BG, McCord CD, Taveras JL (Emory Univ Med Ctr, Atlanta; New York Hosp–Cornell Med Ctr, New York; Tulane Univ Med Ctr, New Orleans)
Ann Ophthalmol 21:129–131, April 1989   5–8

When orbits are imaged with magnetic resonance techniques, paramagnetic effects from heavy metal particles in the pigment base of mascara and eyelining tatoos can alter the normal tissue signals. The results can distort artifactually the globes or simulate true ocular pathology.

Bilateral, focal, hyperintense streaks have been seen in anterior orbits or anterior projections of globes in several women, with no apparent clinical cause. Most brands of mascara contain metallic oxides of iron or titanium or, less often, oxides of bismuth, chromium, or other heavy metals. Other types of eyelid cosmetics and eyelining tattoos have similar effects when heavy metal particles are used as the pigment base. Apart from streak artifacts, there may be false blunting of the globes or appearances mimicking a ciliary body cyst or melanoma (Fig 5–3).

▶ Any patient who wears mascara should be advised to remove thoroughly any and all makeup before having an MRI test. Removal will decrease the number of artifacts, resulting in more reliable MRI interpretations. Patients who have had blepharopigmentation performed obviously cannot remove the pig-

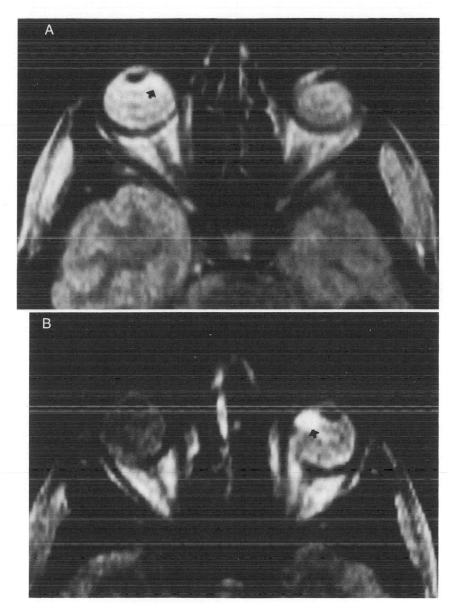

Fig 5–3.—Mascara artifact simulating ciliary body melanoma. **A,** T_2-weighted sequence in the axial plane. TR, 2,150; TE, 32 msec. Focal hyperintensity is noted in the nasal ciliary body region of the right globe (*arrow*) as a result of the mascara artifact. **B,** T_2-weighted image in the axial plane. TR, 1,500; TE, 90 msec. Focal hyperintensity is present in the ciliary body of the left globe as a result of a highly pigmented ciliary body melanoma. Note the similarity of this lesion with the mascara artifact in **A.** (Courtesy of Weiss RA, Saint-Louis LA, Haik BG, et al: *Ann Ophthalmol* 21:129–131, April 1989.)

ment: however, the radiologist should be alerted to this on the MRI protocol. The problems described are simply more good reasons for not having blepharopigmentation performed.—J.C. Flanagan, M.D.

Posterior Lamellar Eyelid Reconstruction With a Hard Palate Mucosal Graft
Bartley GB, Kay PP (Mayo Clinic, Mayo Found, Rochester, Minn)
Am J Ophthalmol 107:609–612, June 1989   5–9

A hard palatal graft is suited especially to repairing cicatricial entropion as well as lining a reconstructed lid after tumor excision. The graft is harvested readily, shrinks minimally, provides a mucosal surface, and supports the eyelid. The palatal graft may be taken under local anesthesia in adults. The palatal donor site heals with minimal care.

A hard palate graft was used in 4 lids of 3 patients with severe cicatricial entropion. There were 2 elderly patients and 1 child. Each of them previously had had 2 or more procedures. The posterior lamella was reconstructed adequately in each instance. Follow-up for 4 to 8 months showed less than 10% shrinkage of the grafts. The only complication was partial ketatinization of a graft in a child with probable Stevens-Johnson syndrome.

The hard palate mucosa is a good substitute for the posterior tarsoconjunctival lamella. It is much sturdier than mucosal grafts from the lip or buccal sulcus. This procedure has several potential applications in ophthalmic plastic surgery.

▶ I would not recommend that an ophthalmologist harvest a hard palate graft himself or herself; however, this procedure may be performed by an ear, nose, and throat or plastic and reconstructive surgeon colleague. A similar graft is nasal septal cartilage with mucosa, which is useful in the same type of case and has withstood the test of time.—J.C. Flanagan, M.D.

Intractable Orbicularis Myokymia: Treatment Alternatives
Jordan DR, Anderson RL, Thiese SM (Univ of Utah, Salt Lake City)
Ophthalmic Surg 20:280–283, April 1989   5–10

Facial myokymia is most frequent in the orbicularis oris and orbicularis oculi regions. Involuntary continuous contractions take place, most often unilaterally. Individual muscle bundles, a whole muscle, or several muscles may be affected. Transient myokymia may affect only the orbicularis oculi of the lower, or occasionally the upper, lid on 1 side. If lid myokymia lasts several months, it may be a sign of impending neurologic disease.

The treatment options include surgical myectomy, botulinum-A toxin, and muscle relaxants. Satisfactory results were obtained from surgery and botulinum A-toxin injections in 5 patients with intractable orbicularis myokymia. Two of the patients had responses to toxin injections, and 3 were operated on when botulinum toxin was refused or was unavailable. A limited myectomy was done with local anesthesia. The functional and cosmetic results were good after 1 year or longer.

Botulinum toxin injection or surgical myectomy is warranted if orbicularis myokymia fails to respond to a muscle relaxant and CNS causes are excluded. Toxin injection should be avoided in the medial aspect of the lower lid because it may cause inferior oblique paresis and diplopia.

▶ Botulinum-A toxin injection is an excellent way to treat intractable orbicularis myokymia. The patients must be informed that this may give only temporary relief, lasting approximately 12 to 16 weeks. However, once the cycle of spasm is interrupted, the result may be permanent. Neuro-ophthalmologic evaluation is essential before treating this condition medically or surgically because of the possibility of CNS abnormalities.—J.C. Flanagan, M.D.

Success of the Fasanella-Servat Operation Independent of Müller's Smooth Muscle Excision
Buckman G, Jakobiec FA, Hyde K, Lisman RD, Hornblass A, Harrison W (Manhattan Eye, Ear & Throat Hosp, New York)
Ophthalmology 96:413–418, April 1989   5–11

The Fasanella-Servat operation often is used to correct minimal ptosis, but the reasons for its effectiveness are uncertain. Of 40 excised tissue strips from 37 patients having this operation, 3 of them bilaterally, all contained tarsus. Thirty percent were classified as having minimal tarsus, and 70%, as having moderate tarsus. Müller's smooth muscle was negligible or absent in 42.5% of specimens, minimal in 45%, moderate in 10%, and large in 2.5%. In all instances, the levator aponeurosis was absent and conjunctiva was present. Accessory lacrimal gland tissue was present in more than 40% of specimens, but tear production was not compromised. Patients in whom smooth muscle resection was lacking or minimal had clinical results as good as those having substantial smooth muscle resected.

Posterior lamellar shortening is a likely mechanism of correction of ptosis by the Fasanella-Servat operation, but other mechanisms also may be operative. In more severe cases, this procedure is suboptimal or ineffective. Whatever the mechanism, smooth muscle resection per se is not necessary for a good outcome.

▶ The Fasanella-Servat operation is a mechanical method of elevating an eyelid 2 mm. If the operation is used for greater amounts of ptosis, it may jeopardize good results after secondary procedures if an undercorrection is present. Past literature has suggested that tear production may be compromised; therefore, preoperative Schirmer testing and other tests for tear production are imperative.—J.C. Flanagan, M.D.

Methylprednisolone Pulse Therapy in Severe Dysthyroid Optic Neuropathy

Guy JR, Fagien S, Donovan JP, Rubin ML (Univ of Florida, Gainesville)
Ophthalmology 96:1048–1053, July 1989
5–12

Dysthyroid ophthalmopathy can be managed conservatively when optic nerve function is not compromised. In severe cases, the enlarged extraocular muscles may compress the optic nerve and result in marked loss of visual acuity. Treatment options include oral corticosteroids, external beam irradiation, or surgical decompression of the bony orbit. In this study, 5 severely affected patients were given methylprednisolone pulse therapy as their initial treatment, a previously unreported strategy.

After 3 days of therapy (1 g daily), all 5 patients had striking improvement in visual acuity (Fig 5–4). Oral prednisone and external beam irra-

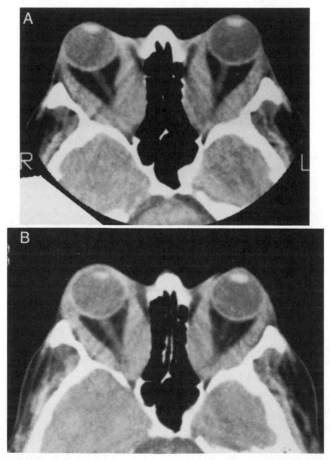

Fig 5–4.—**A**, CT before, and **B**, after pulse therapy; a decrease in extraocular muscle congestion is seen at the posterior orbit. (Courtesy of Guy JR, Fagien S, Donovan JP, et al: *Ophthalmology* 96:1048–1053, July 1989.)

diation of the orbit maintained remission of the disorder. Corticosteroids, as initial treatment, have taken considerably longer to bring about improvement. When prolonged administration of oral corticosteroids causes adverse reactions, supervoltage orbital irradiation is a valuable alternative. Surgical treatment, used as the primary therapy or as an alternative when corticosteroids or irradiation, or both, fail, may be superior to both of these noninvasive methods in long-term outcome.

The choice of pulse methylprednisolone or oral corticosteroids may be governed by the recognition of possible adverse reactions. In this small group of patients, pulse methylprednisolone was an effective method of achieving rapid visual improvement.

▶ Methylprednisolone pulse therapy should be considered for patients with rapid onset of symptoms, particularly that of decreased visual acuity and color perception. It might also be helpful as an adjunct to surgical decompressions for optic neuropathies. In this circumstance, if there are medical contraindications, super voltage irradiation can be substituted for pulsed steroid therapy — J.C. Flanagan, M.D.

Computed Tomographic Features of Nonthyroid Extraocular Muscle Enlargement
Patrinely JR, Osborn AG, Anderson RL, Whiting AS (Baylor College of Medicine, Houston; Univ of Utah Med Ctr, Salt Lake City)
Ophthalmology 96:1038–1047, July 1989   5–13

Although Graves' disease is the most common cause of extraocular muscle enlargement (Fig 5–5), a number of nonthyroid disorders are associated with such enlargements. These include inflammatory disease, primary or locally invasive tumors, metastatic tumors, infection, vascular diseases, and acromegaly. The differential radiographic features of these conditions were examined with a series of CT scans of 60 patients.

One fourth of the patients were found to have inflammatory disease, with myositic pseudotumor accounting for 12 of 15 cases. The majority (53%) of cases involved multiple muscles; bilateral involvement was present in 40%. Single muscle involvement was most common (81%) in cases resulting from primary or locally invasive tumors. Only 2 of 16 cases had bilateral involvement. Rhabdomyosarcoma and lymphoma each accounted for 4 cases.

Seven of the 12 metastatic tumors were adenocarcinoma from various sources; 4 of these patients had breast cancer. Most of these tumors (83%) were unilateral and involved isolated recti (64%). In half of the patients, nodular enlargement was the predominant configuration. All of the 8 vascular cases were unilateral; 75% had multiple muscle enlargement. Most cases (88%) showed distention of the superior ophthalmic vein; 38% had enlargement of the optic nerve sheath.

Infection was the cause of extraocular muscle enlargement in 7 patients. All cases were unilateral; 57% involved a single muscle, most

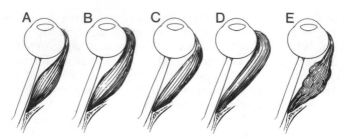

Fig 5–5.—Extraocular muscle enlargement configurations. **A**, fusiform sparing the tendon; **B**, fusiform involving the tendon; **C**, cylindrical sparing the tendon; **D**, cylindrical involving the tendon, **E**, nodular. (Courtesy of Patrinely JR, Osborn AG, Anderson RL, et al: *Ophthalmology* 96:1038–1047, July 1989.)

commonly the medial rectus (86%). Finally, 2 cases of acromegaly produced a diffuse, homogenous, bilateral enlargement of all extraocular muscles. In both patients, the optic nerve sheaths were slightly enlarged and muscle border sharply delineated.

Because extraocular muscle enlargement can have many causes and an overlap of signs occurs, care must be taken to correlate clinical information with radiographic findings and to distinguish Graves' disease radiographically. No single feature is pathognomic for any disorder, although certain tumors exhibit a predilection for certain muscle groups.

▶ As in all medical situations, the treating physician is responsible for making a correct diagnosis. This article again stresses that when ordering any imaging studies, the physician should supply a complete history to the radiologist. It is helpful if the radiologist can examine the patient; likewise, the physician always should review the imaging studies before instituting any therapy or surgery to make sure the findings are compatible with his clinical impression. Optimally, the physician would review the imaging studies with the radiologist to prevent errors in diagnosis.—J.C. Flanagan, M.D.

Levator Aponeurosis Surgery: A Retrospective Review
Berlin AJ, Vestal KP (Cleveland Clinic Found)
Ophthalmology 96:1033–1037, July 1989   5–14

The results of surgical correction of blepharoptosis have been unpredictable. Numerous techniques have been used, such as modified levator aponeurosis surgery using the external approach. Aponeurosis dehiscences at surgery have been described. Ptosis after cataract extraction was caused by aponeurosis disinsertion. Detailed anatomical studies have established the exact attachments of the levator aponeurosis, and aponeurotic repair now is accepted as an anatomically rational approach to involutional ptosis. The ability to surgically adjust eyelid height also has contributed to more consistent results. The efficacy of levator aponeurosis surgery in 1 series was investigated.

All cases of aponeurotic repair done by 1 surgeon since 1980 were reviewed. One hundred forty patients with 174 affected eyelids were treated. Results at 6 weeks were determined. An acceptable outcome was defined as a lid level within 1 mm of the desired level, which was achieved in 74% of eyelids with acquired ptosis. At an average follow-up of 7.9 months, the success rate for initial procedures dropped to 54%. In cases of congenital ptosis, the 6-week success rate was 69%, and the 4.6-month success rate was 52%. The major factor in outcomes was the amount of ptosis present preoperatively. Levator function and type of anesthesia did not influence success rates.

In this series, postoperative drops in lid height occurred 2 to 4 months after surgery and comprised a major cause of unacceptable lid level after aponeurotic repair. These drops may have been caused by disinsertion of the aponeurosis as the absorbable sutures weakened. Nonabsorbable sutures should be used to attach the aponeurosis to the tarsus. The amount of ptosis present before surgery seemed to be the major factor affecting outcomes in this patient group.

▶ Levator aponeurosis resection, plication, or reattachment can provide adequate eyelid elevation with the ability to titrate the lid level on the operating table if the procedure is done with local anesthesia. Lid level is, therefore, fairly predictable; however, the surgeon must advise the patient that exact symmetry cannot be guaranteed. This lack of symmetry is more likely to occur if the procedure is done with general anesthesia where titration is not possible. I believe that nonabsorbable sutures in this type of surgery are well tolerated and more likely to ensure lid elevation.—J.C. Flanagan, M.D.

Transconjunctival Lower Eyelid Blepharoplasty: Technique and Complications
Baylis HI, Long JA, Groth MJ (Jules Stein Eye Inst, UCLA Med Ctr, Los Angeles)
Ophthalmology 96:1027–1032, July 1989   5–15

Various authors recently have expounded on the transconjunctival approach to prolapsed orbital fat and the inferior orbit. Some have suggested that transconjunctival lower eyelid blepharoplasty avoids many complications associated with transcutaneous lower lid blepharoplasty. However, the transconjunctival approach never has been as popular as the transcutaneous. Surgeons tend to be unfamiliar with the transconjunctival approach to the lower lid, and the success of improving lower lid wrinkles by skin excision generally has been overestimated, but increased awareness of the complications and limitations of the transcutaneous procedure has renewed interest in the transconjunctival approach. The current technique and complications of transconjunctival lower eyelid blepharoplasty were described for 122 consecutive transconjunctival blepharoplasties done in a 24-month period.

Procedure.—Topical and infiltrative local anesthesia is used; the anesthetic agent must be injected subconjunctively. One drop of proparacaine HCl 0.5% is placed on the conjunctiva, and a cotton-tipped applicator soaked in 10% cocaine is held for 1–2 minutes in the inferior fornix. The surgeon then injects 2% lidocaine with 1:100,000 epinephrine and Wydase (hyaluronidase) with a 30-gauge needle, passing the needle through the conjunctival fornix directed just posterior to the inferior orbital rim behind the orbital septum. This is done in 3 meridians centrally, medially, and laterally, with a total of 2 to 3 mL in each lower lid. The surgeon applies gentle intermittent pressure to the lids. Fifteen minutes is allowed for the hemostatic properties of epinephrine to take effect.

Four of the 122 patients had skin excision through the pinch technique in conjunction with the transconjunctival fat excision. No patient had lateral canthal resuspensions or other lower lid-tightening techniques. The main complication was underexcision of lower lid fat, which occurred in 9 patients (7.4%). All had additional fat excision through the transconjunctival route.

The transconjunctival lower lid blepharoplasty is effective in decreasing lower lid fullness caused by prominent orbital fat. The primary advantage of this technique is that it avoids the most common complication of transcutaneous lower lid blepharoplasty: lower eyelid retraction.

▶ This technique of performing lower eyelid blepharoplasty is not necessarily more complex than the time-honored external approach. The approach to the orbital fat is not significantly different from the approach used for the cul-de-sac approach to orbital fractures or certain types of thyroid eyelid surgery. It is especially efficacious in dealing with younger patients whose primary problem is anteriorly displaced excess orbital fat.—J.C. Flanagan, M.D.

Sebaceous Carcinoma of the Eyelids: The Role of Adjunctive Cryotherapy in the Management of Conjunctival Pagetoid Spread
Lisman RD, Jakobiec FA, Small P (Manhattan Eye, Ear & Throat Hosp, New York)
Ophthalmology 96:1021–1026, July 1989   5–16

The optimal treatment for sebaceous carcinoma of the ocular adnexa has yet to be established. Exenteration has been advocated by many when this entity extends within the epithelium of the palpebral, forniceal, and bulbar conjunctiva, but this recommendation is debated. A group of patients whose upper lid sebaceous carcinomas were widely but locally excised was described.

Upper lid tumors and varying degrees of epibulbar pagetoid extension in 6 patients were treated with Cutler-Beard procedures and adjunctive cryotherapy to the involved epibulbar surfaces after presurgical map biopsies of the conjunctiva were done. After initial resection of the tumor bulk, cryotherapy was applied during the second-stage Cutler-Beard procedure. The patients were followed up for 12 to 50 months. Conjunctival biopsies were done every 6 months. No recurrence of the pagetoid tumor was found. Adverse effects included dry-eye symptoms, symblepharon, corneal erosion, and vascularization. The patients were willing to tolerate these side effects to avoid radical surgery. Complications were most severe in an elderly patient and a patient who had more than 2 quadrants of epibulbar pagetoid disease.

No patient had a recurrence of pagetoid tumor 12 to 50 months after wide but local excision and adjunct cryotherapy. Intensive and extensive cryotherapy should be limited in elderly patients and in patients with pagetoid intraepithelial extension involving more than half of the epibulbar conjunctiva.

▶ Cryotherapy may be useful as an adjunct treatment to sebaceous carcinoma of the eyelid. It may avoid or delay extensive debilitating surgery in this group of patients. In a 1-eyed patient, it may allow postponement of radical surgery for some time, and may especially allow maintenance of some vision for a period of years. This adjunct method does not negate the importance of complete surgical resection, if possible.—J.C. Flanagan, M.D.

Periorbital Cellulitis in Infancy
Molarte AB, Isenberg SJ (Univ of California, Los Angeles and Torrance)
J Pediatr Ophthalmol Strabismus 26:232–234, September–October 1989
5–17

Periorbital cellulitis is diagnosed more often than orbital cellulitis in younger children, in whom it may differ bacteriologically and anatomically from that in older children. Of 30 infants, all aged less than 1 year with diagnoses of periorbital cellulitis, 7 were neonates.

The usual clinical findings were edema, erythema, warmth, and minimal chemosis with ocular discharge. Infection of the upper respiratory tract was by far the most frequent predisposing factor. Eighteen patients had positive results of cultures; 8 had positive results of blood cultures. *Haemophilus* was the most common isolate, followed by *Staphylococcus* and *Streptococcus*. Only 5 patients had abnormal sinus x-ray films. Patients received ampicillin with oxacillin, or chloramphenicol with either ampicillin or oxacillin intravenously. All infections remained preseptal, and there were no major complications.

The major pathogens in young infants with preseptal cellulitis are *Haemophilus influenzae* and gram-positive cocci. *Streptococcus pneumoniae* and *Staphylococcus aureus* are of major concern in neonates. Because of the high rate of bacteremia, infants with periorbital cellulitis should be treated in the hospital.

▶ Periorbital cellulitis in infants and young children may progress to orbital cellulitis with its many serious problems. This, combined with the high rate of bacteremia, makes it imperative that these patients be treated in the hospital, preferably with intravenous antibiotics, and receive frequent, careful pediatric evaluations.—J.C. Flanagan, M.D.

Spontaneous Repair of Lower Eyelid After Tumour Excision
Hoppenreijs VPT, Cruysberg JRM (Univ of Nijmegen, The Netherlands)
Acta Ophthalmol 67:447–454, 1989   5–18

Twelve patients with clinical diagnoses of basal cell carcinoma of the lower eyelid underwent full-thickness excision of their lower lids, including the margins. Three of the patients had recurrent cancer after partial excision or radiotherapy elsewhere. Apart from cauterization of bleeding vessels, lid excision was the only primary surgical procedure.

The surgical defects ranged from one third to three fourths of the horizontal extent of the lower eyelid, and from 4 to 8 mm in height. All defects healed spontaneously within a few weeks, and cosmetic improvement continued to occur for the next 1–2 months. The final cosmetic and functional results were good in each patient. There were few ocular or palpebral complications, although 1 patient had recurrent basal cell cancer. Minimal notching of the lid was present in 3 patients. The new lid was neither limp not taut, and it conformed adequately to the contours of the globe. A proper fornix was present. The segment without lashes often was considerably smaller than the original defect.

This operation may be done on an outpatient basis under local anesthesia in 10 to 15 minutes. Unlike cryotherapy or radiotherapy, the excision margins can be checked for tumor cells. This approach is simple and inexpensive. If frozen section monitoring is included, the 5-year cure rate is greater than with cryotherapy or radiotherapy.

▶ I do not recommend spontaneous repair for eyelid defects because rapid healing occurs and results are better if defects are repaired primarily, utilizing the appropriate techniques. Occasionally, one is confronted with an early wound dehiscence before suture removal, leaving a small to moderate eyelid notch. In this instance, suture removal and subsequent granulation may lead to satisfactory cosmetic results, and the ophthalmologist need not repair the wound dehiscence immediately upon diagnosis. If a lid notch or other deformity persists, it may be revised with excision, tight closure, and alleviation of tension by way of procedures such as a lateral canthoplasty.—J.C. Flanagan, M.D.

Ptosis Revision
Brown BZ (Univ of Southern California, Los Angeles)
Int Ophthalmol Clin 29:217–218, Winter 1989   5–19

In blepharoptosis the eyelids droop to a cosmetically unacceptable degree or enough to interfere with the field of vision. Although many surgeons have strong opinions on the exact means of placing the lids at the correct level, some experienced ophthalmic plastic surgeons believe that ptosis surgery is unpredictable.

Determining the lid level is especially difficult in operating on children under general anesthesia. In this instance a predetermined amount of revision is done based on preoperative measurements, impressions, and pictures. For adults, however, a surgeon is better able to achieve appropriate lid levels because patients are awake and only mildly sedated. Nevertheless, injected anesthesia can stretch tissues and alter surgical judgments. Cauterization shrinks tissues but promotes fluid migration to the area.

A survey of 10 surgeons showed that repeated surgery was necessary for 18% of 298 patients with congenital ptosis and 12% of 501 patients with acquired ptosis. About 2% of both groups needed a third procedure.

Berris has described a method of placing silk sutures tied with slip-knots for use in making adjustments after surgery. Jordan and Anderson used an early adjustment procedure amounting to reoperation within 3 weeks of the primary operation. Others have proposed adjusting the lid level immediately after operation if significant overcorrection or undercorrection is present.

It seems necessary to make sure that patients and their families know that ptosis surgery is complex and that adjustment or reoperation may be necessary.

▶ This article stresses the all-important fact that ptosis surgery always is difficult and that exact symmetry may not be obtained even after 1 or 2 surgical procedures in a small number of cases. The best results are obtained when the patient has a minimal to moderate ptosis in the presence of fair to good levator function. The use of local anesthesia combined with mild sedation increases the chances of obtaining excellent results. Any significant overcorrection or undercorrection should be adjusted as soon as it is noticed so that the repair may be done before fibrosis, retraction, and scarring occur.—J.C. Flanagan, M.D.

Avulsion of the Canalicular System
Hurwitz JJ, Avram D, Kratky V (Univ of Toronto; Mt Sinai Hosp, Toronto)
Ophthalmic Surg 20:726–728, October 1989   5–20

Canalicular injury usually involves transection of the upper or lower canaliculi, but occasionally both may be lacerated. Avulsion of the common canaliculus from its attachment to the lacrimal sac should be suspected in cases involving deep lacerations on the lateral side of the nose or traumatic telecanthus as part of midfacial injury. These injuries are difficult to manage with intubation alone and often require canaliculo-dacryocystorhinostomy to rejoin the lacrimal drainage paths and relieve epiphora. Confirmatory signs include blunting of the canalicular angle and rounding of the inner canthus.

Seven patients with severe midfacial trauma and avulsion of the canalicular system from the lacrimal sac underwent canaliculodacryocystorhinostomy. In each case a lacrimal probe was seen at the inner canthus when passed through the upper and lower canaliculi, indicating disruption of the common canaliculus. A Silastic stent was left in place for 3 to 4 months. If severe bony injury was present, surgery may have been more easily done after a few months. Individual canalicular lacerations were sutured directly and stented.

▶ If there is disruption of 1 canaliculus, it is my feeling that it is best treated with monocanalicular intubation with silicone tubes, to prevent any manipulation of the uninvolved canaliculus. However, if both canaliculi are involved or if the injury is at the common canaliculus, intubation of the entire lacrimal drainage apparatus through the upper and lower canaliculus is suggested. These silicone tubes are left in place for 6 months or longer to prevent cicatricial closure of the nasal lacrimal drainage apparatus. If any laceration involves the canaliculi and the lacrimal sac, a dacryocystorhinostomy combined with a canalicular reconstruction and silicone intubation should be done at the time of the initial repair.—J.C. Flanagan, M.D.

Orbital Malignant Peripheral Nerve Sheath Tumours
Lyons CJ, McNab AA, Garner A, Wright JE (Moorfields Eye Hosp; Inst of Ophthalmology, London)
Br J Ophthalmol 73:731–738, 1989   5–21

Only 13 cases of malignant nerve sheath tumor of the orbit have been described previously. These tumors are radioresistant and can spread rapidly to the middle cranial fossa. Total excision is the only chance of curing them. One of the authors' 3 patients was well a year after operation, but 1 died within 4 months and 1 was lost to follow-up after refusing exenteration.

This tumor tends to arise from the supraorbital branch of the trigeminal nerve. There often is a history of a preexisting lump, often above the medial canthus, and excision may have been attempted. Radiography has not been diagnostically helpful.

The tumors are radioresistant and therefore need total excision. Early diagnosis and excision may prevent extension into the cranial fossa or metastasis to regional lymph nodes or distant sites such as the lung and mediastinum. Nine of 13 previously reported patients died of disease within 5 years. In cases with extension, radical midfacial surgery with exploration of the middle cranial fossa may offer the only hope of cure.

▶ Orbital malignant peripheral nerve sheath tumors are extremely rare. However, they have a high mortality because of early intracranial invasion or metastasis by way of the lymphatic system. An orbital mass of unknown origin should be biopsied and treated aggressively if this diagnosis is obtained. Early, aggressive surgical excision is the only hope that these patients have for a cure.—J.C. Flanagan, M.D.

6 Oncology

Advances in Retinoblastoma

JAMES J. AUGSBURGER, M.D.
Foerderer Eye Movement Center for Children, Wills Eye Hospital, Philadelphia, Pennsylvania

The most dramatic changes that have occurred in the field of ocular oncology during the past several years have been in the realm of retinoblastoma. In the 1989 YEAR BOOK OF OPHTHALMOLOGY (1), Dr. Ralph Eagle reviewed new developments in the genetics of retinoblastoma in detail in his introduction to the Pathology chapter. In this issue, I would like to comment on some of the practical advances in evaluation and management of retinoblastoma in children.

Clinical Genetics

The nature of the retinoblastoma gene and its current evaluation by recombinant DNA techniques were reviewed in detail by Dr. Eagle in his introduction last year (1). I refer the reader to the excellent recent papers by Albert and Dryja (2), Wiggs and Dryja (3), and Yandell and co-workers (4) for updated information on the genetics of retinoblastoma.

The methodology involved in assessment of the DNA sequence of normal and affected cells currently is complex, time-consuming, and expensive. Consequently, the effectiveness of recombinant DNA technology in predicting the clinical risk of retinoblastoma has been determined to a large extent only in families with known hereditary retinoblastoma (3). However, recent technical advances have shown promise for the identification of DNA abnormalities as small as one base pair even in simplex cases of retinoblastoma (4).

At present, because of its cost, labor-intensive nature, and predictive limitations, recombinant DNA technology should not, in my opinion, be regarded as an indicated evaluation for every family having a child with retinoblastoma. This recommendation may change in the not too distant future, of course, if automated and less costly applications of recombinant DNA technology can be developed for the study of the retinoblastoma gene.

Management of Retinoblastoma

The management of retinoblastoma in children has been advanced for both intraocular disease and extraocular extension of the tumor. The principal advances in management of intraocular retinoblastoma have occurred in episcleral plaque radiotherapy, photocoagulation with the laser indirect ophthalmoscope, and focal tumor treatment with photodynamic therapy.

Episcleral plaque radiotherapy has been used in one form or another for many years to treat retinoblastoma in selected children. Improvements in radiation dosimetry and plaque construction and the use of shieldable radioisotopes have increased the likelihood of effectively delivering a satisfactory radiation dose to the tumor while simultaneously reducing the risk of severe radiation-induced ocular complications. Episcleral plaque radiotherapy using Ru 106 or I 125 shielded plaques (5, 6) has been shown to be effective for treating intraocular tumors larger than those conventionally managed with photocoagulation or cryotherapy.

Retinal photocoagulation with the laser indirect ophthalmoscope (7) is a technical advance that has been needed for some time. Although retinal photocoagulation with the xenon arc photocoagulator has been used for quite a number of years in selected children with retinoblastoma, the technique is difficult to master. With the laser indirect ophthalmoscope, clinicians can treat retinal tumors and monitor burn placement simultaneously. To get an effect with the laser indirect ophthalmoscope that is similar to that obtained with xenon arc photocoagulation, a surgeon must defocus the beam slightly to increase the burn diameter on the retina, lengthen the exposure duration to 1 second or more, and use relatively low energy settings on the instrument panel. Thus, photocoagulation burns can be quite similar in both size and intensity to those obtained with xenon arc photocoagulation. One can occlude retinal feeder vessels quite effectively with the laser indirect ophthalmoscope, and one also can treat tumors anterior to the equator quite easily.

Photodynamic therapy with a photosensitizing drug and subsequent exposures of the tumor to long duration sessions of low-energy laser light (8) have been used effectively to destroy some intraretinal retinoblastomas. The relative effectiveness of this therapy as compared with conventional photocoagulation has not yet been determined. Treatment of retinoblastoma by photodynamic therapy requires a laser light delivery system in the operating room. Experience with this technique consists almost exclusively of treatments involving a specially modified slit lamp laser delivery system and a fundus contact lens in the operating room with the anesthetized child positioned on his or her side. Whether the laser indirect ophthalmoscope will be suitable and effective for photodynamic therapy currently is unknown.

Monitoring Children With Retinoblastoma

It has long been known that some children with apparently successfully eradicated intraocular retinoblastoma eventually have viable intraocular tumors years after their treatment. A more recent observation by several clinicians around the world is that "retinomas" (spontaneously arrested retinoblastomas) can and occasionally do become viable and progressive retinoblastomas months to years after their initial detection (9). The implication of these observations are that one must monitor persons with clinically inactive retinoblastoma (either regressed after treatment or spontaneously arrested) for evidence of reactivation later in life.

My recommendations for follow-up of children with retinoblastoma are dependent on several factors, including age at onset or detection, laterality of disease, status of disease at last evaluation, and method of treatment. Considering these factors, I currently recommend the following follow-up schedule:

- For children with unilateral nonfamilial retinoblastoma managed with enucleation for whom pathologic evaluation of the globe showed no extraocular tumor extension, I recommend evaluation every 6 months postenucleation until the second postenucleation year and then yearly thereafter.
- For children with bilateral or familial retinoblastoma, or both, treated in at least one eye with a conservative ("eye-preserving") therapy, I recommend reevaluation every 2 to 4 weeks after completion of treatment (with retreatment if needed at that time) until no clinical evidence of viable tumor exists, every 3 months thereafter as long as there is no clinical tumor recurrence for at least 2 posttreatment years, approximately every 6 months until age 6 years, and yearly thereafter for life.

I recommend *examination under anesthesia* for all follow-up evaluations of children with bilateral or familial retinoblastoma, or both, during the first 2 posttreatment years. Thereafter, I perform almost all ophthalmic examinations in the office, unless some extenuating circumstance compels me to continue with examinations under anesthesia. In contrast, I generally recommend examination with anesthesia only for the 6-month follow-up evaluation of children with unilateral nonfamilial disease that is managed with enucleation. I perform all subsequent follow-up examinations in the office, unless some clinical circumstances are extenuating or unless my outpatient assessment reveals unexpected changes in the fundus.

Although the true incidence of nonretinoblastoma cancers in retinoblastoma survivors and the precise impact of prior radiotherapy and chemotherapy on the development of such tumors are still controversial there is virtually no disagreement that children with genetic retinoblastoma are at increased risk for development of nonretinoblastoma malignancies later in life (10, 11). Consequently, it is essential that all children with bilateral, familial, or otherwise genetic retinoblastoma be followed up regularly for life in search of nonretinoblastoma cancers. This tendency for nonretinoblastoma malignancies does not appear to extend to any great degree to survivors of true somatic retinoblastoma. At present, many genetic retinoblastoma survivors succumb to their second malignancies. Only with earlier detection do we have any likelihood of being able to improve the survival of such persons.

As a practical matter, I currently recommend at least yearly systemic follow-up examinations for life for all children with retinoblastoma. I also advise the parents to bring their young children to their pediatricians if any unusual or unexplained neurologic symptoms, constitutional symptoms, or unexplained bony or soft tissue lumps or bumps develop. I similarly advise juveniles and young adults to seek prompt medical attention should similar symptoms and signs occur later in life.

118 / Ophthalmology

References

1. Eagle RC: New developments in the genetic of retinoblastoma, in Laibson PR (ed): 1989 YEAR BOOK OF OPHTHALMOLOGY. Chicago, Year Book Medical Publishers, Inc, pp 125–128, 1989.
2. Albert DM, Dryja TP: Recent studies of the retinoblastoma gene. _Arch Ophthalmol_ 106:181–182, 1988.
3. Wiggs JL, Dryja TP: Predicting the risk of hereditary retinoblastoma. _Am J Ophthalmol_ 106:346–351, 1988.
4. Yandell DW, Campbell TA, Dayton SH, et al: Oncogenic point mutations in the human retinoblastoma gene: Their application to genetic counseling. _N Engl J Med_ 321:1689–1695, 1989.
5. Amendola BE, Markoe AM, Augsburger JJ, et al: Analysis of treatment results in 36 children with retinoblastoma treated by scleral plaque irradiation. _Int J Radiat Oncol Biol Phys_ 17:63–70, 1989.
6. Lommatzsch PK: Experience with beta-irradiation (106Ru/106Th) of patients suffering from retinoblastoma: Report on 33 patients. _Jpn J Ophthalmol_ 22:424–430, 1978.
7. Mizuno K: Binocular indirect argon laser photocoagulator. _Br J Ophthalmol_ 65:425–428, 1981.
8. Ohnishi Y, Yamana Y, Minei M: Photoradiation therapy using argon laser and a hematoporphyrin derivative for retinoblastoma: A preliminary report. _Jpn J Ophthalmol_ 30:409–419, 1986.
9. Eagle RC, Shields JA, Donoso LA, et al: Malignant transformation of spontaneously regressed retinoblastoma, retinoma/retinocytoma variant. _Ophthalomology_ 96:1389–1385, 1989.
10. Schwarz MB, Burgess LPA, Fee WE, et al: Postirradiation sarcoma in retinoblastoma: Induction of predisposition? _Arch Otolaryngol Head Neck Surg_ 114:640–644, 1988.
11. Roarty JD, McLean IW, Zimmerman LE: Incidence of second neoplasms in patients with retinoblastoma. _Ophthalmology_ 95:1583–1587, 1988.

Clinicopathologic Characteristics of Premalignant and Malignant Melanocytic Lesions of the Conjunctiva
Jakobiec FA, Folberg R, Iwamoto T (Manhattan Eye, Ear & Throat Hosp, New York; Columbia–Presbyterian Med Ctr, New York; Univ of Iowa; New York Hosp–Cornell Med Ctr)
Ophthalmology 96:147–166, February 1989   6–1

Primary acquired melanosis (PAM) is a proliferative condition of the melanocytes that normally populate the conjunctival epithelium. It is characterized by a flat, variably brown conjunctival blemish and is seen most often in middle-aged to elderly white persons. The most important light microscopic features of PAM are the pattern of intraepithelial growth and the presence or absence of cytologic atypia. Primary acquired melanosis with atypia has a strong tendency to progress to conjunctival malignant melanoma.

Small lesions can be managed with excisional biopsy. Larger lesions must be evaluated with incisional biopsies, which may number 10 or more If cytologic atypia is present, the entire lension must be removed. When large areas of conjunctiva are affected, treatment must be directed at the most atypical regions first.

Conjunctival malignant melanoma may arise within PAM or evolve directly without preceding PAM. About three fourths of conjunctival melanomas are believed to arise from preexisting PAM. The interval between initial appearance of PAM and development of conjunctival melanoma in such cases is usually less than 6 years. Any degree of invasion of the substantia propria connotes malignancy. Pathologic factors predictive of an unfavorable outcome are found in patients with conjunctival melanoma cell type, thickness greater than 0.8 mm, and pagetoid growth pattern.

Both PAM and malignant melanoma of the conjunctiva have a strong tendency to recur after surgical excision. Consequently, if histopathologic study of the excised conjunctiva reveals PAM with atypia or malignant melanoma at the resection margins, wide reexcision and cryotherapy are usually necessary. Cryosurgery alone can be used for flat lesions but is not adequate primary treatment for nodular disease. Patients must be followed closely for the rest of their lives for local and regional nodal recurrence and systemic metastasis. Enucleation is not indicated for epibulbar melanoma unless the globe is invaded. Bulky tumors invading the anterior orbit may be treated with exenteration, but this aggressive intervention in no way ensures survival.

▶ This comprehensive article on the clinical and pathologic features of conjunctival PAM and malignant melanoma is a landmark discussion of an important oncologic ophthalmic disorder. The authors are comprehensive and yet clear about the clinical and pathologic distinctions between PAM without atypia, PAM with atypia, and malignant conjunctival melanoma. They provide the reader with a reasoned approach to the diagnosis and management of these potentially fatal melanocytic conjunctival disturbances.—J.J. Augsburger, M.D.

Metastatic Eyelid Disease in 49 Cases
Mansour AM (Univ of Texas Med Branch, Galveston)
Orbit 7:245–248, 1988   6–2

Metastatic carcinoma to the eyelid is an uncommon tumor that must be included in the differential diagnosis of lid lesions, particularly in the elderly. The typical metastatic carcinoma to the eyelid is a painless, rapidly enlarging mass occurring in an elderly woman with a history of mastectomy. Bilateral or multifocal lid involvement also suggests metastatic disease. Metastasis may be the first sign of occult malignancy or the first sign of recurrence in a patient whose known malignancy has been treated.

The author reviews the clinical features and differential diagnosis of 49 patients with metastatic carcinoma to the eyelid seen during the interval 1967–1986. The most frequent incorrect referring diagnoses were chalazion, cyst, xanthoma, and basal cell epithelioma. The most frequent known sites of primary carcinoma in this series were breast, skin (melanoma), kidney. The lid was the first identified site of metastasis in 7 of 29 patients who had a known primary malignancy.

▶ Although this article is relatively brief, it reminds us that a rapidly arising eyelid lesion in an elderly adult may be a metastatic carcinoma. One should include metastatic carcinoma in the differential diagnosis of eyelid tumors, particularly those occurring in elderly women with a history of primary breast carcinoma.—J.J. Augsburger, M.D.

Recurrence of Posterior Uveal Melanoma After ^{60}Co Episcleral Plaque Therapy
Karlsson UL, Augsburger JJ, Shields JA, Markoe AM, Brady LW, Woodleigh R (Hahnemann Univ; Thomas Jefferson Univ, Philadelphia)
Ophthalmology 96:382–388, March 1989   6–3

The authors investigated the rate of local intraocular tumor relapse in 277 patients with primary choroidal or ciliary body melanoma treated by ^{60}Co plaque radiotherapy in 1976 to 1982. Local intraocular tumor relapse requiring consideration of supplemental therapy was observed in 39 of the 277 patients. The actuarial 5-year local relapse rate was 12%. Patients with larger and more posteriorly located tumors (relative to the optic disk) had the highest risk of local tumor relapse. The actuarial 5-year melanoma-specific survival probability was 82% for patients with sustained local tumor control vs. 58% for those with local tumor relapse.

▶ This article emphasizes that a substantial proportion of patients followed up for 5 years or more after ^{60}Co plaque radiotherapy for a primary choroidal or ciliary body melanoma will have local tumor relapse in the uvea of the treated eye. The actuarially estimated 5-year local tumor relapse probability of 12% is substantially higher than proponents of episcleral plaque radiotherapy generally would like to admit. Although the authors detected a substantial difference between the 5-year survival curves of patients with and without local tumor relapse, they were unable to determine whether the local tumor relapse was directly responsible for the higher tumor mortality or was merely an associated feature in patients with unfavorable baseline prognoses for death from metastatic disease.—J.J. Augsburger, M.D.

Ophthalmic Manifestations of Leukemia
Schachat AP, Markowitz JA, Guyer DR, Burke PJ, Karp JE, Graham ML (Johns Hopkins Med Institutions, Baltimore)
Arch Ophthalmol 107:697–700, May 1989   6–4

Newly diagnosed leukemia in 120 patients was studied prospectively to determine the frequency of ocular manifestations of the disease. Sixty-seven patients had myeloid leukemia, and 53 had lymphoid leukemia.

Fifty-one (42.5%) of the 120 patients had ocular abnormalities related to leukemia. Four patients (3%) had leukemic infiltrates in the fundus, which appeared as preretinal white clumps or masses. Focal white lesions within retinal hemorrhages (Roth's spots) were not considered leukemic

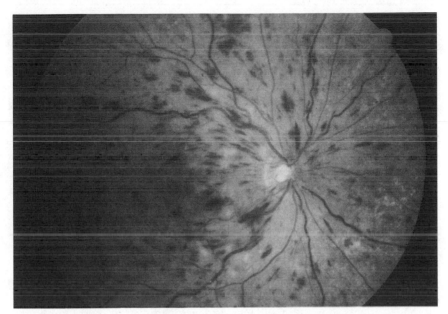

Fig 6–1.—Right fundus of a patient with marked hyperviscosity and a mild central retinal vein occlusion. The left fundus had a similar appearance. (Courtesy of Schachat AP, Markowitz JA, Guyer DR, et al: *Arch Ophthalmol* 107:697–700, May 1989.)

infiltrates. Forty-seven patients had 1 or more secondary ophthalmic features, including subconjunctival hemorrhage, retinal hemorrhages, cotton-wool spots, and central retinal vein obstruction (Fig 6–1).

The biases of the particular patient group were discussed, and the findings were compared and contrasted with the results of prior retrospective studies.

▶ A knowledge of the ocular manifestations of leukemia is important because the eye often reflects the systemic status of the disease. Most previous reports of ocular manifestations of leukemia have been retrospective in nature. Such studies are likely to overestimate the frequency of some ocular manifestations of the disease while underestimating the frequency of others. In contrast, this report describes ocular features identified on the basis of a well-designed prospective study. Consequently, the frequency of the various ocular manifestations observed in this cross-sectional study of newly diagnosed leukemic patients appears to be a reasonable estimate of the true prevalence of these features.—J.J. Augsburger, M.D.

Ten-Year Experience With Primary Ocular "Reticulum Cell Sarcoma" (Large Cell Non-Hodgkin's Lymphoma)

Siegel MJ, Dalton J, Friedman AH, Strauchen J, Watson C (Mt Sinai School of Medicine, New York)
Br J Ophthalmol 73:342–346, May 1989   6–5

Reticulum cell sarcoma (RCS) is a rare form of non-Hodgkin's lymphoma that causes 2 characteristic patterns of ocular involvement in some affected patients: (1) a systemic form, which typically is associated with uveal infiltrates, and (2) a neurologic form, which tends to be characterized by vitreous cells, subretinal pigment epithelial deposits, and CNS lesions. Experience with 14 patients with ocular RCS was summarized.

The mean age of the patients at presentation was 65 years. All had vitritis, and half of them had retinal or subretinal pigment epithelial lesions, or both. Three patients had anterior uveitis. Ocular involvement was bilateral in 10 of the patients. Two patients had CNS involvement at presentation, and 4 had it later.

Reticulum cell sarcoma was confirmed by vitreous aspiration in 11 of the patients. In each of these patients, the vitreous was aspirated with a 19-gauge needle introduced into the vitreous body via a puncture in the pars plana region. Approximately 0.5 mL of fluid vitreous was aspirated in most patients.

Treatment modalities employed in this group of patients included ocular and orbital irradiation (9 of the 14 patients), CNS irradiation (7 patients), and chemotherapy (5 patients). In spite of aggressive treatment, 5 of the 6 patients in whom CNS lesions developed died of their lymphoma within 6 months after diagnosis. Reticulum cell sarcoma should be considered whenever chronic posterior uveitis persists and the cause is uncertain. If the diagnosis of RCS is entertained, diagnosis easily can be confirmed by means of a vitreous aspiration.

▶ This summary report of RCS is a useful reminder to clinicians. This unusual but potentially fatal disorder commonly appears as a nonspecific intraocular inflammation in middle-aged to older adults. If it is recognized, appropriate treatment instituted promptly may substantially improve prognosis for both survival and visual preservation. The authors are correct in stressing a high degree of clinical suspicion for this entity in patients with chronic posterior uveitis of obscure etiology. Whether vitreous aspiration using a 19-gauge needle, as advised by the authors, is as safe and effective as standard posterior vitrectomy for recovery of cells sufficient for cytologic diagnosis of intraocular lymphoma remains to be seen.—J.J. Augsburger, M.D.

Episcleral Plaque Radiotherapy for Retinoblastoma
Shields JA, Giblin ME, Shields CL, Markoe AM, Karlsson U, Brady LW, Amendola BE, Woodleigh R (Thomas Jefferson Univ; Hahnemann Med Ctr, Philadelphia)
Ophthalmology 96:530–537, April 1989   6–6

External beam radiotherapy, although effective in many cases of retinoblastoma, carries a rather high risk of serious complications, including delayed secondary cancers. Fifty selected patients received episcleral plaque radiotherapy with ^{60}Co, ^{192}Ir, ^{106}Ru, and ^{125}I. A total of 97 plaque applications were made to 51 affected eyes, primarily in 15 eyes and as secondary treatment after external beam therapy, photocoagulation, or cryotherapy had failed in 36 eyes. The plaques were removed after delivery of about 3,500 to 4,000 cGy to the tumor apex.

Iodine 125 was the most commonly used isotope. Nearly all treated tumors had a dramatic response, visibly regressing within 3 to 4 weeks. Thirteen of 15 eyes treated primarily with plaque irradiation retained useful vision, as did 22 secondarily treated eyes. Sixteen eyes were blind or required enucleation; all of them had advanced tumor with extensive vitreous seeding. Metastatic retinoblastoma developed in 3 patients.

Plaque radiotherapy currently is used for most solitary retinoblastomas more than 4 to 12 mm in diameter and all those with vitreous seeding from a solitary tumor mass. Tumors occupying more than half the retina are managed with external beam therapy or enucleation. The risks of extensive radiation retinopathy, cataract, and delayed orbital bone development probably are less with plaque therapy.

▶ The authors of this paper are overly optimistic about the benefit-risk ratio of episcleral plaque radiotherapy in retinoblastoma. They present their thoughts on the potential advantages of plaque radiotherapy but omit any in-depth discussion of the potential risks of this therapy. This omission is particularly glaring with regard to their advocacy of the technique of sequential parallel opposed plaques. Although not mentioned by the authors, this form of treatment delivers a very high radiation dose (about 12,000–20,000 cGy) to more than 70% of the retina! Consequently, the authors' comment that "there is probably less chance for . . . radiation retinopathy" is not likely to be borne out in longer-term analysis. Although this treatment may be appropriate for the remaining eye of a child in whom a course of conventional external beam radiation therapy (in which the retinal dose is generally about 4,500 cGy) already had failed, the potential benefits of sequential parallel opposed plaque therapy relative to external beam irradiation (shorter duration of treatment, lower radiation dose to the orbit) certainly do not appear to justify its application as a primary treatment of retinoblastoma, particularly of children with unilateral disease.— J.J. Augsburger, M.D.

Malignant Transformation of Spontaneously Regressed Retinoblastoma, Retinoma/Retinocytoma Variant

Eagle RC Jr, Shields JA, Donoso L, Milner RS (Wills Eye Hosp, Thomas Jefferson Univ, Philadelphia; Med Ctr of Delaware, Wilmington)
Ophthalmology 96:1389–1395, September 1989   6–7

Girl, 7 years, had been found at age 4 years to have unilaterally reduced vision and a retinal lesion resembling a retinoma (Figs 6–2 and 6–3). After 3 years the tumor began growing rapidly and seeded the vitreous, leading to enucleation (Fig 6–4). The newer elevated part of the tumor was an undifferentiated retinoblastoma, but the tumor base had the changes of retinoma—retinocytoma, including bland nuclei, a fibrillar eosinophilic stroma, and no mitoses. Immunoreactivity

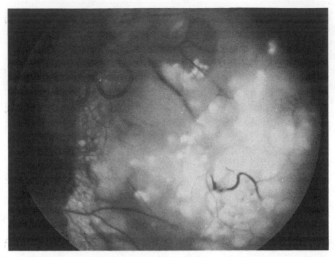

Fig 6–2.—March 1984. Zone of retinal pigment epithelium (RPE) atrophy (**left**) marks posterior border of heavily calcified translucent retinal tumor consistent clinically with retinoma or "spontaneously regressed retinoblastoma." A dilated and tortuous superotemporal vein appears to drain the mass. (Courtesy of Eagle RC Jr, Shields JA, Donoso L, et al: *Ophthalmology* 96:1389–1395, September 1989.)

for retinal S antigen, S-100 protein, and glial fibrillary acidic protein was limited to cells in the basal part of the tumor.

It appears that tumors resembling this patient's original lesion are benign variants of retinoblastoma that arise de novo, not retinoblastomas that have undergone spontaneous regression. Retinomas rarely undergo

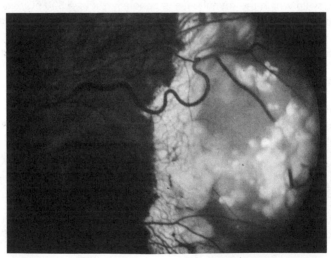

Fig 6–3.—May 1985. Fourteen months later, the retinoma is essentially unchanged. The fovea is normal. (Courtesy of Eagle RC Jr, Shields JA, Donoso L, et al: *Ophthalmology* 96:1389–1395, September 1989.)

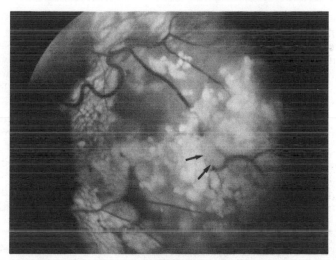

Fig 6–4.—July 1986. *Arrows* denote area of subtle vascular obscuration by tumor tissue suggestive of early growth. (Courtesy of Eagle RC Jr, Shields JA, Donoso L, et al: *Ophthalmology* 96·1389–1395, September 1989.)

malignant transformation after a period of clinical benignancy. Patients presumed to have regressed retinoblastoma should be followed up closely.

▶ Ophthalmologists have been taught in the last few years that "retinoma" is a benign clinical variant of retinoblastoma; now they learn that lesions of this type are not always as benign as they appear at initial evaluation. In view of the observations in this case, patients with a retinal lesion consistent with "retinoma" should be followed up at regular periodic intervals.—J.J. Augsburger, M.D.

Thermoradiotherapy of Choroidal Melanoma: Clinical Experience
Finger PT, Packer S, Paglione RW, Gatz JF, Ho TK, Bosworth JL (Cornell Univ, Manhasset, NY, and New York; Brookhaven Natl Lab; David Sarnoff Research Ctr Inc)
Ophthalmology 96:1384–1388, September 1989   6–8

Previous studies have shown that when hyperthermia is added to ionizing radiation in the treatment of cancer, the combined effectiveness is more than additive. To assess the effectiveness of a combination of radiation therapy and hyperthermia delivered by means of a specially designed episcleral plaque in the treatment of intraocular tumors, iodine 125 plaque irradiation together with microwave hyperthermia was given to 18 patients, 15 of whom had a medium-sized choroidal melanoma and 3 of whom had large choroidal melanoma. A thermocouple system was used to monitor temperatures induced at the scleral surface. However, internal tumor temperature was not monitored directly. The average follow-up period was 13.3 months.

No heat-associated ophthalmic complications outside the targeted treatment zone that might preclude the use of hyperthermia were observed, nor was any evidence of scleral damage noted. One patient died of myocardial infarction 12 months after thermoradiotherapy. However, none of the patients had metastatic disease. Clinical observations included 6 patients who had at least partial resolution of preexisting vitreous opacities and 3 patients with preexisting retinal detachments of whom 2 had partial resolution. Visual acuity improved in 7 of these 9 patients. All tumors responded to treatment, but 1 tumor regrew 20 months later and the eye was enucleated.

Use of the microwave plaque technique successfully delivered hyperthermic radiation to 18 human choroidal melanomas with no evidence of damage to normal ocular structures outside the targeted zone.

▶ Virtually all methods of "conservative treatment" for choroidal melanomas appear successful when the duration of posttreatment follow-up is approximately 1 year, as is the case in this study. The advantages and disadvantages of the combined radiotherapy-hyperthermia method advocated by these authors probably will take many years to determine. Clinicians who advocate such interventions are strongly encouraged to design an appropriate randomized clinical trial early in the course of that therapy rather than continuing with treatment of selected patients according to a nonrandomized protocol.—J.J. Augsburger, M.D.

The Risk of Enucleation After Proton Beam Irradiation of Uveal Melanoma
Egan KM, Gragoudas ES, Seddon JM, Glynn RJ, Munzenreider JE, Goitein M, Verhey L, Urie M, Koehler A (Harvard Med School; Massachusetts Gen Hosp, Boston; Harvard Cyclotron Lab, Cambridge, Mass)
Ophthalmology 96:1377–1383, September 1989   6–9

Many patients with diagnoses of uveal melanoma prefer radiation therapy over enucleation because they wish to retain both the eye and the possibility of useful vision after therapy. Recent reports have shown that most patients irradiated with cobalt 60, iodine 125, and Ru-106 plaques and helium ion beam retain the eye after irradiation. The risk of enucleation after proton beam irradiation in the treatment of uveal melanoma was studied.

During a 10-year study period, 1,006 patients with melanomas of the uveal tract in 1,007 eyes underwent proton beam irradiation. Follow-up data were available for 994 patients who form the basis of this analysis. After a median follow-up period of 2.7 years, 64 (6.4%) of the 994 eyes had been enucleated. The median time between proton beam irradiation and enucleation was 13 months. None of the patients had enucleation later than 5.5 years post treatment. The overall probability of retaining the eye was 95% at 2 years and 90% at 5 years after irradiation.

Multivariate analyses identified clinical characteristics that were independent risk factors for enucleation, including tumor involvement of the ciliary body, tumors greater than 8 mm, and distance of the tumor within 2 disk diameters from the edge of the fovea.

To examine further the risk of enucleation in this population, categories of risk were defined according to the levels of leading prognostic factors. Risk was classified as high if the tumor had 2 or more of the above-cited characteristics, as moderate if only 1 of these characteristics was present, and as low if none of the characteristics was present. The 5-year eye retention rates were 99% for the low-risk group, 92% for the moderate-risk group, and 76% for the low-risk group. Neovascular glaucoma and continued tumor growth were the primary reasons for enucleation after proton beam irradiation.

Thus, the probability of eye retention after proton beam irraiation in the treatment of uveal melanoma is high, even among patients who are at the greatest risk of enucleation.

▶ Preliminary reports led clinicians to believe that proton beam irradiation of choroidal melanomas was substantially better than other available treatment modalities in terms of visual and ocular preservation rates. Now we are starting to coo that the longer term success rates are not as good as the short term results. Despite the impressive total number of patients described by the authors, the median follow-up in their group is still only about 2.5 years. The cumulative proportion of treated patients coming to enucleation probably will continue to increase steadily in this population as the length of follow-up increases.—J.J. Augsburger, M.D.

Case-Control Study of Female Hormones and Eye Melanoma
Hartge P, Tucker MA, Shields JA, Augsburger J, Hoover RN, Fraumeni JF Jr (Natl Cancer Inst, Bethesda, Md: Thomas Jefferson Univ, Philadelphia)
Cancer Res 49:4622–4625, Aug 15, 1989   6–10

It has been suggested that hormones may play a role in the development of melanomas, including ocular melanomas. Several data surveys have shown higher rates of eye cancer in premenopausal women than in men at similar ages. To estimate the risk of eye melanoma according to various hormonal factors, a case-control study of intraocular melanoma was carried out.

The study population consisted of 238 women with a mean age of 58 years who had diagnoses of intraocular malignant melanoma and 223 matched controls with a mean age of 59 years who had had treatment for detached retina. All participants were white.

An increased risk for intraocular malignant melanoma was observed among women who had been pregnant and among those who used replacement estrogens. However, no association was found between the number of pregnancies and the level of risk. Pregnancy was associated with increased risk, regardless of whether the outcome was live birth, stillbirth, or miscarriage. A decreased risk was observed for oophorectomy. No influence of oral contraceptives, age at menarche, age at menopause, or a history of breast cancer was detected. The strength of the associations between the hormonal factor evaluated in this study and the occurrence of intraocular melanoma was weaker and less consistent than that between these factors and tumors of the reproductive organs; this relationship suggests that hormonal factors may have a limited role in causing melanomas of the eye.

▶ With all the information that is currently in newspapers and magazines about environmental risks and possible hormonal relationships to malignancies, physicians dealing with patients having intraocular malignant melanoma frequently are asked about these potential relationships. This case-control study provides at least some evidence that hormonal status may have some role to play in the development of human intraocular malignant melanoma in women. As pointed out by these authors, however, the weakness of the associations between the hormonal factors evaluated in this study and the occurrence of intraocular melanoma signifies that these factors probably have a limited role in the cause of this ocular malignancy.—J.J. Augsburger, M.D.

Clinical Parameters Predictive of Enlargement of Melanocytic Choroidal Lesions
Augsburger JJ, Schroeder RP, Territo C, Gamel JW, Shields JA (Wills Eye Hosp, Jefferson Med College, Philadelphia; Univ of Louisville)
Br J Ophthalmol 73:911–917, 1989   6–11

Fundus photography and ultrasonography were used to follow up 197 melanotic choroidal lesions. Sixty-two of them were classified as benign nevi; 76, as suspicious nevi; 41, as dormant melanomas; and 18, as active melanomas. The patients, all white, had a mean age of 58 years. Fifty-one of the lesions were associated with visual symptoms. Retinal detachment was present in 35 patients and was more than localized in 9 of them. Orange pigment clumps were seen in 9% of cases; drusen, in 42%; and black retinal pigment epithelial pigment clumps, in 13%.

Thirty-nine lesions became enlarged during the study: the actuarial proportion becoming enlarged within 5 years was 26%. Larger lesions and those located near the optic disk were most likely to become enlarged. In addition, more enlarging lesions had associated subretinal fluid, prominent orange pigment clumps, and related symptoms. The use of lesion thickness, extent of retinal detachment, and symptoms classified the cases into 160 low-risk lesions with a 5-year enlargement rate of 11% and a high-risk group of 37 lesions with a 86% risk of enlarging (table).

It remains uncertain whether merely following up lesions is appropriate when choroidal melanoma is suspected. The risk factors for enlargement that were identified in this study will allow clinicians to specify frequent follow-up assessments where appropriate.

Cumulative Actuarial Proportion of 197 Melanocytic Choroidal Lesions That Enlarged During Follow-Up as a Function of the Presence of Identified Prognostic Factors

Symptoms	Thickness of lesion >1.5 mm	Retinal detachment	Number of prognostic factors present	2.5-year incidence of lesion enlargement (percentage)		5-year incidence of lesion enlargement (percentage)	
				rate	standard error	rate	standard error
			0	4.1	2.3	5.8	2.8
Yes			1	38.0	7.1	40.7	7.3
	Yes		1	35.8	6.5	54.1	7.7
		Yes	1	66.1	8.5	81.0	7.4
Yes	Yes		2	64.6	10.9	74.5	11.2
Yes		Yes	2	62.5	10.0	78.6	9.0
	Yes	Yes	2	82.1	9.3	88.1	7.9
Yes	Yes	Yes	3	81.3	11.9	90.6	8.9

(Courtesy of Augsburger JJ, Schroeder RP, Territo C, et al: *Br J Ophthalmol* 73:911–917, 1989.)

► It always seems a bit arrogant for a reviewer to comment on his own article. Nevertheless, at the risk of seeming immodest, I have selected this article for review. The authors identify not only the individual clinical variables associated with subsequent lesion enlargement but also the combination of these factors that best predicts lesion growth. Note that the authors mention 3 distinct limitations of their results. First, they indicate that lesion enlargement (the end point assessed in the study) is not necessarily equivalent to lesion malignancy. Second, they note that the combination of clinical variables they identified for predicting lesion enlargement is not necessarily the best combination for every patient or all series of patients. Third, they comment that their study does not address whether observation of melanocytic choroidal lesions suspected of being choroidal melanomas before intervention is appropriate management. The principal value of this article is its potential usefulness to ophthalmologists who deal infrequently with patients having a melanocytic choroidal lesion. The information contained in this article and in the table reproduced from it can be used to estimate the probability of lesion enlargement during follow-up and to determine an appropriate interval for reevaluation of the lesion if the decision is made to manage the patient by observation.—J.J. Augsburger, M.D.

Evaluation of Tumor Regression and Other Prognostic Factors for Early and Late Metastasis After Proton Irradiation of Uveal Melanoma
Glynn RJ, Seddon JM, Gragoudas ES, Egan KM, Hart LJ (Massachusetts Eye and Ear Infirmary, Harvard Med School)
Ophthalmology 96:1566–1573, October 1989   6–12

Can the change in tumor height that follows proton beam irradiation predict the risk of metastasis of uveal melanoma? Seven hundred patients were followed up after irradiation of melanoma of the choroid or ciliary body or both in 1975 to 1986. The annual actual and percentage changes in tumor height were calculated.

The rate of metastasis within 2 years after treatment was highest in patients with the greatest percentage change in tumor height. Among patients who were free of metastasis for the first 2 years, those with the greatest percentage change in tumor height had the lowest rate of metastasis in the next 3 years, whereas those with the slowest decrease in tumor height had the highest rate of metastasis. When pretreatment tumor features were taken into account, both a rapid annual decline and a greater percentage decrease in tumor height were correlated with a higher risk of metastasis within 2 years.

Early metastasis of uveal melanoma is predicted by large tumor diameter, involvement of the ciliary body, and rapid initial tumor regression. In contrast, tumors spreading several years after treatment tend to regress slowly initially. A large pretreatment height also characterizes these tumors. Rapid tumor regression may be concurrent with metastasis, rather than being a risk factor for subsequent metastasis.

▶ This article makes 2 important points. First, it confirms some previously published information on the adverse prognostic impact of early, pronounced regression of choroidal and ciliary body melanomas after tumor irradiation. These authors showed that patients having tumors that regressed markedly during the first few months after proton beam irradiation were more likely to have early metastatic disease (metastasis occurring within the first 2 years after treatment) than were patients whose tumors (matched statistically for tumor size, location of the tumor's anterior margin, and age of the patient at the time of treatment) regressed slowly and minimally. Second, the article suggests that patients having tumors that failed to regress substantially within the first months to years after irradiation were more likely to have late metastatic melanoma (metastasis occurring after the second posttreatment year) than were the surviving patients whose tumors regressed rapidly and substantially. This latter point will need to be verified in other data sets.—J.J. Augsburger, M.D.

Local Extraocular Extension of Retinoblastoma Following Intraocular Surgery

Stevenson KE, Hungerford J, Garner A (Moorfields Eye Hosp; Inst of Ophthalmology, London)
Br J Ophthalmol 73.739–742, 1989   0–13

Three patients were encountered within 1 year who had local extraocular extension of retinoblastoma after intraocular surgery done via a transscleral approach.

Case 1.—Girl, 8 years, underwent a pars plana lensectomy for presumed panophthalmitis after failing to respond to medical treatment. Cells from an area of white friable tissue overlying the inferior pars plana were highly suspicious of retinoblastoma, and the eye was removed 3 weeks later. The poorly differentiated retinoblastoma had seeded the anterior vitreous, but the retinal component was confined to the anterior periphery. Orbital swelling and pain developed 6 months after enucleation, and an excisional biopsy showed tumor extending to the resection margins. Radiotherapy and chemotherapy were given, and the patient was free of disease 21 months after the orbital recurrence.

Case 2.—Girl, 5 years, had preauricular node metastasis of retinoblastoma 3 months after enucleation of the right eye. A vitreous biopsy had been carried out 2 months before enucleation. No tumor mass was found in the orbit on CT scanning. Radiotherapy was given, followed by 6 courses of chemotherapy; the patient was free of tumor 18 months later.

Case 3.—Girl, 6 years, had had an intraocular biopsy beneath a partial-thickness scleral flap that demonstrated retinoblastoma. Enucleation was done 4 days later. Tumor extended into the optic nerve head, and a large scleral perforation was present through which necrotic tumor tissue had prolapsed. An orbital recurrence was present 3 months later; an excisional biopsy specimen was positive for retinoblastoma. Radiotherapy and chemotherapy were given, and the patient was well 11 months later.

Orbital or nodal recurrence of retinoblastoma carries a very poor prognosis. Only 1 of 16 previously reported patients from the authors' center was a long-term survivor. The benefit of diagnosing intraocular inflammation by biopsy must be weighed against the very serious effects of releasing tumor cells into the orbit should retinoblastoma be present.

If retinoblastoma is diagnosed at intraocular biopsy, vitrectomy, or lensectomy, the eye should be removed as soon as possible and a detailed histologic study carried out, giving special attention to sclerostomy sites. An orbital implant should not be placed so that the socket can be examined at frequent intervals. Orbital radiotherapy is recommended if local extraocular extension is present. It may be a good precaution even if tumor cells are not found at the sclerostomy site.

▶ Children in whom retinoblastoma recurs in or around the orbit after enucleation generally are considered doomed to die of their malignancy. These authors show that such an outcome is not always inevitable. The 3 children they describe all had management with an aggressive approach consisting of debulking of the orbital tumor, systemic chemotherapy, and orbital irradiation. This regimen proved effective in eradicating the disease and prolonging life. The other important point made by this article concerns the fact that the 3 children they describe had all undergone intraocular surgery before the diagnosis of retinoblastoma. As pointed out by the authors, retinoblastoma must be considered in the differential diagnosis of any case of unilateral leukokoria with signs of intraocular inflammation, even in children aged more than 6 years and without evident intraocular calcification on ultrasonography or CT.—J.J. Augsburger, M.D.

7 Pathology

Immunohistochemistry in Ophthalmic Pathology

Ralph C. Eagle, Jr., M.D.
Department of Pathology, Wills Eye Hospital, Philadelphia, Pennsylvania

The increasingly widespread use of immunohistochemistry is quietly revolutionizing the practice of ophthalmic pathology and other branches of surgical pathology. "Immuno" has become an integral part of surgical pathologic practice because it provides important new data that allows the pathologist to make easier and more accurate diagnoses. Routine histopathologic diagnosis had rested solely on the microscopic appearance of the tissue in routine hematoxylin and eosin histologic sections, supplanted on occasion by relatively nonspecific histochemical "special stains." Unfortunately, it occasionally is difficult to distinguish between cells of widely disparate lineages using light microscopic criteria alone. For example, it may be nearly impossible to determine whether cells in an orbital biopsy are from a poorly differentiated lymphoma or represent an amelanotic melanoma or poorly differentiated carcinoma metastatic to the orbit. Such diagnoses had been "judgment calls" based largely on a pathologist's expertise and clinical experience, or necessitated costly and time-consuming electron microscopy. Today, thanks to the advent of special immunohistochemical stains, pathologists can be reasonably confident that an unknown orbital tumor is a metastatic carcinoma if they know that its cells react with antibodies against the epithelial marker cytokeratin and are not immunoreactive with leukocyte or melanoma markers.

A wide variety of commercially available monoclonal antibodies directed against fairly specific cellular antigenic components (or epitopes) are employed in clinical immunohistochemistry. Most of these give excellent results in routinely processed paraffin-embedded tissue. Tissue sections are prepared and made to react with a primary antibody. The binding, if any, of the primary antibody to the tissue is shown by a second antibody of a different class (made in another species) that is directed against the first class of antibody. Although techniques and reagents vary, the second, or occasionally third, antibody is labeled with an enzyme (usually peroxidase) that reacts with a substrate called a chromogen to produce a colored reaction product (usually brown) that is deposited in the tissue where the primary antibody binds to the antigen. Appropriate negative and positive controls are mandatory to ensure that results are accurate and meaningful.

An important group of monoclonal antibodies that are widely used in clinical immunohistochemical diagnosis is directed against cellular components called intermediate filaments. Intermediate filaments are fibrous

133

polypeptide molecules that are cytoskeletal components in most eukaryotic cells. They are called intermediate filaments because their diameter, characteristically 8 nm to 10 nm, is intermediate between that of actin microfilaments (4 nm) and microtubules. Different types of cells harbor distinctive classes of intermediate filaments that vary in their chemical composition and immunoreactivity. Intermediate filaments are useful markers in diagnostic immunohistochemistry because the filaments tend to be specific to cell type, and that relative specificity is retained after neoplastic transformation. Five distinct classes of intermediate filaments are recognized. Epithelial cells and carcinomas contain a large class of intermediate filaments called cytokeratins. Vimentin is found in mesenchymal cells and sarcomas. Striated and smooth muscle cells and neoplasms contain desmin (in association with vimentin). Glial filament protein, also called glial fibrillary acidic protein (GFAP) occurs in glial cells and gliomas. Neurons and paraganglia cells contain neurofilaments.

Other antibodies that are used frequently in the ophthalmic pathology laboratory include those directed against leukocyte common antigen (LCA), melanoma specific antigen (HMB-45), S-100 protein, Leu-7, epithelial membrane antigen (EMA), factor VIII, and the Ulex lectin. Leukocyte common antigen is expressed by all types of inflammatory and lymphoid cells and is used to determine whether a tumor is lymphocytic in nature. Melanoma specific antigen is a fairly new antibody that appears to be an excellent marker for malignant melanoma cells. In our experience HMB-45 seems to be a better marker for melanomas than S-100 protein, which was widely used for that purpose in the past. It is particularly helpful in the evaluation of metastatic foci of poorly differentiated amelanotic tumor. The protein S-100 remains an important marker for neural lesions such as orbital schwannomas and neurofibromas. Leu-7 is another excellent marker for neural tumors; it binds to natural killer lymphocytes, but also reacts with myelin proteins. Epithelial membrane antigen is derived from human milk globule membranes on the surfaces of many epithelial cells. When used in conjunction with antibodies against cytokeratins (the intermediate filaments found in the cytoplasm of epithelial cells), antibodies against EMA can confirm that a tumor is a carcinoma. Because the antigen is associated with the cell membrane, EMA stains the periphery of cells, not their cytoplasm. Factor VIII and the Ulex lectin are markers for vascular endothelial cells. Ulex lectin is a plant protein that binds nonimmunologically to the H substance of the ABO system.

A host of antibodies directed against specific types of lymphocytes and immunologic markers are used in evaluating lymphoid infiltrates and neoplasms. Some of these antibodies are used to determine whether the lymphoid tumor is composed largely of B or T lymphocytes. Most ocular lymphomas are composed of B lymphocytes, whereas T cells predominate in reactive infiltrates. Other antibodies are used to determine whether the lymphocytes' immunoglobulin molecules all share the same kind of light chains (either kappa or lambda). If they do, the infiltrate is monoclonal and is more likely to constitute a neoplastic proliferation. If the lymphoid infiltrate is composed mainly of T cells that harbor a mixture of kappa and lambda light chains (i.e., are polyclonal) the infiltrate is probably reactive and is not a lymphoma. Although the best results are still obtained if "immuno" is performed on fresh frozen tissue, several antibodies now available can differentiate between B and T lymphocytes in paraffin embedded tissues.

Several examples that illustrate how immunohistochemistry is used in ophthalmic pathology follow. We have already alluded to the use of "immuno" in the evaluation of poorly differentiated orbital tumors. In elderly patients, the great majority of orbital tumors are either lymphomas or metastatic carcinomas. In this clinical scenario a panel of multiple antibodies is used: EMA and several cytokeratins of varying molecular weight and acidity to detect epithelial cells, and LCA and HMB-45 to rule out lymphoma and melanoma, respectively. If the tumor is positive for cytokeratin and EMA and proves to be a carcinoma, additional stains occasionally can help to identify the primary. Specific markers that can identify primary tumors include a marker for breast and other apocrine tumors called gross cystic disease protein; chromogranin, which is found in the granules of neuroendocrine carcinomas; thyroglobulin; prostate specific antigen; and carcinoembryonic antigen (CEA), a marker for gastrointestinal tumors. Even the type of cytokeratin expressed by the cells can be suggestive; for example, squamous cell carcinoma generally expresses basic cytokeratins of high molecular weight. It is unfortunate that immunohistochemical identification of the primary tumor actually is possible in very few cases.

Orbital tumors composed of spindle cells are common diagnostic problems that frequently are examined with immunohistochemistry. The differential diagnosis of an orbital spindle cell lesion includes primary neural tumors such as schwannoma and neurofibroma; fibrous histiocytoma, the most common mesenchymal orbital tumor found in adults; and sarcomatous lesions including rhabdomyosarcoma, fibromyosarcoma, and leiomyosarcoma. The pathologist also must exclude an invasive spindle melanoma as well as spindle cell carcinoma, a rare variant of squamous cell carcinoma that originates in the skin and can invade the orbit secondarily.

In practice, immunohistochemical diagnosis relies on a tumor's pattern of reactivity to a panel of different antibodies. For example, both a schwannoma and a malignant melanoma usually will express S-100 protein, but the melanoma should be positive for HMB-45 and negative for Leu-7 and the opposite true for schwannoma. A spindle cell carcinoma should express cytokeratin. Rhabomyosarcoma and leiomyosarcoma both express the mesenchymal marker vimentin and desmin, the intermediate filament found in smooth and striated muscle. Most childhood rhabdomyosarcomas are embryonal tumors that lack cross striations in routine light microscopy. Transmission electron microscopy (EM) had been necessary to confirm the presence of striated muscle differentiation. Now the immunohistochemical demonstration of the muscle marker desmin, or occasionally myoglobin, readily establishes the diagnosis. Immunohistochemistry rapidly is supplanting diagnostic EM in this area because it is quicker and less expensive. It is less helpful in cases of fibrosarcoma and fibrous histiocytoma, which largely remain light microscopic diagnoses of exclusion.

Immunohistochemistry is required less often in the diagnosis of intraocular tumors because it generally is possible to distinguish between primary uveal melanoma and metastatic carcinoma, which constitute the great majority of lesions, in routine sections. "Immuno" occasionally is done when this determination must be performed on the relatively small number of cells obtained by fine-needle aspiration biopsy. We also have successfully employed the smooth muscle marker SMA (smooth muscle actin) on several occasions to confirm that a ciliary body tumor was leiomyoma, an exceedingly rare type of uveal tumor, rather than bland amelanotic melanoma. Electron microscopy confirmed that the results of the immunohistochemistry were accurate.

I emphasize the need to interpret immunohistochemical data with caution. As pathologists gain more experience it is becoming evident that many markers initially touted as "magic bullets" are less specific than originally thought. If results are puzzling, unexpected, or totally discordant with routine light microscopic data, the fault also may lie in the immunohistochemical preparations themselves. Immunohistochemistry is definitely an art. Artifacts and nonspecific staining abound, and the attainment of accurate, consistent, and meaningful results is dependent on competent technical personnel who are skilled and experienced and who perform immunohistochemistry "full-time."

References

1. Warhol MJ: *Current Surgical Pathology*. Philadelphia, Dekker, 1990.
2. Enzinger FM, Weiss SW: Immunohistochemistry of soft tissue lesions, in *Soft Tissue Tumors*. St Louis, CV Mosby, 1988, p 83.

A Clinical, Histopathologic, and Electron Microscopic Study of *Pneumocystis carinii* Choroiditis

Rao NA, Zimmerman PL, Boyer D, Biswas J, Causey D, Beniz J, Nichols PW (Univ of Southern California, Los Angeles)
Am J Ophthalmol 107:218–228, March 1989   7–1

Pneumocystis carinii is the most frequent infection in AIDS patients and often is the initial manifestation. Ocular involvement, however, is rarely reported. Three patients with AIDS were evaluated; in 2 a provisional diagnosis of disseminated *P. carinii* infection was made by ophthalmologic examination.

Numerous slightly elevated yellow-white plaquelike lesions were present in the choroid without signs of intraocular inflammation. Vitreous cells were virtually absent. The lesion may resemble those of reticulum cell sarcoma, metastatic cancer, atypical mycobacterial infection, or sarcoid granuloma. Intraretinal hemorrhage may be associated with the choroidal lesions.

Histopathologic study showed eosinophilic, acellular, frothy choroidal infiltrates. Cystic and crescentic organisms were apparent on methenamine silver staining, and electron microscopy revealed thick-walled cystic organisms and trophozoites. Organisms also were present within vessels and the choriocapillaries.

Both the clinical and histologic characteristics of *P. carinii* choroiditis are distinctive. Intravenous or oral trimethoprim-sulfamethoxazole or pentamidine should be used for treatment. Other agents such as dapsone and trimetrexate also are available. Close ophthalmic monitoring may promote the timely treatment of this infection.

▶ Pentamidine inhalation, used prophylactically to prevent pneumocystis pneumonia, may be a factor in this new ocular manifestation of AIDS. Although inhaled pentamidine prevents fatal pneumocystis pneumonia, it has little effect on disseminated disease in the choroid and other organs, which probably results from subclinical pulmonary infection. The striking yellow-white choroidal infiltrates visible ophthalmoscopically are composed of myriad protozoa that do not stimulate an inflammatory response.—R.C. Eagle, Jr., M.D.

Immunophenotypic Analysis of the Inflammatory Infiltrate in Ocular Cicatricial Pemphigoid: Further Evidence for a T Cell-Mediated Disease
Sacks EH, Jakobiec FA, Wieczorek R, Donnenfeld E, Perry H, Knowles DM Jr (Manhattan Eye, Ear & Throat Hosp, New York; Columbia Presbyterian Med Ctr, New York; North Shore Univ Hosp, Manhasset, NY)
Ophthalmology 96:236–243, February 1989   7–2

Ocular cicatricial pemphigoid (OCP), a presumably autoimmune disorder, is a chronic scarring disease that produces chronic conjunctivitis and forniceal foreshortening that can lead to legal blindness. In most cases there is immunoglobulin or complement deposition, or both, along the basement membrane zone of affected tissues. Conjunctival tissue has a mononuclear-cell infiltrate within the substantia propria.

Monoclonal antibody studies showed a threefold increase in epithelial T lymphocytes and a 20-fold increase in the substantia propria in 6 specimens of OCP compared with normal tissues. Activated interleukin 2 receptor-positive lymphocytes were present at both sites. Macrophages also were increased in the substantia propria, as were plasma cells. Dendritic cells that process antigen locally were much more prevalent that in control specimens.

The T cells in OCP may be effector cells through releasing cytokines that promote fibroplastic change. They also may underlie an immunoregulatory defect that permits local B lymphocytes to produce autoantibodies to the basement membrane zone. The clinical results of scarring conjunctival inflammation include lacrimal duct obstruction, conjunctival epithelial metaplasia, altered mucus production, and depletion of the aqueous tear film.

▶ Standard textbooks state that ocular cicatricial pemphigoid is an immune complex-mediated hypersensitivity reaction in which autoantibodies directed against basement membrane components combine with the conjunctival basement membrane and fix complement, which mediates the inflammatory response and subsequent scarring. The authors suggest that pemphigoid is actually a T lymphocyte-mediated disease. Although the anti–basement membrane antibodies appear to be a secondary epiphenomenon, they still remain useful in the immunohistochemical diagnosis of the disorder.— R.C. Eagle, Jr., M.D.

Optic Nerve Involvement in Retinoblastoma
Magramm I, Abramson DH, Ellsworth RM (Manhattan Eye, Ear & Throat Hosp, New York; New York Hosp–Cornell Med Ctr)
Ophthalmology 96:217–222, February 1989   7–3

Survival in retinoblastoma presumably reflects the degree of optic nerve involvement. Of 814 cases of retinoblastoma, 240 had tumor extension into the optic nerve. Involvement was graded from I (superficial invasion of the optic nerve head) to IV (involvement up to and including the surgical margin). Grade II involvement is up to and including the lamina cribrosa.

About 30% of patients in this series had optic nerve involvement. Mortality in patients without such involvement was 9%. Survival declined with advancing grade of optic nerve involvement, most markedly between grades III and IV. Mortality ranged from 10% in grade I cases to 78% in grade IV cases. All grade IV patients who survived received aggressive radiotherapy, and some received chemotherapy as well.

Once tumor cells reach the lamina cribrosa they have access to the pia-arachnoid system and can spread rapidly via the CSF. Invasion can occur even with minimal invasion of the optic nerve head. Choroidal extension, in contrast, does not correlate with increased mortality. Prolonged survival may depend on aggressive radiotherapy and chemotherapy.

▶ Involvement of the surgical margin by retinoblastoma can be minimized by obtaining a long segment of optic nerve during enucleation. Eyes with known or suspected retinoblastomas should be enucleated by experienced ophthalmic surgeons, not by first-year residents. I have reviewed sections from 1 eye with retinoblastoma that was "button-holed" intraoperatively by an ophthalmologist-in-training (from another institution, of course!). Despite intensive radiotherapy and chemotherapy, the child died several months later.— R.C. Eagle, Jr., M.D.

Epithelial Downgrowth: A 30-Year Clinicopathological Review
Weiner MJ, Trentacoste J, Pon DM, Albert DM (Harvard Med School; Bascom-

Palmer Eye Inst; Univ of Chicago)
Br J Ophthalmol 73:6–11, 1989

7–4

The clinical and pathologic findings for 124 patients with epithelial downgrowth, seen in a 30-year period, were reviewed. Epithelial downgrowth followed surgery in 108 cases and ocular trauma in 18 others. The incidence after cataract surgery was 0.12% but fell to 0.08% in the most recent decade.

More than 80% of postoperative patients had epithelial downgrowth within a year of surgery (Fig 7–1). They frequently reported decreasing vision, redness, and pain. Retrocorneal membrane was apparent in 45% of patients, and glaucoma, in 43%. Corneal edema and a positive Seidel test result were less frequent findings. When complications were noted at or just after surgery, vitreous loss was frequent. About half the postsurgical patients eventually had enucleation. The figure was much lower for

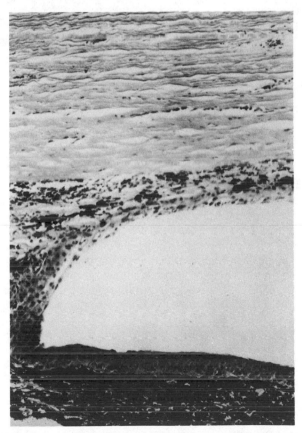

Fig 7–1.—Epithelium growing on posterior surface of cornea, across the angle, and onto the anterior surface of the iris. Hematoxylin and eosin; original magnification, ×65. (Courtesy of Weiner MJ, Trentacoste J, Pon DM, et al: *Br J Ophthalmology* 73:6–11, 1989.)

patients with surgical excision and iridectomy or penetrating kerato-plasty.

Improved surgical techniques and instrumentation may have contrib-uted to a decreased occurrence of epithelial downgrowth. A fistulous wound often disposes to downgrowth by facilitating the invasion of epi-thelial tissue. In organ culture, the presence of endothelium inhibits epi-thelial growth, and endothelium is disrupted or attenuated in most cases where epithelium has migrated to the posterior cornea. The prognosis re-mains poor, but treatment does improve the outcome in some cases.

► Although the incidence of epithelial downgrowth has decreased markedly in recent years, modern cataract surgical techniques have not totally obliterated this dreaded postoperative complication. I recently have examined tissue from several cases of epithelial downgrowth that followed intraocular lens implanta-tion. One patient had epithelial downgrowth after secondary implantation of an anterior chamber lens in a 20/20 eye.—R.C. Eagle, Jr., M.D.

Idiopathic Epiretinal Membranes: Ultrastructural Characteristics and Clini-copathologic Correlation
Smiddy WE, Maguire AM, Green WR, Michels RG, de la Cruz Z, Enger C, Jae-ger M, Rice TA (Johns Hopkins Univ, Baltimore)
Ophthalmology 96:811–821, June 1989   7–5

Current views of the development of idiopathic epiretinal membrane (ERM) focus on a glial tissue origin. The clinical and ultrastructural find-ings in 101 cases of idiopathic ERM were reviewed. The median age of patients was 66 years. The median duration of preoperative symptoms was 15 months, and the median preoperative acuity was 20/200. A cello-phane membrane was present in 44 of 100 evaluable cases.

The predominant cell type was retinal pigment epithelium in 51 cases (Fig 7–2), fibrous astrocytes in 29, fibrocytes in 14, and myofibroblasts in 7. Features of myofibroblastic differentiation were present in nearly two thirds of cases. These changes were most frequent in younger pa-tients with symptoms for a shorter time. Fibrous astrocytes were more common in females. Patients with myofibrocytes tended to have a shorter duration of symptoms than those with retinal pigment epithelial cells, but the difference was not significant.

The chief finding of this study is the high rate of retinal pigment epi-thelial cells in idiopathic ERM. The cells could migrate through occult breaks or through the retina. Alternately, developmental rests of RPE cells could be activated, or transformation from other cell types might oc-cur.

► Two thirds of the idiopathic ERMs examined in this study contained sheets of polarized epithelial cells presumably originating in the retinal pigment epithe-lium (RPE). To explain this puzzling finding, the authors postulate that RPE cells

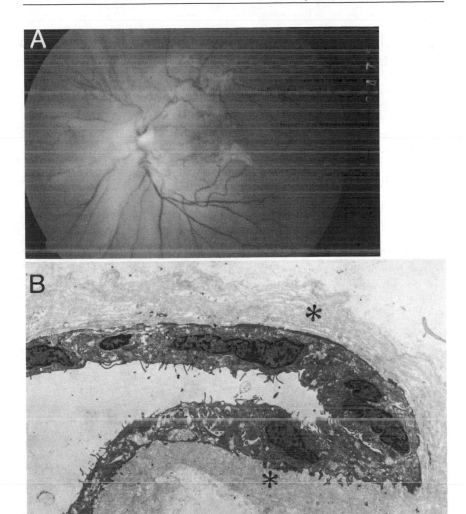

Fig 7–2.—**A,** preoperative appearance of 35-year-old man with idiopathic ERM. **B,** ERM consists of a monolayer of RPE cells on a multilaminated base of basement membrane (*asterisks*). Original magnification, ×4,200. (Courtesy of Smiddy WE, Maguire AM, Green WR, et al: *Ophthalmology* 96:811–821, June 1989.)

may migrate through intact retina or occult retinal breaks or may transdifferentiate from other types of cells. The epithelial cells illustrated appear nonpigmented. I question whether the nonpigmented ciliary epithelium could be another potential source for these cells.—R.C. Eagle, Jr., M.D.

Dual Infection of Retina With Human Immunodeficiency Virus Type 1 and Cytomegalovirus

Skolnik PR, Pomerantz RJ, de la Monte SM, Lee SF, Hsiung GD, Foos RY, Cowan GM, Kosloff BR, Hirsch MS, Pepose JS (New England Med Ctr, Boston; Harvard Med School; Washington Univ, St Louis; Yale Univ; Univ of California, Los Angeles; et al)

Am J Ophthalmol 107:361–372, April 1989

7–6

Cytomegalovirus is a common pathogen in patients with AIDS, and cytomegalovirus retinitis is the most frequent cause of blindness in these patients. Retinal tissue from 8 HIV-1-positive patients with AIDS or AIDS-related complex was examined for evidence of concomitant cytomegalovirus infection.

Both cytomegalovirus and HIV-1 were isolated in 2 of 13 retinal tissue specimens from patients with AIDS. Human immunodeficiency virus type 1 alone was isolated in 6 specimens. Examination of cytomegalovirus-infected eyes showed severe, full-thickness retinitis as well as acute and chronic choroidal inflammation. Intranuclear and cytoplasmic inclusions typical of cytomegalovirus infection were present in retinal and pigment epithelial cells (Fig 7–3). Cytomegalovirus antigen was found in cells in all retinal layers but not in retinal vascular endothelial cells. Human immunodeficiency virus type 1 antigen was present in the cytoplasm of cells in all retinal layers and also in retinal vascular endothelial cells. This an-

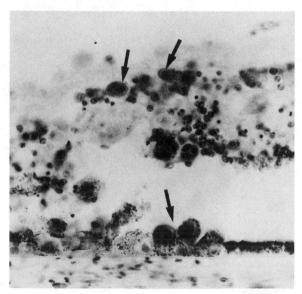

Fig 7–3.—Microscopic appearance of the retina at the edge of a necrotic plaque. The retina and pigment epithelium centrally are severely degenerated but show only mild inflammation. Several retinal and pigment epithelial cells (*arrows*) show both the intranuclear and cytoplasmic inclusions characteristic of cytomegalovirus infection. The choroid contains only a few inflammatory cells. Hematoxylin and eosin; original magnification, ×750. (Courtesy of Skolnik PR, Pomerantz RJ, de la Monte SM, et al: *Am J Ophthalmol* 107:361–372, April 1989.)

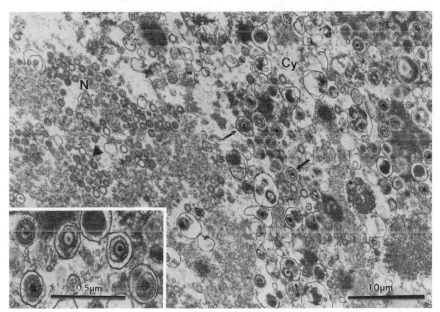

Fig 7—4.—Electron micrograph of glutaraldehyde-fixed retinal specimen showing an aggregate of herpesvirus nucleocapsids *(arrowhead)* and scattered capsids throughout the nucleus *(N)*. Mature virions with dense cores are present within cytoplasmic *(Cy)* vacuoles *(arrows)*. **Inset,** higher magnification of cytoplasmic vacuoles containing virions. (Courtesy of Skolnik PR, Pomerantz RJ, de la Monte SM, et al: *Am J Ophthalmol* 107:361—372, April 1989.)

tigen also was found in the cytoplasm of cytomegalic cells. Particles of herpesvirus morphology were found in both the nuclear matrix and cytoplasic vacuoles of retinal tissue (Fig 7—4). No retroviral particles were observed.

Infection of the retina with HIV-1 occurs, but HIV-1 may not by itself cause acute retinal necrosis. The retina may be a protected site of persistent HIV-1 replication because of the effect of zidovudine or the limiting blood-retinal barrier. Human immunodeficiency virus type 1 and cytomegalovirus can coexist in vivo, raising the possibility of direct viral interactions.

▶ The most common intraocular infection in AIDS patients, cytomegalovirus retinitis totally and irrevocably destroys involved portions of the neurosensory retina, a tissue that is incapable of regeneration or repair. The authors have confirmed that HIV-1, the AIDS virus, also infects the retina. Although HIV-1 does not appear to cause retinal necrosis, the clinical course of cytomegalovirus retinitis may be accelerated by dual infection of retinal cells.—R.C. Eagle, Jr., M.D.

The Association of Posterior Capsular Lens Opacities With Bilateral Acoustic Neuromas in Patients With Neurofibromatosis Type 2

Kaiser-Kupfer MI, Freidlin V, Datiles MB, Edwards PA, Sherman JL, Parry D, McCain LM, Eldridge R (Natl Eye Inst; Uniformed Services Univ of Health Sciences; National Cancer Inst; National Inst of Neurologic and Communicative Disorders and Stroke, Bethesda, Md)

Arch Ophthalmol 107:541–544, April 1989   7–7

Neurofibromatosis type 2 (NF 2), or bilateral acoustic neurofibromatosis, usually appears during the teen years or 20s with hearing loss or tinnitus. Schwann cell tumors develop on the vestibular nerves and there may be Schwann cell tumors of the spinal cord, meningiomas, or gliomas. Posterior capsular lens opacities were sought in 47 patients from 11 families with NF 2.

Posterior capsular lens opacities were closely associated with NF 2, but no such association was found for other types of lens opacities. Posterior capsular opacities were present in 1 or both eyes in significant association with NF 2, as diagnosed with magnetic resonance imaging or a history of known tumor.

All patients with NF 2 should have careful biomicroscopic examination of the lens. Lens examination should be part of the screening of all persons at 50% risk for NF 2. The presence of posterior capsular opacities may be the initial clinical sign of NF 2.

▶ Ophthalmologists are generally familiar with the ocular manifestations of type 1, or peripheral, neurofibromatosis, which include Lisch nodules, plexiform neurofibromas of the lid, choroidal infiltration, secondary glaucoma, and optic nerve gliomas. The presenile posterior capsular lens opacities described in this report are found in patients who have type 2, or central, neurofibromatosis. These patients are at risk for bilateral acoustic neuromas.—R.C. Eagle, Jr., M.D.

Benign Conjunctival Melanocytic Lesions: Clinicopathologic Features

Folberg R, Jakobiec FA, Bernardino VB, Iwamoto T (Univ of Iowa, Iowa City; Manhattan Eye, Ear & Throat Hosp, New York; Wills Eye Hosp, Philadelphia, New York Hosp–Cornell Med Ctr, New York)

Ophthalmology 96:436–461, April 1989   7–8

Common acquired conjunctival nevi usually mature progressively and only exceptionally give rise to conjunctival melanoma. Pure junctional nevi are rare after childhood, but this lesion may be histologically indistinguishable from primary acquired melanosis with atypia, which tends to evolve into melanoma. Nevi in adolescents may be confused with a regressing nodule of melanoma, which occurs chiefly in adults. Congenital conjunctival nevi rarely are found, sometimes in patients having adjacent congenital nevi of the eyelid. The clinical features of conjunctival melanocytic lesions are compared in the table.

Comparison of the Clinical Features of Conjunctival Nevi, Episcleral Melanosis, Primary Acquired Melanosis, and Malignant Melanoma*

Feature	Common Congenital and Acquired Nevus	Blue Nevus	Episclera Melanosis	PAM	Melanoma with PAM
Location	Not in fornix or palpebral conjunctiva	Anywhere	Superficial sclera	Anywhere	Anywhere
Color	Flesh, tan, or brown	Brown, uniformly pigmented	Slate gray	Golden or chocolate brown	Pigmented or nonpigmented
Cysts	May be present in compound and subepithelial nevi	Absent	Absent	Absent	May be present
Thickness	Compound and sub-epithelial nevi may be raised	Mild placoid thickening without nodularity	Flat	Flat	Elevated or nodular
Movability over globe	Always movable	Always movable	Always nonmovable	Always movable	Usually movable but rarely fixed to sclera
Edges	Well outlined	Distinct	Spiculated	Indistinct	Indistinct
Focality	Unifocal	Unifocal	Multifocal	Unifocal or multifocal	Unifocal or multifocal

*PAM, primary acquired melanosis.
(Courtesy of Folberg R, Jakobiec FA, Bernardino VB, et al: *Ophthalmology* 96:436–461, April 1989.)

Common conjunctival nevi are most frequent in the juxtalimbal region and other epibulbar sites. Nevi may be focal or diffuse but generally are not multifocal. Nevi are quite exceptional in the palpebral and forniceal conjunctiva, where any pigmented lesion should be suspected of being a melanoma or melanoma precursor. Any pigmented lesion at the lumbus that straddles onto the peripheral cornea should be considered a malignant melanoma. Up to one third of conjunctival nevi lack pigment almost entirely. Cysts are distinctive features of conjunctival nevi. A melanocytic lesion limited to the epithelium in a patient aged more than 30 years probably is primary acquired melanosis.

Most nevi need not be excised and can be observed, especially if they have been stable for many years or since childhood. However, a biopsy should be done on all pigmented lesions of the forniceal or palpebral conjunctiva. Any excised conjunctival pigmented lesion should be evaluated pathologically.

▶ This thoughtful, comprehensive, informative, literate, and handsomely illustrated review of benign conjunctival melanocytic lesions is highly recommended. A brief abstract cannot do justice to its wealth of clinical and pathologic data. It is the perfect sequel and companion to the definitive review of conjunctival melanoma and primary acquired melanosis published previously by the authors (*Ophthalmology* 96:147, 1989), which is equally recommended.—R.C. Eagle, Jr., M.D.

Ocular Manifestations of Acquired Immune Deficiency Syndrome

Jabs DA, Green WR, Fox R, Polk BF, Bartlett JG (Johns Hopkins Univ, Baltimore)
Ophthalmology 96:1092–1099, July 1989   7–9

Patients with AIDS have a number of ocular complications, including noninfectious microangiopathy, opportunistic infections, ophthalmic neoplasms, and neuro-ophthalmic lesions. The incidence of these complications was studied in 200 patients with AIDS (table), 35 with AIDS-related complex (ARC), and 232 asymptomatic HIV-infected persons. Subjects were drawn from outpatient clinics or an inpatient service of the Johns Hopkins Hospital.

The mean age of the AIDS patients was 38 years; 92% were men and 73.5% were homosexual or bisexual men. Common systemic manifestations of the disease included *Pneumocystis carinii* pneumonia (76.5%), atypical mycobacterial infection (15.5%), Kaposi's sarcoma (13.5%), and cryptococcal infection (13.5%).

Retinopathy associated with AIDS was found in 66.5% of AIDS patients, in 40% of ARC patients, but in none with asymptomatic HIV infection. Microaneurysm formation, telangiectatic vessels, and focal capillary nonperfusion could be demonstrated in affected eyes when fluorescein angiography was performed, though the disorder was generally asymptomatic. Cotton-wool spots were a common finding.

Prevalence of Ocular Findings in 200 Patients With AIDS*

Ocular Manifestation	Frequency (%)
"AIDS retinopathy"	66.5
Cotton-wool spots	64.0
Intraretinal hemorrhages	12.0
Opportunistic ocular infections	
CMV retinitis	28.0
Herpes zoster ophthalmicus	4.0
Presumed varicella zoster retinitis	0.5
Presumed cryptococcal choroiditis	0.5
Toxoplasma retinitis	1.0
Bacterial corneal ulcers	1.0
Ocular neoplasms	
Eyelid Kaposi's sarcoma	1.5
Conjunctival Kaposi's sarcoma	1.0
Neuro-ophthalmic lesions	8.0
Optic neuropathy	2.5
Papilledema	1.5
Cranial nerve palsy or motility disturbance	4.0

*CMV, cytomegalovirus.
(Courtesy of Jabs DA, Green WR, Fox R, et al: *Ophthalmology* 96:1092–1099, July 1989.)

The most common intraocular infection among AIDS patients was cytomegalovirus (CMV) retinitis (28%), a progressive and potentially blinding disorder when untreated. Ganciclovir effects a high rate of remission in patients with CMV retinitis. Other opportunistic ocular infections appeared infrequently in AIDS patients, as well as in those with ARC or asymptomatic HIV infection. Only 2% of AIDS patients had ocular involvement by Kaposi's sarcoma. Sixteen AIDS patients (8%) had neuro-ophthalmic lesions, most commonly (56%) a result of cryptococcal meningitis. Involvement included cranial nerve palsies, papilledema, and visual loss.

Although microangiopathic changes are common in AIDS patients, they appear infrequently in asymptomatic HIV-infected patients. Thus, the development of AIDS retinopathy appears to be related to the patient's increasing immunologic dysfunction.

▶ There is little doubt that the steadily growing AIDS epidemic will have a major impact on the delivery and financing of medical care in the future. If these data from Baltimore are representative, CMV retinitis will be the major challenge facing ophthalmology; 28% of AIDS patients in this study had this potentially blinding opportunistic infection.—R.C. Eagle, Jr., M.D.

Sebaceous Carcinoma of the Eyelids: The Role of Adjunctive Cryotherapy in the Management of Conjunctival Pagetoid Spread

Lisman RD, Jakobiec FA, Small P (Manhattan Eye, Ear & Throat Hosp, New York)
Ophthalmology 96:1021–1026, July 1989   7–10

The significance of conjunctival pagetoid spread remains unresolved in treatment of sebaceous carcinoma of the eyelid. Recommendations range from no additional therapy to exenteration. In this report, 6 patients who had undergone wide but local excision of upper eyelid sebaceous carcinomas had adjunctive cryotherapy for residual intraepithelial pagetoid spread.

All patients had long histories of ocular complaints. Pagetoid spread was extensive; in 3 patients, the area went below the midline into the inferior bulbar conjunctiva. After resection of the tumor bulk and eyelid reconstruction, cryotherapy was administered in an additional procedure. The cryoprobe was applied to areas of the conjunctiva previously mapped by biopsy, with care taken to minimize contact with the sclera. Edema of the eyelids resulting from cryotherapy was treated with systemic or topical corticosteroids.

After surgery, follow-up biopsies were done at 6-month intervals for 3 years. No recurrence of pagetoid tumor occurred. Complications, which included dry-eye symptoms, symblepharon, corneal erosion, and vascularization, were most severe in an elderly patient and in a patient with widespread epibulbar involvement. Treatment of dry-eye symptoms and the maintenance of a good fornix with a conformer shell were found to be the most important aspects of postoperative care.

Strictly intraepithelial pagetoid extension does not worsen the prognosis for metastasis when this extension is removed completely. Cryotherapy will not be curative, however, if the entire conjunctival sac is affected by pagetoid spread.

▶ Pagetoid involvement of the conjunctival epithelium by sebaceous carcinoma is similar in many respects to the in situ form of conjunctival melanoma called primary acquired melanosis (PAM). The authors have successfully applied the cryotherapy techniques that they developed to treat PAM to this equally challenging conjunctival malignancy. Although cryotherapy is not without complications, it certainly appears preferable to orbital exenteration, an extremely radical form of therapy for an in situ neoplasm.—R.C. Eagle, Jr., M.D.

Metastatic Melanoma Within and to the Conjunctiva

Jakobiec FA, Buckman G, Zimmerman LE, La Piana FG, Levine MR, Ferry AP, Crawford JB (Manhattan Eye, Ear & Throat Hosp; Columbia-Presbyterian Med Ctr, New York; Armed Forces Inst of Pathology; Walter Reed Army Med Ctr, Washington, DC; Case Western Reserve Univ, Cleveland; et al)
Ophthalmology 96:999–1005, July 1989   7–11

Conjunctival metastases are an unusual manifestation of malignant melanoma. This form of the disease, infrequently discussed in the ophthalmic literature, might prove to be more common were thorough ocular examinations performed on patients with metastatic melanoma. Seven patients are described here; 2 with epibulbar juxtalimbal primary conjunctival melanomas and 5 with cutaneous melanomas in whom metastasis developed to the conjunctiva. All lesions were in the substantia propria and were separated from the overlying epithelium by a thin mantle of collagen.

Case 1.—Woman, 55, had a malignant melanoma removed from the bulbar conjunctiva in her right eye. Three years later a metastatic malignant melanoma was excised from the inferior cul-de-sac of the same eye. Over several years, 2 more recurrences of the tumor were removed. The woman since has remained free of metastatic disease.

Case 2.—Woman, 51, died of metastatic melanoma after a number of apparently successful excisions of conjunctival masses.

Case 3.—Man, 38, had a nodular melanoma with invasion to Clark's level III excised from the skin of his back. Metastatic melanoma was discovered in 1 of 11 right axillary lymph nodes. Several months later, in addition to cutaneous spread, nodules were found in the inferior fornix and in skin just above the inner canthus. The patient died soon after of widespread metastatic disease.

Conjunctival metastases may result from primary conjunctival melanoma or from metastases of cutaneous melanoma. In all 5 cases of the latter reported here, the primary cutaneous lesions were deeply infiltrating and located on the truncal skin: the back, chest, or abdomen. Four patients died less than a year after discovery of the cutaneous and ocular adnexal metastases.

▶ The development of metastases within the conjunctiva after excision of a primary conjunctival melanoma is less ominous than conjunctival metastases from a primary skin melanoma. Patients with skin melanomas that metastasize to the conjunctiva usually die within 1 year after conjunctival metastases develop.—R.C. Eagle, Jr., M.D.

Orbital Optic Nerve Glioma in Adult Life
Wulc AE, Bergin DJ, Barnes D, Scaravilli F, Wright JE, McDonald WI (Univ of Pennsylvania; Southeast Eye Ctr, Greensboro, NC; Inst of Neurology; Moorfields Eye Hosp, London)
Arch Ophthalmol 107:1013–1016, July 1989   7–12

Optic nerve glioma is an uncommon finding, especially after childhood. Seven rare cases of an orbital mass indicating optic nerve glioma in adults are described. The patients were seen at 2 hospitals in London; all were found to have visual loss and proptosis of varying severity. Their mean age at onset of symptoms was 28.7 years.

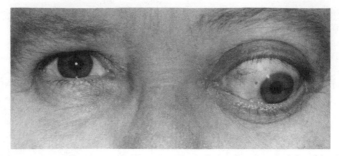

Fig 7–5.—A 64-year-old woman at presentation. She had poor vision in the left eye for 3 years and progressive proptosis for 1 year. (Courtesy of Wulc AE, Bergin DJ, Barnes D, et al: *Arch Opthalmol* 107:1013–1016, July 1989.)

Woman, 64, had a 3-year history of decreasing vision in her left eye. Although the right eye was normal, the left eye was blind and displaced inferiorly and temporally (Fig 7–5). A grossly enlarged orbital optic nerve was seen with CT (Fig 7–6). The woman underwent surgery with excision of the orbital portion of the optic nerve. Histologic examination revealed a grade II astrocytoma. After 4 years, the left eye again showed proptosis. A recurrent tumor, identical histologically to the previous specimen, was removed. The patient was well at 1-year follow-up.

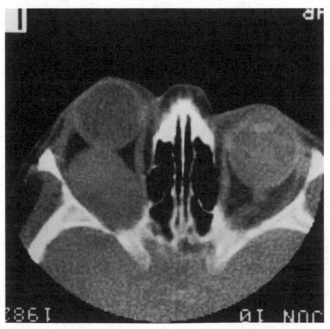

Fig 7–6.—Axial computed tomographic scan shows grossly enlarged orbital portion of the left optic nerve. (Courtesy of Wulc AE, Bergin DJ, Barnes D, et al: *Arch Opthalmol* 107:1013–1016, July 1989.)

Histologic findings in each patient were typical of optic nerve glioma. Areas of cystic degeneration occurred, as well as areas in which spindle-shaped or elongated cells formed bundles. In each of 4 cases, the tumor capsule was invaded by cells and Rosenthal's fibers. These tumors in adults did not differ in morphology or immunohistochemistry from optic nerve gliomas of childhood.

Unlike malignant gliomas, the tumors found in these patients had a relatively benign course. The prognosis was good for all but 1 patient, a 31-year-old woman with neurofibromatosis who later had a frontal glioma. Surgery should be postponed until the affected eye lacks useful vision, and radiotherapy reserved for patients with expanding residual intracranial tumor.

▶ The median age for optic nerve glioma is 5 years. Although "juvenile pilocytic astrocytomas" occur preferentially in children, 1 previously reported series found that nearly one third of patients become symptomatic after age 20 years; 57% of the patients in this report were aged 22 years or younger.—R.C. Eagle, Jr., M.D.

Diabetic-Like Retinopathy in Rats Prevented With an Aldose Reductase Inhibitor
Robison WG Jr, Nagata M, Laver N, Hohman TC, Kinoshita JH (Natl Eye Inst, Bethesda, Md)
Invest Ophthalmol Vis Sci 30:2285–2292, November 1989   7–13

Diabetic retinopathy is chiefly a vascular disorder. The earliest signs include a selective loss of intramural pericytes and thickened capillary basement membranes, lesions prevented by aldose reductase inhibitors in animal models. In this study, rats received a 50% galactose diet with or without tolrestat, an aldose reductase inhibitor, for 28 months.

Control animals had an extensive loss of intramural capillary pericytes that was prevented by inclusion of 0.05% tolrestat in the diet (Fig 7–7). The aldose reductase inhibitor also prevented endothelial-cell proliferation, diffuse dilatation, luminal occlusion, and microaneurysm formation. Clusters of complex microvascular abnormalities resembling those seen in human diabetic retinopathy were not present in rats given tolrestat. Tolrestat did not significantly alter blood glucose or galactose levels.

Long-term galactosemia produces retinal microangiopathic changes in rats that are very like those seen in human beings with background diabetic retinopathy. The lesions are prevented by an aldose reductase inhibitor. Early treatment with such agents may help delay or even prevent changes of diabetic retinopathy in human beings.

▶ The experimental retinal microvascular abnormalities in this study are identical to those found in human eyes with diabetic retinopathy. If the aldose reductase inhibitor tolrestat works equally as well in diabetic persons as it does in

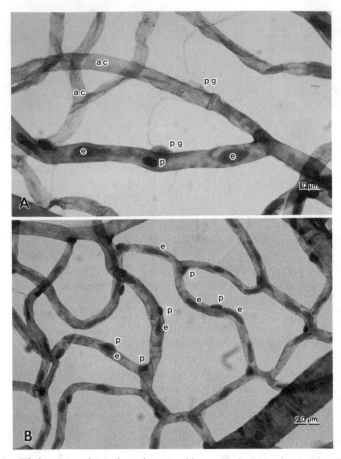

Fig 7–7.—Whole mounts of retinal vessels prepared by trypsin digestion, showing the effects of an aldose reductase inhibitor. Intramural pericytes and endothelial cells degenerated, leaving pericyte ghosts *(pg)* and acellular capillaries *(ac)* in rats fed a diet with 50% galactose for 28 months (**A**). However, the changes were prevented when 0.05% tolrestat was added to the diet (**B**). In treated rats, mainly normal-appearing endothelial cell *(e)* and pericyte *(p)* nuclei were found in an approximately normal ratio. Original magnifications, ×1,170 (*bar* = 10 μm, **A**) and ×653 (*bar* = 20 μm, **B**). (Courtesy of Robison WG Jr, Nagata M, Laver N, et al: *Invest Ophthalmol Vis Sci* 30:2285–2292, November 1989.)

galactosemic rats, it could become an important new prophylactic agent against diabetic retinopathy.—R.C. Eagle, Jr., M.D.

Human Papillomavirus DNA in a Recurrent Squamous Carcinoma of the Eyelid
McDonnell JM, McDonnell PJ, Stout WC, Martin WJ (Univ of Southern California, Los Angeles)
Arch Ophthalmol 107:1631–1634, November 1989   7–14

Human papillomaviruses (HPVs) are implicated in the pathogenesis of proliferative squamous lesions of the male and female genital tracts and the respiratory tract. Previous studies with the polymerase chain reaction (PCR) technique demonstrated HPV type 16 DNA in conjunctival dysplasias. Polymerase chain reaction methodology was used to demonstrate HPV 16 DNA in a recurrent infiltrating, well-differentiated squamous carcinoma of the eyelid (Fig 7–8).

Human papillomavirus type 16 is associated with a majority of uterine cervical malignancies and is considered to have a major causative role. It also may be pathogenetically important in squamous malignancies of the conjunctiva, cornea, and eyelid skin. As in the female genital tract, the finding of HPV 16 in an in situ process may serve to alert the clinician to possible future invasive disease unless adequate treatment is ensured. Preoperative measures such as recombinant interferon alfa, which shrinks HPV-related laryngeal papillomas, may help reduce the size of

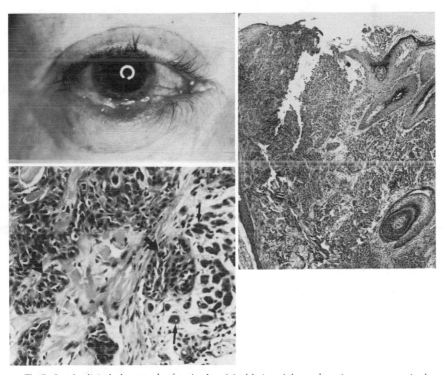

Fig 7–8.—A, clinical photograph of patient's original lesion. A large ulceration was present in the center of the right lower eyelid, involving the skin and eyelid margin, with loss of lashes. Purulent material drained from the surface of the lesion. Elsewhere, the patient had numerous pigmented areas suggesting extensive solar exposure. **B** and **C,** histopathologic features of the original lesion disclose neoplastic cells extending from surface epithelium into the deep connective tissue. The tumor infiltrated in the form of individual cells and small nests *(large arrows)*. Nests extended to involve the orbicularis muscle *(small arrows)*. Hematoxylin-eosin, ×157 (**B**), ×393 (**C**). (Courtesy of McDonnell JM, McDonnell PJ, Stout WC, et al: *Arch Ophthalmol* 107:1631–1634, November 1989.)

large cancers of the eyelids, allowing tissue-sparing excision to be carried out.

▶ Human papillomavirus 16, a major cause of cervical cancer, has been demonstrated with the chain reaction technique in a recurrent squamous cell carcinoma of the eyelid. Researchers using PCR must be extremely meticulous to avoid extraneous contamination of their specimens. This new research tool is so powerful that it theoretically can amplify and detect the nuclei acid in a single virus.— R.C. Eagle, Jr., M.D.

Chronic Orbital Inflammatory Disease: Parasitisation of Orbital Leucocytes by Mollicute-Like Organisms
Wirostko E, Johnson L, Wirostko B (Columbia–Presbyterian Med Ctr; Columbia Univ, New York)
Br J Ophthalmol 73:865–870, 1989   7–15

Chronic orbital inflammatory disease usually is considered noninfectious. An appropriate search, however, often reveals mollicute-like organisms (MLO) parasitizing and destroying vitreous leukocytes and producing chronic uveitis. Mollicutes are cell wall-deficient bacteria that are easily overlooked or confused with viruses. Extracellular mollicutes are fastidious, lipid-rich organisms containing a variety of potent cytotoxic substances, including nucleases. They are detected by transmission electron microscopy within parasitized cells.

Electron microscopic study of samples from 3 patients with chronic orbital inflammation showed undulating intracytoplasmic filaments and pleomorphic trilaminar membrane-bound tubulospherical bodies in 2% to 10% of leukocytes. Lymphocytes, monocytes, and polymorphonuclear leukocytes all are parasitized. Forms may develop into sporelike cocci through deposition of electron-dense material within trilaminar membranes.

Inoculation of MLO into mouse eyelids produces chronic uveitis and exophthalmic orbital inflammation. Disease caused by extracellular mollicutes is characterized by lymphoid infiltration, immunosuppression, and autoantibody production. Rifampicin significantly reduces morbidity and mortality in experimentally infected mice. Empirical rifampicin therapy may be considered in patients with progressive chronic orbital inflammation if MLO cannot be ruled out by electron microscopic study of tissue leukocytes.

▶ The authors believe that strange mycoplasma-like organisms called mollicutes cause orbital pseudotumor and other poorly understood inflammatory diseases such as sarcoidosis. These exciting and somewhat provocative new observations must be confirmed by other laboratories; they could have major therapeutic implications. Laboratory tests for these elusive microrganisms besides transmission electron microscopy are needed.— R.C. Eagle, Jr., M.D.

8 Pediatrics

Anterior Transposition of the Inferior Oblique: Its Use in Strabismus Surgery*

LEONARD B. NELSON, M.D.
Pediatric Ophthalmology Service, Wills Eye Hospital, Philadelphia, Pennsylvania

Numerous weakening procedures for the inferior oblique muscle have evolved since the first reported myotomy operations in 1908 by Posey (1). The overacting inferior oblique muscle may be weakened effectively by myectomy (2), disinsertion (3), recession (4), and, more recently, denervation and extirpation (5). Each procedure has strong proponents for its effectiveness and low rate of complications.

Even though the recession procedure is more difficult to perform than either myectomy or disinsertion, a surgeon can grade the amount of recession according to the extent of overaction. Parks found that significant overaction recurred less frequently with the recession technique (15%) than with myectomy (37%) or disinsertion (57%). To further reduce the incidence of residual overaction of the inferior oblique muscle, Apt and Call suggested anteriorly displacing the posterior portion of the muscle along the temporal border of the inferior rectus (6).

Scott, using a computer model, showed that a greater weakening effect could be achieved by transposing the entire insertion of the inferior oblique muscle to a position adjacent to the temporal insertion of the inferior rectus muscle (7). From this position anterior to the equator, the inferior oblique muscle continues posteriorly and parallel to the inferior rectus muscle. It then passes beneath the inferior rectus muscle at Lockwood's ligament near the equator. Under these circumstances, contraction of the inferior oblique muscle produces forces that depress the eye (8). Therefore, anterior transposition of the inferior oblique muscle not only weakens it, but converts it from an elevator to a depressor.

Elliott and Nankin compared the surgical results of 64 anterior transpositions to 90 standard recessions varying from 8 to 14 mm in magnitude (9). Of the anterior transposition procedures, 31% (20 of 64) were performed on +1 to +2 overacting inferior oblique muscles and 69% (44 of 64) were performed for +3 to +4 overactions. Of the recession procedures, 89% (80 of 90) were accomplished on +1 to +2 overacting muscles with 11% (10 of 90) performed on +3 to +4 overactions. The authors found a −3.0 net change in the amount of overaction of the inferior oblique after anterior transposition as compared with a −2.0 net change for all standard recession procedures. A pronounced bias was in-

*This study was supported in part by a grant from Fight for Sight, Inc., New York, to the Fight for Sight Children's Eye Center of Wills Eye Hospital.

155

troduced in the study because the majority of anterior transpositions were reserved for the most markedly overacting inferior oblique muscles. However, the results do indicate that both procedures are effective in significantly reducing oblique overactions.

Seven patients for whom anterior transposition was performed had previously recessed inferior oblique muscles. None of these seven oblique muscles overacted after the anterior transposition procedure.

Elliott and Nankin also found that both procedures were effective in decreasing primary position hypertropia when present preoperatively. In 5 of 16 unilateral recessions in which a primary position hypertropia was present preoperatively, an average reduction of 5 prism D occurred. In 6 of 15 unilateral anterior transposition procedures in which a preoperative vertical deviation was present in the primary position, an average reduction in the hypertropia of 15 prism D occurred.

Bremer and co-workers (10) and Mims (11) each reported 3 cases of hypotropia with limitation of elevation after unilateral anterior transposition of an inferior oblique muscle. Elliott and Nankin found a −1 to −2 primary position elevation deficiency postoperatively in 73% of unilateral anterior transposition procedures, but in only 25% of unilateral recession surgeries (9). However, the authors do not state that any primary position hypotropia occurred postoperatively. Converting the inferior oblique muscle into a depressor was detrimental in these cases, but Bremer and co-workers (10) and Mims (11) suggested that anterior transposition may be beneficial in treating dissociated vertical deviations (DVDs).

Mims and Wood expounded on the benefits of anterior transposition of the inferior oblique muscles (12). Not only did they find this procedure effective in eliminating overaction of the inferior oblique muscles, but in preventing or substantially reducing the incidence of DVD in children with congenital esotropia. The authors reported on 61 children with congenital esotropia who had bilateral anterior transposition of the inferior oblique muscles. One patient subsequently needed surgery for DVD, and another needed denervation and extirpation for recurrent overaction of an inferior oblique muscle. Nine patients had profound reductions of their DVDs after bilateral anterior transposition. The primary indication for surgery in all nine cases was overaction of the inferior oblique muscles.

Mims and Wood reported an additional 60 children of similar ages who had bimedial recessions for congenital esotropia but little or no overaction of the inferior oblique muscles. None of these patients needed surgery on her or his inferior oblique muscle. Nine of these patients eventually needed surgery for DVD.

Successful surgical treatment of DVD requires the changing of the sum of forces on the eye in favor of depression. Three surgical approaches have been advocated to correct DVD: recession of the superior rectus (13, 14), recession of the superior rectus combined with a posterior suture (15), and resection of the inferior rectus (16). Each procedure has had its enthusiastic proponents.

Because of the depression force of anterior transposition of the inferior oblique muscle, Kratz and co-workers tested the effectiveness of this procedure as a treatment for DVD (17). They also graded the anteriorization of the posterior part of the inferior oblique muscle relative to the insertion of the inferior rectus. The placement of the posterior fibers varied according to the amount of preoperative DVD. The results from the graded group were compared with a group of patients with DVD that received the same amount of anteriorization regardless of the degree of preoperative DVD. This study showed that anteriorization of the inferior oblique muscle was an effective primary procedure in the treatment of DVD. Grading the anteriorization of the posterior fibers improved the results.

Anterior transposition has been shown to be a safe and effective procedure in reducing overaction of the inferior oblique muscle. It also has produced excellent results in patients for whom inferior oblique muscle overaction had persisted after previous standard recessions. A potential benefit of this procedure is the prevention or substantial reduction of DVD. The incidence of DVD in patients with congenital esotropia is high, ranging from 46% to 90% (18). Therefore, if a patient with congenital esotropia has overaction of the inferior oblique muscles that requires surgical correction, it makes sense to perform anterior transposition. This procedure certainly will reduce the overaction, and if it does reduce the incidence of DVD, it may ultimately prevent further surgery for the vertical deviation.

The role of anterior transposition as a primary procedure for DVD needs further study. A prospective randomized study with long-term follow-up is needed to evaluate the effect of grading the placement of the posterior fibers of the inferior oblique muscle in the treatment of DVD.

References

1. Posey WC: *Ophthalmic Record.* 1908, p 346.
2. Daniel G, McNeer KW, Spencer PF: Myectomy of the inferior oblique muscle. *Arch Ophthalmol* 104:855, 1986.
3. Dyer LA: Tenotomy of the inferior oblique muscle at its scleral insertion. *Arch Ophthalmol* 68:56, 1962.
4. Parks MM: A study of the weakening surgical procedure for eliminating overaction of the inferior oblique. *Am J Ophthalmol* 73:107, 1972.
5. DelMonte MA, Parks MM: Denervation and extirpation of the inferior oblique. *Ophthalmology* 90:1178, 1983.
6. Apt L, Call NB: Inferior oblique muscle recession. *Am J Ophthalmol* 85:95, 1978.
7. Scott AB: Planning inferior oblique muscle surgery, in Reinecke RD (ed): *Strabismus.* New York, Grune and Stratton, 1978, pp 347–354.
8. Goldstein HP, Scott AB, Nelson LB: Ocular motility, in Tasman W, Jaeger EA (eds): *Duane's Biomedical Foundations of Ophthalmology.* Philadelphia, JB Lippincott, 1989.
9. Elliott RL, Nankin SJ: Anterior transposition of the inferior oblique. *J Pediatr Ophthalmol Strabismus* 18:35, 1981.
10. Bremer DL, Rogers GL, Quick LD: Primary-position hypotropia after anterior transposition of the inferior oblique. *Arch Ophthalmol* 104:229, 1986.

11. Mims JL: Benefits of bilateral anterior transposition of the inferior obliques. *Arch Ophthalmol* 104:800, 1986.
12. Mims JL, Wood RC: Bilateral anterior transposition of the inferior obliques. *Arch Ophthalmol* 107:41, 1989.
13. Raab EL: Dissociated vertical deviation. *Int Ophthalmol Clin* 25:119–131, 1985.
14. Braverman DE, Scott WE: Surgical correction of dissociated vertical deviation. *J Pediatr Ophthalmol Strabismus* 14:337, 1977.
15. Sprague JB, Moore S, Eggers H, et al: Dissociated vertical deviation: Treatment with the Faden operation of Coppers. *Arch Ophthalmol* 98:465, 1980.
16. Noel LP, Parks MM: Dissociated vertical deviation associated findings and results of surgical treatment. *Con J Ophthalmol* 17:10, 1982.
17. Kratz RE, Rogers GL, Bremer DL, et al: Anterior tendon displacement of the inferior oblique for DVD. *J Pediatr Ophthalmol Strabismus* 26:212, 1989.
18. Nelson LB, Wagner RS, Simon JW, et al: Congenital esotropia. *Surv Ophthalmol* 31:363, 1987.

Screening for Uveitis in Juvenile Chronic Arthritis

Kanski JJ (Canadian Red Cross Mem Hosp, Taplow; Northwick Park Hosp, Harrow, England)

Br J Ophthalmol 73:225–228, 1989   8–1

About one fifth of patients with juvenile chronic arthritis (JCA) have anterior uveitis, which typically is asymptomatic and can lead to severe loss of vision unless treated at a relatively early stage. In a series of 315 patients with JCA and anterior uveitis, girls predominated in a ratio of 3:1. Uveitis was diagnosed after arthritis developed in all but 6% of cases. The risk was quite small when 7 years had elapsed after the onset of arthritis. Patients with a pauciarticular onset of JCA were at greatest risk, whereas those with a systemic onset had the lowest risk of uveitis. Circulating antinuclear antibody also increased the risk.

Girls are more at risk of chronic anterior uveitis than boys, regardless of whether they have JCA. The risk of uveitis diminishes 7 years after the onset of arthritis. Annual screening will suffice for patients with a systemic onset of JCA. The activity of the arthritis and that of the ocular inflammation are not correlated.

Patients positive for antinuclear antibodies should be screened at 2- to 3-month intervals from the time of onset of JCA, for at least 7 years.

▶ Anterior uveitis associated with JCA may be present asymptomatically. If the intraocular inflammation is not detected early, serious intraocular complications may occur. It is imperative that all patients with JCA have a slit-lamp examination at regular intervals. Those patients with pauciarticular onset and a positive ANA need to be screened ophthalmologically every few months for approximately 7 years.—L.B. Nelson, M.D.

Congenital Adduction Palsy and Synergistic Divergence: A Clinical and Electro-Oculographic Study

Cruysberg JRM, Mtanda AT, Duinkerke-Eerola KU, Huygen PLM (Univ of Nijmegen, The Netherlands)
Br J Ophthalmol 73:68–75, 1989   8–2

Two patients were encountered who had a congenital disorder of ocular motility in which horizontal movements of the left eye always were opposite to the expected direction. The common features were congenital

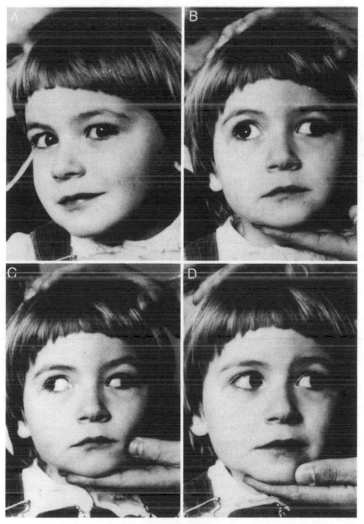

Fig 8–1.—A, looking forward with permanent head turn to the right. B, exotropia on forced straightening of the head. C, extreme exotropia on attempted gaze to the right. Note that the left eye moves further into abduction, and there is narrowing of the left palpable fissure. D, decreased exotropia of the left eye on gaze to the left. Note that the exotropia of the left eye is maximal on gaze to the right and minimal on gaze to the left. (Courtesy of Cruysberg JRM, Mtanda AT, Duinkerke-Eerola KU, et al: *Br J Ophthalmol* 73:68–75, 1989.)

monocular adduction palsy and exotropia of the left eye; divergence on attempted dextroversion (Fig 8–1); ocular torticollis with the head turned to the right; and inverse nystagmus of the left, both spontaneous and on optokinetic and vestibular testing.

Congenital adduction palsy with synergistic divergence usually is noted in childhood as an adduction deficit. The left eye is involved in three fourths of cases. In the primary position the affected eye is exotropic. In 1 case the lateral rectus was absent, which most likely reflected past surgery. Nevertheless, the synergistic abduction did not result from lateral rectus innervation alone, but as a secondary action of the inferior rectus or inferior oblique, or both.

Synergistic divergence is similar to Duane's retraction syndrome, and probably also is a developmental anomaly caused by absence of the abducens nucleus and subsequent innervation of the lateral rectus by the inferior branch of the oculomotor nerve.

▶ Congenital adduction palsy and synergistic divergence is a rare disorder that has clinical and electromyographic similarities to Duane's retraction syndrome (DRS). In 2 recent autopsy cases of DRS, the abducens nuclei and nerves were absent and the lateral recti were innervated by a branch from the inferior division of the oculomotor nerve. These anatomical findings in DRS would help explain the clinical findings in congenital adduction palsy and synergistic divergence. However, in case 2, the lateral rectus at the time of surgery could not be found, yet when the patient attempted to adduct the involved eye there was abduction instead. The authors suggested that in this case the abduction movement probably was carried out by a secondary action of the inferior rectus or inferior oblique muscles, or both.—L.B. Nelson, M.D.

Acute Comitant Esotropia in Children With Brain Tumors
Williams AS, Hoyt CS (Univ of California, San Francisco)
Arch Ophthalmol 107:376–378, March 1989   8–3

Acute comitant esotropia without divergence insufficiency has been considered a benign disorder. Six children with acute comitant esotropia subsequently were found to have a brainstem or cerebellar tumor (table). No child had incomitant esotropia with deficient abduction. Diagnostic delay ranged from 3 to 71 weeks; detailed neurologic assessment was avoided initially because of the ostensibly benign presentation. Four patients had strabismus surgery after neurologic treatment, but ocular motor fusion never was reestablished.

Comitancy does not ensure that a patient's strabismus is not associated with neurologic disease, including CNS tumor. Hydrocephalus may have a role in some cases, but is not always present. Intensive work-up is indicated if ocular motor fusion is not restored after neurosurgical or optical treatment.

Summary of 6 Patients With Acute Onset of Comitant Esotropia

Patient No./Sex/ Age at Onset of Esotropia, year	Delay in Diagnosis of Brain Tumor, week	Angle of Esotropia: Far/Near, Prism Diopters	Refraction	Other Neuro-oph-thalmologic Signs	Diagnosis
1/M/4.3	3	25/25	OD +1.75 / OS +1.25	Upbeating nystagmus	Cerebellar astrocytoma
2/M/6.1	4	18/20	OD -25 +0.75 x090 / OS plano +0.50 x090	Torsional nystagmus	Cerebellar astrocytoma
3/M/10.4	21	30/35	OD +75 +0.50 x090 / OS +50 +25 x090	...	Cerebellar medullo-blastoma
4/F/5.4	6	15/20	OD +1.75 +0.25 x080 / OS +1.50 +0.50 x110	...	Pontine glioma
5/M/3.1	71	25/25	OD +2.25 / OS +2.20	...	Cerebellar astrocytoma
6/F/7.3	4	35/35	OD -1.75 +0.50 x090 / OS -1.50 +0.2T x090	Torsional nystagmus	Cerebellar astrocytoma

(Courtesy of Williams AS, Hoyt CS: Arch Ophthalmol 107:376–378, March 1989.)

▶ Acute comitant esotropia, a rare condition that usually occurs in older children and adults, is characterized by a dramatic onset of a relatively large angle of esotropia with diplopia and mild hyperopic refractive error. Patients in whom this condition develops must have a careful motility analysis to rule out a paretic deviation. The authors clearly show that even patients who are comitant may still have an intracranial tumor. Therefore, all patients with acute comitant esotropia should have a neuroradiologic evaluation.—L.B. Nelson, M.D.

Preservation of the Anterior Ciliary Vessels During Extraocular Muscle Surgery

McKeown CA, Lambert HM, Shore JW (Lackland Air Force Base; Univ of Texas Health Science Ctr, San Antonio)

Ophthalmology 96:498–507, April 1989   8–4

The anterior ciliary vessels are disrupted in the course of conventional full-tendon rectus muscle surgery, and this may produce anterior segment ischemia if anterior segment blood flow is sufficiently compromised. Both clinical and histologic studies indicate that it is feasible to dissect and preserve the anterior ciliary vessels. It might be possible to avoid staging surgery when several extraocular muscles are tenotomized (Fig 8–2).

Attempts were made to dissect and preserve 35 clinically apparent anterior ciliary vessel groups on 15 rectus muscles during strabismus surgery. The rate of unplanned vessel destruction was 9.5%. Twelve recessions, 2 full-tendon transpositions, and 1 resection were carried out.

It might be useful to repeat this study by performing standard tenotomy of 3 or 4 rectus muscles on 1 eye and tenotomy with preservation of the anterior ciliary vessels on the other. Anterior segment ischemia would be detected by slit-lamp examination and anterior segment blood flow monitored by iris fluorescein angiography.

▶ Anterior segment ischemia may result in serious ocular sequelae. Interruption of the anterior ciliary vessels at the time of rectus muscle tenotomy generally is accepted as the cause of anterior segment ischemia after strabismus surgery. Preservation of the anterior ciliary vessels during strabismus surgery may reduce the risk of anterior segment ischemia. However, this complication after strabismus surgery is rare enough so that a valid statistical study of human beings would be difficult to obtain. As the authors suggest, animal experimentation using this technique ultimately may demonstrate its validity.— L.B. Nelson, M.D.

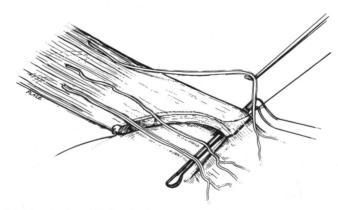

Fig 8–2.—Diagram of partially completed tenotomy with suture in place and 1 vessel suspended on a retinal hook. The *dashed line* marks the proposed site of completion of the tenotomy. (Courtesy of McKeown CA, Lambert HM, Shore JW: *Ophthalmology* 96:498–507, April 1989.)

Follow-Up and Diagnostic Reappraisal of 75 Patients With Leber's Congenital Amaurosis
Lambert SR, Kriss A, Taylor D, Coffey R, Pembrey M (Hosps for Sick Children; Inst of Child Health, London)
Am J Ophthalmol 107:624–631, June 1989   8–5

Seventy-five children with a diagnosis of Leber's congenital amaurosis were reviewed. Thirty were found to have ocular or systemic disorders other than Leber's congenital amaurosis. The most frequent alternate diagnoses were congenital stationary night blindness, achromatopsia, infantile-onset retinitis pigmentosa, Joubert's syndrome, Zellweger syndrome, and infantile Refsum's disease (table). The diagnostic criteria for Leber's disease included an unrecordable or highly attenuated electroretinogram, a severe visual deficit present since infancy, and absence of other specific retinal or multisystemic disease.

Evaluation of a child presumed to have congenital retinal dystrophy should include an electroretinogram and visual-evoked potential recording. The latter provides useful information on macular function even when the electroretinogram is unrecordable. In addition, children suspected of having Leber's congenital amaurosis should be carefully assessed for signs of developmental delay. The diagnosis should be made reluctantly for children with moderately preserved visual acuity.

▶ Severe visual impairment with a normal retinal appearance in infancy should be evaluated with an electroretinogram and visual-evoked potential. It is important to differentiate Leber's congenital amaurosis from other ocular conditions because the visual programs differ markedly. Any child with severe visual impairment should be evaluated carefully by a pediatrician for developmental de-

Revised Diagnoses	
DIAGNOSES	NO. OF PATIENTS
Congenital stationary night blindness	5
Joubert's syndrome	5
Retinitis pigmentosa	4
Achromatopsia	4
Infantile Refsum's disease	2
Zellweger syndrome	2
Senior syndrome	2
Idiopathic retinal dystrophy and myopia	2
Cone-rod degeneration	1
Dandy-Walker malformation and retinal dystrophy	1
Alström's syndrome	1

(Courtesy of Lambert SR, Kriss A, Taylor D, et al: *Am J Ophthalmol* 107:624–631, June 1989.)

lay. If the child apppears more delayed than expected for a visually impaired child, a neurodegenerative or other systemic condition should be excluded carefully.—L.B. Nelson, M.D.

Expanded Binocular Peripheral Visual Fields Following Surgery for Esotropia

Wortham EV, Greenwald MJ (Children's Mem Hosp; Northwestern Univ, Chicago)

J Pediatr Ophthalmol Strabismus 26:109–112, May–June 1989   8–6

The horizontal extent of the binocular peripheral visual field was measured in 10 adult esotropes before and after strabismus surgery using Goldmann perimetry. An increased horizontal dimension of the field was documented in each case, after corrections ranging from 5 to 30 degrees. The degree of expansion accorded fairly well with the change in the angle of strabismic deviation, regardless of the presence of amblyopia or the recovery of binocular fusion. A number of patients noted subjective improvement in peripheral vision.

Expansion of the peripheral visual field is a valid indication for correcting esotropia. A contracted peripheral visual field has special relevance to operating a motor vehicle. Expansion of the peripheral field may be a major benefit even in patients with severe amblyopia. In contrast, exotropes may be dissatisfied with the outcome of successful surgery because the supernormal visual field is smaller after surgery.

▶ Surgical correction of esotropia in older children and adults with poor prognoses for binocularity often is performed for cosmetic reasons. This study has demonstrated that after surgery for esotropia, the visual field was expanded; subjective improvement in the peripheral field was appreciated by a number of patients. Expansion of the peripheral visual fields has obvious functional significance even in patients with severe amblyopia.—L.B. Nelson, M.D.

Adrenal Suppression After Corticosteroid Injection of Periocular Hemangiomas

Weiss AH (Univ of South Florida, Tampa)

Am J Ophthalmol 107:518–522, May 1989   8–7

Hemangiomas of the eyelids and orbit that threaten vision usually are treated with localized or systemic corticosteroids. Intralesional corticosteroid injections have caused many complications, including central retinal artery occlusion and blindness.

Two infants with symptomatic periocular hemangiomas had adrenal suppression after receiving 1-mL intralesional injections of a 50:50 mixture of triamcinolone acetonide (40 mg/mL) and betamethasone (8 mg/mL). The serum levels of cortisol and adrenocorticotropic hormone were depressed immediately. One patient remained suppressed for 5 months and had declines in weight and growth rate to below the fifth percentile.

Adrenal suppression is a complication of corticosteroid injection of periocular hemangioma. This still is a valuable treatment, but it is important to monitor pituitary-adrenal function on a monthly basis until it recovers fully. Pharmacologic doses of corticosteroids might be needed during clinical stress states such as infection and surgery.

▶ As intralesional corticosteroid injections have replaced the systemic route to treat periocular hemangiomas, more complications have been reported. Most of the complications for intralesional corticosteroid injections primarily have been ocular. Doctor Weiss has shown that this treatment modality may result in adrenal suppression. It is important for the clinical who uses intralesional corticosteroid injections for significant periocular hemangiomas to be aware of this potential systemic complication and to monitor pituitary-adrenal function after treatment.—L.B. Nelson, M.D.

Delayed Visual Maturation: A Longitudinal Clinical and Electrophysiological Assessment
Lambert SR, Kriss A, Taylor D (Hosp for Sick Children, London)
Ophthalmology 96:524–529, April 1989   8–8

Delayed visual maturation is a disorder of unknown cause characterized by visual inattention during infancy. Nine children with this diagnosis were followed up and their electroretinographic and visual evoked potential (VEP) findings were compared with those of age-matched control children. Eight of the patients had consistently normal VEP responses to flash and pattern stimulation. All of the children had normal electroretinograms (ERGs). Visually mediated behavior gradually developed at ages 3 to 8 months. Five of them also had delay in general developmental milestones.

Recording of VEP is helpful in making a visual prognosis for children with delayed visual maturation. This term is applicable only to infants with visual inattention of unknown origin. The mechanism of the disorder is uncertain, but macular immaturity and delayed myelination are not likely causes. Delayed visual maturation may be secondary to immaturity of the visual association areas that mediate visual attention. However, all of the present patients were full-term infants.

▶ Delayed visual maturation or idiopathic visual inattention in infancy is an uncommon clinical entity. However, the use of the VEP and the ERG can assist clinicians in establishing the diagnosis and giving an appropriate prognosis. Many children with delayed visual maturation also will have a delay in general developmental milestones.—L.B. Nelson, M.D.

The Pupils of Term and Preterm Infants
Isenberg SJ, Dang Y, Jotterand V (Harbor–UCLA Med Ctr, Los Angeles and Torrance, Calif)
Am J Ophthalmol 108:75–79, July 1989   8–9

The pupils of newborn infants have received little attention. Pupil responses might be used to indicate the intactness of the visual system and aid in the diagnosis of neonatal neurologic disorders. Therefore, the nature of the pupil in term and preterm infants was studied.

One hundred term and preterm infants, aged 26.5 to 46 weeks, comprised the study group. In a dark environment, the mean pupil diameter was 3.6 mm. Nine infants had anisocoria of 0.5 to 1 mm. Before 32 weeks of age, pupils did not consistently respond to 600 foot-candles of light. Pupils responded increasingly after that age. The progressive light response was significantly correlated with postconceptual age, weight, Apgar scores, and corneal diameter. Neurologic or radiologic assessment in the perinatal period may be warranted if the pupil diameter in the dark is less than 1.8 mm or more than 5.4 mm or if pupils do not respond to light challenge after the infant is 31 weeks' postconceptual age.

Neonate pupils assume a mean diameter of 3.6 mm in less than 10 foot-candles of light. This value does not change significantly in the first few weeks of life. Clinicians can consider a pupil diameter of more than 2 standard deviations from this mean as an indicator of possible neurologic abnormality.

▶ Pupillary abnormalities in all age groups may indicate a neurologic problem. Few data have been available on the pupil responses of newborns. The authors have given the reader clear guidelines as to when pupillary responses in newborns may warrant neurologic or radiologic evaluation.—L.B. Nelson, M.D.

Ocular Manifestations in Pediatric Patients With Acquired Immunodeficiency Syndrome
Dennehy PJ, Warman R, Flynn JT, Scott GB, Mastrucci MT (Univ of Miami)
Arch Ophthalmol 107:978–982, July 1989   8–10

Ocular findings in children with AIDS may or may not differ from those reported in adult patients. The incidence, type, and natural history of ocular problems in pediatric AIDS were reported.

Forty children who were seropositive for HIV antibody underwent eye examinations. Eighty-seven assessments were performed. Twenty percent of the children had ocular findings. Two had cytomegalovirus retinitis, 1 had isolated retinal cotton-wool spots, 1 had toxoplasmosis retinochoroiditis, and 3 had external infections of adnexal structures. Unusual peripheral retinal findings were noted in 1 child. Although the incidence of ocular manifestations in these children was considerably less than that reported in several adult series, ophthalmic screening should be done in all children with AIDS with encephalopathy or disseminated opportunistic infections or when symptoms suggest ophthalmic manifestation.

In this series, a large number of ophthalmic examinations yielded normal results, despite the presence of severe clinical problems. The incidence of ocular manifestations was much lower than that in adult series. Therefore, extensive ophthalmic screening of children who are HIV seropositive is not needed. However, children known to have encephalopathy, disseminated opportunistic infections, or clinical signs and symptoms suggesting ocular involvement should be examined by an ophthalmologist.

▶ The incidence of ocular manifestations in pediatric patients with AIDS is much less than in several series of adult patients with AIDS. These findings are similar to those of other investigations, yet the reason remains unknown. All children with HIV antibody seropositivity with CNS involvement, disseminated opportunistic infections, or clinical signs and symptoms suggestive of an ophthalmic problem should have a careful and thorough ophthalmologic evaluation.—L.B. Nelson, M.D.

Complications After Surgery for Congenital and Infantile Cataracts
Keech RV, Tongue AC, Scott WE (Univ of Iowa Hosps and Clinics, Iowa City, Oregon Health Sciences Univ, Portland)
Am J Ophthalmol 108:136–141, August 1989   8–11

Removal of the lens and anterior vitreous is the most common cataract procedure done in young children. The complications of such surgery were reviewed.

The records of 78 children undergoing 128 surgical procedures for congenital or infantile cataracts were studied. All children had undergone surgery before 30 months of age. Operations done included 92 limbal lensectomies and anterior vitrectomies, 13 pars plicata lensectomies, 20 aspirations, and 3 additional procedures. Twenty-one of the 105 lensectomy and anterior vitrectomy procedures resulted in complications (table). Ten percent of the eyes needed additional operations for a secondary membrane, glaucoma developed in 11%, and retinas became detached in 1%. Infants who had surgery by 8 weeks of age suffered significantly more complications.

In this series, a higher rate of complications was associated with lensectomy and vitrectomy techniques than has been reported previously. A child's age at the time of surgery seemed to be the most important factor

---

Complications After Surgery for Congenital and Infantile Cataracts

COMPLICATION	ASPIRATION (N = 17)	LIMBAL LENSECTOMY AND ANTERIOR VITRECTOMY (N = 19)	PARS PLICATA LENSECTOMY AND ANTERIOR VITRECTOMY (N = 2)	TOTAL (N = 38)
Secondary membrane	15	10	0	25
Chronic closed-angle glaucoma	2	3	0	5
Pupillary block glaucoma	1	0	0	1
Open-angle glaucoma	1	2	1	4
Anomalous angle	0	5	1	6
Retinal detachment	1	1	0	2

(Courtesy of Keech RV, Tongue AC, Scott WE: *Am J Ophthalmol* 108:136–141, August 1989.)

contributing to the high complication rate. Children undergoing cataract surgery as infants should be assessed routinely for possible glaucoma development. The extensive removal of the lens cortex, posterior capsule, and anterior vitreous seems to be the best way to reduce secondary membrane formation and some types of glaucoma.

▶ Cataract surgery in the pediatric age group is not without complications. The authors found a higher rate of complications than in previously reported series, which they suggest may result from a longer follow-up. However, they include many patients who had an aspiration technique in which the posterior capsule was left intact. It is not surprising that the rate of secondary membrane formation was high. The authors also included patients with systemic conditions known to be associated with glaucoma such as Lowe's syndrome and congenital rubella.

The number of complications in patients operated on by 2 months of age was significantly increased. This has been the finding of other pediatric ophthalmologists as well. The authors suggest that the higher complication rate may result from technical difficulties associated with operating on small eyes as well as the marked inflammation and scarring that may occur.—L.B. Nelson, M.D.

Chemodenervation of Strabismic Children: A 2- to 5-Year Follow-Up Study Compared With Shorter Follow-Up
Magoon EH (Northeastern Ohio College of Medicine, Canton)
Ophthalmology 96:931–934, July 1989   8–12

The short-term results of botulinum chemosurgery for incisional strabismus in infants and children have been good. A longer follow-up study was done to compare long-term results with previously reported short-term results.

Eighty-five children aged less than 14 years were followed up. All had been treated from 1982 to 1984. Defining successful motor alignment as 10 prism D (PD) deviation or less, the short- and long-term results were

Residual Deviation Noted After Follow-Up		
No. of Patients	Residual Deviation (PD)	Follow-up
Total 70*		
10	>10	>6 mos
60	≤10	>6 mos
Total 62†		
9	>10	>2 yrs
53	≤10	>2 yrs

*60/70 = 85.7% of patients with "satisfactory" alignment.
†53/62 = 85.5% of patients with "satisfactory" alignment.
(Courtesy of Magoon EH: *Ophthalmology* 96:931–934, July 1989.)

comparable at 85% (table). Fifty esotropes meeting the 2-year criteria for follow-up had average PDs of 35 before treatment and 5 after treatment. Twelve exotropes had an average of 30 and 5 PD, respectively. There were no long-term complications.

Botulinum chemosurgery can substantially correct eye alignment. The good result persists at 2 to 5.5 years after injection. Generally, the treatment undercorrects the deviation, which can be managed with reinjection. However, very few patients in this series needed reinjection after 2 years. This procedure is beneficial for older children, who can undergo the injection in an office setting without sedation.

▶ Ophthalmologists usually can achieve a satisfactory ocular alignment within several weeks after surgery for horizontal strabismus. The advantages of using either topical or ketamine anesthesia for botulinum injection and not having to intubate a child is outweighed by the frequency of reinjection and complications such as hypertropia and ptosis. These complications can cause amblyopia in young children, although the author did not find these complications severe enough to cause amblyopia. However, the author did not include preoperative and postoperative visions, and more than 25% of his patients were lost to follow-up. The author used the distance deviation in this study. However, in treating patients with a large esodeviation at near fixation than distance fixation (high AC/A ratio), botulinum injections may cause further undercorrections.— L.B. Nelson, M.D.

Management of Strabismus With Botulinum A Toxin
Biglan AW, Burnstine RA, Rogers GL. Saunders RA (Univ of Pittsburgh; Northeast Med School of Ohio, Akron; Ohio State Univ, Columbus; Med Univ of South Carolina, Charleston)
Ophthalmology 96:935–943, July 1989   8–13

Many researchers are optimistic that botulinum A toxin can be used routinely to treat infantile esotropia, comitant strabismus, acute cranial nerve palsies, dysthyroid myopathy, and vertical strabismus, but few have studied the long-term effects of this treamtent for strabismus. A 5-year experience of using botulinum A toxin to treat ocular deviations was reported.

Three hundred eight patients with strabismus underwent chemodenervation with botulinum A toxin. One hundred fifty-three patients were followed up for at least 6 months. Ninety-seven received botulinum A toxin injections as their primary treatment, and 56 received injections after traditional extraocular muscle surgery. Botulinum A toxin was found to be useful for treating patients with recent surgical overcorrections and some patients with sixth cranial nerve palsy. However, chemodenervation of an extraocular muscle was not as successful as traditional strabismus surgery for patients with infantile esotropia and other comitant deviations. Injection of botulinum A toxin was not effective in the treatment of restrictive strabismus.

Chemodenervation of extraocular muscles with injections of botulinum A toxin has limited use in treating strabismus. The best results occurred in patients with overcorrections after traditional surgery for repositioning muscles and in patients with acute mild sixth cranial nerve palsies. Other forms of strabismus improved with treatment, but too many patients needed reinjection or additional strabismus surgery.

▶ With more experience and longer follow-ups, many investigations have found the use of botulinum for the treatment of strabismus to be less than satisfactory. Many of the patients in the present study needed multiple reinjections and, ultimately, strabismus surgery. I agree with the authors that botulinum injections have limited use in patients with strabismus. The drug may be helpful in treating undercorrections for traditional strabismus surgery and for patients with acute sixth nerve palsy to prevent medial rectus contractions.— L.B. Nelson, M.D.

Long-Term Stability of Alignment in the Monofixation Syndrome
Arthur BW, Smith JT, Scott WE (Queen's Univ, Kingston, Ont; Univ of Iowa, Iowa City)
J Pediatr Ophthalmol Strabismus 26:224–231, September–October
1989   8–14

Of 328 patients with congenital esotropia, 80 were followed up for 4 years or longer after surgical alignment within 8 prism D of orthophoria. Thirty-eight of these patients had monofixation syndrome (MS), whereas 42 lacked monofixation. Three fourths of the MS patients maintained alignment within 8 prism D of orthophoria after 17.5 years. Only 45% of patients without monofixation maintained good alignment after 14 years. The latter patients lost stability significantly more rapidly.

Achievement of the MS promotes stable ocular alignment, but it does not ensure it. About one fourth of monofixators in this study deteriorated, compared with more than half of patients without monofixation. Monofixation syndrome is more likely to be achieved if ocular alignment is normalized at a young age. Subnormal binocular vision can, however, be achieved in older children.

▶ One of the important features of the monofixation syndrome is that the range of the horizontal fusional vergence amplitudes is similar to that for patients with bifixation. It is this characteristic that helps stabilize the alignment of patients with the monofixation syndrome over the years. The authors clearly have demonstrated that although the stability of alignment in the monofixation syndrome is not permanent, it is certainly better than if monofixation is absent.— L.B. Nelson, M.D.

Changes in the Aphakic Refraction of Children With Unilateral Congenital Cataracts

Moore BD (Children's Hosp, Boston)
J Pediatr Ophthalmol Strabismus 26:290–295, November–December 1989
8–15

The treatment of unilateral congenital cataract has been greatly improved by advances in surgical technique, contact lens correction, and amblyopia management. However, the availability and cost of contact lenses for infants and the difficulty of long-term successful amblyopia treatment are obstacles to good outcomes. Longitudinal changes in the spherical equivalent of the refractive error of patients with unilateral congenital cataracts in the first 4 years of life were reported.

Forty-two infants who had cataract surgery by 6 months of age received 369 serial refractions of the aphakic eye for the first 4 years of life. The 14 children followed up most intensively had a rapid reduction in mean spherical equivalent in the first years from +30.75 D to +26.36 D, with a less rapid reduction thereafter. The rate of monthly change dropped from 0.43 D between 1 and 6 months, 0.37 D between 6 and 12 months, 0.30 D between 12 and 18 months, 0.24 D between 18 and 24 months, to less than 0.19 D a month thereafter (Fig 8–3).

The refractive error of the aphakic eye of children treated for unilateral congenital cataracts decreases most rapidly in infancy and less rapidly through the next few years of childhood. These data can be used to estimate expected changes and to predict contact lens corrections at various early ages.

▶ Most ophthalmologists use contact lenses for the optical correction of unilateral pediatric aphakia. These lenses can be replaced easily or modified if adjust-

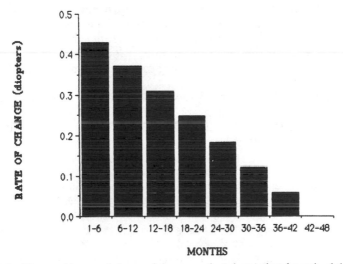

Fig 8–3.—The monthly rate of change of the mean spherical equivalent for each of the eight 6-month intervals. No. = 14. (Courtesy of Moore BD: *J Pediatr Ophthalmol Strabismus* 26:290–295, November–December 1989.)

ments in power or fitting become necessary. The author has demonstrated the rapid decrease in mean spherical equivalent of the aphakic eye of infants during the first year of life, with a less rapid decrease thereafter. Because of the rapidity of change in refraction found especially in the first year of life, the use of intraocular lenses or epikeratophakia are less practical alternatives to the correction of pediatric aphakia.—L.B. Nelson, M.D.

Long-Term Results of Bifocal Therapy for Accommodative Esotropia
Ludwig IH, Parks MM, Getson PR (Mary Imogene Bassett Hosp, Cooperstown, NY; Children's Hosp Natl Med Ctr; George Washington Univ, Washington, DC)
J Pediatr Ophthalmol Strabismus 26:264–270, November–
December 1989   8–16

The use of bifocals to correct the residual esodeviation or near in distance-corrected accommodative esotropes is well established, but the long-term course of these patients is not well documented. A group of accommodative esotropes who needed bifocals to maintain alignment at near was followed up for an average of 10.5 years.

Sixty-five patients were studied. Forty patients could stop using their bifocals after a mean of 5.5 years. After a mean 9.7 years, 38.5% continued to wear bifocals. Surgical correction of deteriorated accommodative esotropia was done in 50% of the patients who discontinued bifocal use and in 36% of those who did not. Surgery produced a mean decrease in the accommodative convergence relationship (AC/A) of about 10 prism D in both groups. Patients who underwent surgery and who were unable to discontinue bifocal wear began with a clinically higher AC/A than those who did discontinue bifocal wear. The nonsurgical patients who discontinued bifocal use had spontaneous improvement of the AC/A over time. On average, this did not happen in the patients who continued use. Surgical patients had significantly lower hyperopia than nonsurgical patients and had an earlier age of beginning bifocal wear. The average age of bifocal discontinuation among surgical and nonsurgical patients was 9.7 and 9.3 years, respectively.

Bifocals may be discontinued successfully by most patients at a mean age of 9.5 years, but a significant proportion need long-term bifocals, some despite surgery. A relatively high AC/A was the only factor that predicted long-term bifocal wear.

▶ Over the past several years, controversy over the best way to manage a high AC/A ratio has arisen. Many pediatric ophthalmologists attempt to correct the esodeviation at near with bifocals, provided the distant deviation is less than 10 prism D. This study showed the high success with bifocal use; however, Pratt-Johnson and Tillson found in a retrospective study that bifocals offered little advantage in the management of high AC/A ratio in which fusion is present in the distance (1). They suggested that a carefully planned, prospective, and randomized multicenter study involving large numbers of patients with high AC/A ratios should be organized with regard to bifocal therapy.—L.B. Nelson, M.D.

Reference

1. Pratt-Johnson JA, Tillson G: The management of esotropia with high AC/A ratio (convergence excess). *J Pediatr Ophthalmol Strabismus* 22:238, 1988.

Anterior Tendon Displacement of the Inferior Oblique for DVD

Kratz RE, Rogers GL, Bremer DL, Leguire LE (Ohio State Univ; Children's Hosp, Columbus)
J Pediatr Ophthalmol Strabismus 26:212–217, September–October 1989

8–17

Successful surgical treatment of dissociated vertical deviation (DVD) includes changing the sum of forces on the eye in favor of depression. Relative strengthening of depression would be primary in any new procedure. To test the efficacy of inferior oblique muscle tension anteriorization as a treatment in itself for DVD, 10 girls and 15 boys aged 11–14 months had treatment.

All children had congenital esotropia, and all but 3 had overactive inferior oblique muscles. The anteriorization of the posterior part of the inferior oblique muscle tendon fibers were graded relative to the insertion of the inferior rectus. The placement of fibers varied according to the degree of preoperative DVD. The results from the graded group were compared with those from a group with DVD who received the same amount of anteriorization, irrespective of the degree of preoperative DVD. Generally, anteriorization of the inferior oblique muscle tendon fibers to the level of insertion of the inferior rectus was effective. Grading the anteriorization of the posterior part of the inferior oblique muscle tendon fibers significantly reduced residual postoperative deviation.

Anterior displacement of the inferior oblique tendon is a successful treatment for DVD. Grading the procedure improves outcomes. The role of grading to tailor the procedure to the severity of DVD merits further study.

► The successful treatment of DVD remains an enigma. A variety of surgical techniques are available, all with enthusiastic proponents. In a well-controlled study, Mimms has shown that not only does anteriorization of the inferior oblique reduce the incidence of DVD, but it adequately corrects overaction of the inferior oblique muscle. The authors of this study show that grading the anteriorization of the posterior part of the inferior oblige muscle significantly reduces the residual postoperative vertical deviation. As the authors suggest, a prospective, randomized study with long-term follow up is needed to evaluate the effect of grading the placement of the posterior fibers of the inferior oblique muscle in the treatment of DVD.—L.B. Nelson, M.D.

9 Refractive Surgery

Intraocular Lenses and Pseudophakic Bullous Keratopathy

PETER R. LAIBSON, M.D.
Cornea Service, Wills Eye Hospital, Philadelphia, Pennsylvania

Corneal transplantation is performed most often today for pseudophakic bullous keratopathy (1). Numerous articles in the world's literature implicate certain styles of intraocular lenses as the primary cause of this corneal problem. Waring has called it an epidemic of pseudophakic corneal edema (2). Fortunately, most of the offending intraocular lenses (IOLs), such as the iris fixed and anterior chamber lenses (e.g., the Azar 91Z, the Leiske lens, the Stableflex, and the Hessburg lenses) have been withdrawn voluntarily either by the manufacturer or by the Food and Drug Administration (FDA).

It has been estimated that more than 1 million of these offending iris fixed and anterior chamber lenses were inserted. Significant corneal edema may develop in approximately 5% to 10% of these patients, and therefore, 100,000 patients may be at risk for corneal edema and need corneal transplantation for pseudophakic bullous keratopathy. The problem has been recognized and is being dealt with by ophthalmologists who will advise and treat those patients destined to have pseudophakic bullous keratopathy and those already afflicted with the problem.

For those with early pseudophakic bullous keratopathy who still have good vision, one is concerned with the rapidity of corneal deterioration and the possibility of acquiring cystoid macular edema also. The question for the treating ophthalmologists is, should he or she remove the offending IOL and replace it with another IOL, remove it and do not replace it, or do nothing and wait for significant edema to occur, then perform a penetrating keratoplasty. If the IOL is not removed, how likely is the patient to have cystoid macular edema that may not respond later when the IOL finally is removed? Once the decision to replace the IOL is made, the surgeon is faced with several more choices. Is the IOL replaced with a single-piece polymethylmethacrylate anterior chamber lens, which has the advantage of easier placement and shorter surgical time, or a posterior chamber lens? The posterior chamber lens usually is placed in the ciliary sulcus and sutured to the iris or placed behind the iris and sutured through the sclera just beyond the limbus. The long-term results of lens replacement do not favor either the anterior chamber lens site or the posterior chamber lens site. The trend today is toward placing the posterior chamber lens in the sulcus, but the long-term outcome is not yet clear. A collaborative study prospectively evaluating anterior chamber versus posterior chamber sutered lens replacement is now under way.

An important question must be faced. Why were so many offending anterior chamber lenses inserted before the problem of pseudophakic bullous keratopathy was recognized? How did these lenses get by the system of checks and balances, the manufacturers' scrutiny, and FDA diligence? Is the current system that is used to investigate and screen new developments vigorous enough to weed out bad technology and yet allow medical progress by promoting good technology? It is certain that ophthalmologists do not want to delay significant medical advances that will benefit humankind, but neither do they wish to prematurely apply technology in a widespread manner before it is tested thoroughly and proved efficacious with minimal and acceptable side effects.

References

1. Brady SE, et al: *Am J Ophthalmol* 108:118, 1989.
2. Waring GO III: *Arch Ophthalmol* 107:657, 1989.

Five-Year Results of Radial Keratotomy
Sawelson H, Marks RG (Univ of Florida, Gainesville)
Refract Corneal Surg 5:8–20, January–February 1989   9–1

Follow-up data at 5 years were obtained for 68% of 198 radial keratotomy operations done in 1980–1981. The average keratometry reading at 5 years was 40.7 D, compared with 41.2 D at 18 months. The keratometric results seemed to be less stable than the refractive outcome. Seventeen percent of eyes gained at least 1 D of refraction between 18 months and 5 years, compared with 13% at 18 to 36 months, and 13% at 12–24 months. Those eyes with the most evident refractive gain had a continued reduction in residual myopia. One patient had vascularization of incisions in both eyes at 5 years, and both eyes of another patient had stromal haze. Nine eyes had incisional cysts.

The refractive results of radial keratotomy are relatively stable at 5 years. Acuity shows some loss, but the ongoing change in keratometry measurements is of most concern. The center of the cornea becomes flatter and a knee develops, beyond which the cornea is steeper. The central area continues to flatten over time as the knee becomes more accentuated (Fig 9–1). The area of cornea between the center and the knee probably becomes more aspheric, and may neutralize the hyperopic shift expected from central corneal flattening. How long the cornea will continue to change its shape and what effect this will have on vision remain to be seen. At present it is not possible to prove these other theories as technology to accurately measure the changes in corneal topography that follow radial keratotomy still is evolving.

▶ The 5-year follow-up of only 68% of 198 patients undergoing radial keratotomy is low for this prospective study. Were those not seen at 5 years unsatisfied, and did they seek ophthalmic care elsewhere? For those patients who

Preop Corneal Shape

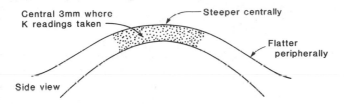

Immediate Postop RK Corneal Shape

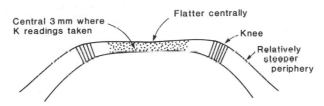

Postulated 5 Year Postop RK Corneal Shape

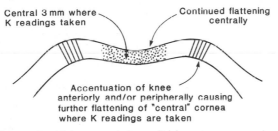

Fig 9–1.—Cross section of the cornea before radial keratotomy surgery, immediately after, and about 5 years later illustrate the new aspheric shape of the cornea, which makes the keratotomy readings difficult to interpret after radial keratotomy surgery. (Courtesy of Sawelson H, Marks RG: *Refract Corneal Surg* 5:8–20, January–February 1989.)

were followed up for 5 years, that there is an ongoing change in keratometry even 5 years later continues to be discouraging. The long-term keratometric results are less stable than the refractive results, which would indicate that corneal wound healing still is not completed. Corneal modeling machines and other new technology may help us discover why corneal wound healing has not stabilized completely 5 years after radial keratotomy.—P.R. Laibson, M.D.

Analysis of Astigmatic Keratotomy

Agapitos PJ, Lindstrom RL, Williams PA, Sanders DR (Univ of Minnesota, Minneapolis; Univ of Illinois, Chicago)
J Cataract Refract Surg 15:13–18, January 1989   9–2

The efficacy of 82 keratotomy procedures done for idiopathic, postsurgical, or myopic astigmatism was assessed by vector and linear regression analysis. About half the patients had had penetrating keratoplasty (table). Delta keratometry values were compured for each case as delta K in the desired axis of effect.

The greatest shifts occurred with trapezoidal procedures. Results were most predictable after relaxing incision–compression suture procedures. Correction of preoperative cylinder was greatest in the nonintersecting trapezoidal astigmatic keratotomy group. However trapezoidal keratotomy gave the largest shift only for post-penetrating keratoplasty patients. The smallest standard deviation of mean delta K values was in patients having relaxing incisions and compression sutures. A mean hyperopic shift was noted in all groups except those having intersecting trapezoidal astigmatic keratotomy or relaxing incisions.

Astigmatic keratotomy can produce significant changes in corneal astigmatism, but the accuracy of these techniques is highly variable.

▶ Six different operations for astigmatism were evaluated for 3 different causes of astigmatism in a total of 82 keratotomy procedures. Few studies on astigmatism have detailed this number of surgical procedures. Even so, the

	Number of Patients	Etiology of Astigmatism		
Procedure		Idiopathic	Post-cataract	Post PKP
Trapezoidal keratotomy (intersecting)	30	8	2	20
Trapezoidal keratotomy (nonintersecting)	7	---	1	6
Relaxing incisions with compression sutures	10	---	---	10
T cuts	10	3	2	5
T cuts with radial keratotomy	20	20	---	---
Radial keratotomy with elliptical optical zones	5	5	---	---

Etiology of Preoperative Astigmatism

(Courtesy of Agapitos PJ, Lindstrom RL, Williams PA, et al: *J Cataract Refract Surg* 15:13–18, January 1989.)

numbers are small, and as the authors state, this is an evolving process. Relaxing incisions with compensation sutures were performed on 10 postoperative corneal transplant patients with astigmatism and were the most predictable of all the operations. All groups had a high degree of variability and poor predictibility. To better predict the outcome for astigmatic keratotomy, the ophthalmologists who brought us the PERK study are trying to organize the PEAK: Prospective Evaluation of Astigmatic Keratotomy. It is hoped that such a study will provide more data and long-term follow-up of patients with surgically correctable astigmatism.—P.R. Laibson, M.D.

Contrast Sensitivity Testing: A More Complete Assessment of Vision
Jindra LF, Zemon V (Wills Eye Hosp, Philadelphia; Rockefeller Univ, New York)
J Cataract Refract Surg 15:141–148, March 1989   9–3

Snellen acuity measurements, although the standard measure in common clinical practice, provide limited information on the visual system and are influenced by psychological factors. Contrast sensitivity testing is an alternative approach to assessing visual function. The procedure (Fig 9–2) measures the least amount of contrast needed to detect a visual stimulus when grating patterns of varying size are presented, either in a stationary manner or dynamically by reversing the contrast at different rates.

In many instances losses of contrast sensitivity are detected where visual acuity is normal. Such findings have been obtained in amblyopia, retinal diseases, anterior segment diseases, neuro-ophthalmologic disorders, and glaucoma. The contrast sensitivity function (CSF) correlates more closely with subjective complaints than does visual acuity. Losses in

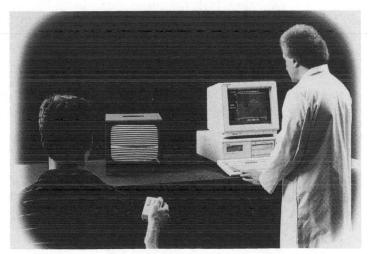

Fig 9–2.—A computerized contrast sensitivity testing apparatus that is used to determine the CSF. (Courtesy of Jindra LF, Zemon V: *J Cataract Refract Surg*15:141–148, March 1989.)

contrast sensitivity to low and intermediate spatial frequency patterns may indicate glaucoma or optic nerve injury. Losses in sensitivity to high spatial frequency patterns may indicate anterior segment disease or refractive error.

There is a different between vision and visual acuity. Testing of CSF allows the diagnosis of selective defects in visual processing at an earlier stage than conventional methods and when visual acuity is normal.

▶ The assessment of vision to most of us is the Snellen acuity measurement. Contrast sensitivity is an additional and perhaps better way to assess vision than the standard Snellen acuity charts. With government agencies and insurance companies demanding better evaluation of visual function before cataract surgery, contrast sensitivity should become an important and perhaps primary means of evaluating visual function. This article reviews visual assessment and contrast sensitivity well.— P.R. Laibson, M.D.

Recovery After Loss of an Eye

Linberg JV, Tillman WT, Allara RD (West Virginia Univ, Morgantown; Pittsburgh)

Ophthalmic Plast Reconstr Surg 4:135–138, 1988   9–4

How well does a patient recover after losing an eye? Recovery involves both adjustment to monocular vision and resolution of serious emotional trauma. Data for 125 monocular patients, including 49 adults who had suddenly lost a sighted eye, were reviewed.

Eighty-five persons reported that loss of an eye had not altered their lives in any permanent respect. Only 7 patients described persistent visual problems, whereas 12 had problems at work. Twenty-one persons had anxiety or a poor self-image. Half the adults with sudden loss of an eye reported that they had required less than a month to adjust to driving, work, home activities, or walking. A large majority believed that their adjustment was complete within 1 year.

These findings do not support the AMA Guide's estimate that loss of an eye constitutes a 25% disability of the "whole man." Employment problems are more prevalent than visual problems. Difficulties in self-image also may need attention.

It is important to ensure a supportive relationship among the patient, oculist, and ophthalmologist. Particularly important are recommendations that patients use protective eyewear.

▶ Ophthalmologists who perform enucleation would be well served to read this article. Completing the operation successfully and supervising the fitting of a cosmetic prosthesis certainly is not all there is to enucleation. The emotional adjustment necessary and the socioeconomic problems encountered are as important as the operation itself.— P.R. Laibson, M.D.

Corneal Preservation

Wilson SE, Bourne WM (Mayo Clinic Found, Rochester, Minn)
Surv Ophthalmol 33:237–259, January–February 1989   9–5

The supply of donor corneas for use in transplantation still is inadequate. It is up to an operating surgeon to make sure that proper guidelines are followed so that all recipients are given tissue of the highest quality, and that potential donors are free of disorders that could be transmitted (table). Among the chief exclusions related to transmissibility

---

Eye Bank Association of America Donor Selection Criteria

1. Age. Lower limit, full-term birth. Upper limit left to the discretion of the eye bank medical director.
2. Interval between death and enucleation. Left to the discretion of the eye bank medical director. Generally recommended, however, that death to enucleation time not exceed 6 hours.
3. Absolute exclusions
   a. Death of unknown cause
   b. Death from central nervous system diseases of unknown etiology
   c. Jakob-Creutzfeldt disease
   d. Subacute sclerosing panencephalitis
   e. Congenital rubella
   f. Progressive multifocal leukoencephalopathy
   g. Reyes syndrome
   h. Subacute encephalitis, cytomegalovirus brain infection
   i. Septicemia
   j. Hepatitis
   k. Rabies
   l. Intrinsic eye disease — retinoblastoma, conjunctivitis, iritis, glaucoma, corneal disease, and malignant tumors of the anterior segment
   m. Blast-form leukemia
   n. Hodgkin's disease
   o. Lymphosarcoma
   p. Acquired immunodeficiency syndrome (AIDS)
   q. High risk for AIDS groups including known or suspected intravenous drug abusers, known or suspected male homosexuals or bisexuals, prostitutes, hemophiliacs, infants of mothers with AIDS, and sexual contacts of high risk groups.
4. Negative donor serologies for Hepatitis B surface antigen and Human Immune Virus.

(Courtesy of Wilson SE, Bourne WM: *Surv Ophthalmol* 33:237–259, January–February 1989.)

of disease are bacterial, fungal, and viral infections and malignancy. Donors aged less than 3 years are not accepted because of the difficulty of handling tissue and the rapid changes in corneal power that occur in infancy. In addition, fitting a contact lens may be difficult when steep donor tissue is grafted to a relatively flat recipient cornea.

Current upper age limits for corneal donation are arbitrary. It may be that cell density and morphological characteristics of the individual cornea are the important factors. If so, specular microscopy could serve to screen potential donors without regard to age.

▶ This excellent, detailed review of corneal preservation should be read by surgeons who perform corneal transplants. Among other things, it details the history of preservation methods of assessing corneal endothelial viability, donor selection, and methods of preserving donor tissue. I would argue with few statements; however, the authors elect not to transplant tissue from donors aged less than 3 years. Most corneal surgeons would use tissue from donors as young as 2 years or even younger. The upper age of corneal tissue used is still open to question, although these days all surgeons prefer younger tissue. Tissue even from donors in their 70s or 80s can be used on similar-aged patients if the endothelium looks healthy on specular microscopy and the cell count is adequate. I agree with the authors that further investigation is needed to determine how old tissue may be before it is used for corneal transplantation.—P.R. Laibson, M.D.

What We Have Learned About Corneal Wound Healing From Refractive Surgery
Binder PS (Univ of California, San Diego)
Refract Corneal Surg 5:98–120, March–April 1989   9–6

When Bowman's layer is cut during refractive surgery, the curvature of the cornea changes permanently. Optical interfaces tend to degrade the visual image because the potential space created can serve as a site for foreign material, keratocytes (Fig 9–3), and epithelium. Freezing and lyophilization produce severe morphological changes, and operations that utilize fresh tissue are safer. All thermal collagen-shrinking procedures produce severe, permanent stromal damage. Corneal wound healing must be controlled if photorefractive keratectomy is to succeed.

Laser sculpting eventually may replace lamellar refractive procedures. The results of radial keratotomy may improve with pharmacologic control of wound healing and with better incisional techniques. Intrastromal implants may be clinically applicable if the microkeratome can be eliminated and a biocompatible polymer found. The key to refractive corneal surgery will be a better understanding of the molecular interactions that control and inhibit wound healing. Computer modeling of the refractive system also will be helpful, as will new instrumentation such as the tandem scanning confocal microscope.

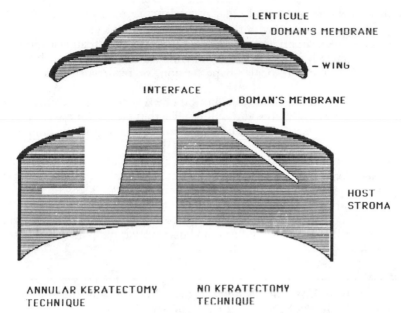

LENTICULE
BOMAN'S MEMBRANE
WING
INTERFACE
BOMAN'S MEMBRANE
HOST
STROMA

ANNULAR KERATECTOMY
TECHNIQUE

NO KERATECTOMY
TECHNIQUE

Fig 9–3.—Computer diagram of epikeratoplasty wound performed with *(left)* and without *(right)* a keratectomy to show potential routes for keratocyte repopulation. Less stromal surface is available for the cells to enter the donor lenticule in the nonkeratectomy technique. (Courtesy of Binder PS: *Refract Corneal Surg* 5:98–120, March–April 1989.)

▶ This third Barraquer lecture sponsored by the International Society for Refractive Keratoplasty is a lengthy but readable recital of Dr. Binder's extensive experience in refractive surgery. It is also a review of the histopathology of most refractive surgical procedures, including excimer laser photoablation and intrastromal lenses. The principles of corneal wound healing as applied to refractive surgery are well covered, and the author uses his crystal ball to try to predict which refractive surgery procedures would be most beneficial for patients in the future. This 23-page review with 173 references should be read by anyone interested in refractive surgery.—P.R. Laibson, M.D.

Effect of Factors Unrelated to Tissue Matching on Corneal Transplant Endothelial Rejection
Boisjoly HM, Bernard P-M, Dubé I, Laughrea P-A, Bazin R, Bernier J (Laval Univ, Québec)
Am J Ophthalmol 107:647–654, June 1989   9–7

Data on 348 consecutive adult corneal transplant recipients were reviewed for clinical evidence of endothelial rejection. The 5 important risk factors identified were a primary diagnosis of herpetic, interstitial, or traumatic keratitis; a graft measuring 8 mm or more; more than 1 previous transplant; age less than 60 years; and corneal vascularization in the recipient.

Other workers have found older transplant recipients to have a higher rejection rate, a contrast with the present finding. One explanation is that some may look primarily at transplant failures rather than rejection episodes. Apart from rejection, transplant failure may be caused by poor-quality donor material, ocular hypertension, or recurrent ocular inflammation.

To properly interpret the contribution of HLA tissue matching for the prevention of rejection episodes will require that concurrent and possibly confounding risk factors not related to tissue watching be accounted for.

▶ It is still not apparent how important HLA tissue matching is in preventing graft failure for high-risk keratoplasty. At least 5 factors were found to be important risks for immunologic rejection in this study. Even some of these factors are controversial. This study and the still uncompleted National Eye Institute–funded study of HLA-matched grafts make clear that multiple factors in addition to HLA matching are critical in determining the potential for immunologic rejection.— P.R. Laibson, M.D.

Implantation of Posterior Chamber Intraocular Lenses in the Absence of Lens Capsule During Penetrating Keratoplasty
Soong HK, Musch DC, Kowal V, Sugar A, Meyer RF (Univ of Michigan)
Arch Ophthalmol 107:660–665, May 1989   9–8

Corneal endothelial cell counts were reviewed for 133 consecutive placements of iris-sutured posterior chamber (PC) intraocular lenses (IOLs) during penetrating keratoplasty, without lens capsular support. The placement of polypropylene sutures is illustrated in Figure 9–4. Patients were followed for 3 to 24 months; 82 were observed for 1 year or longer.

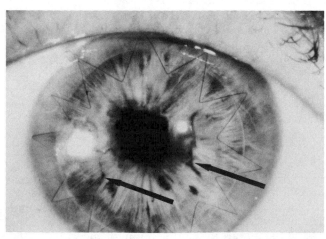

Fig 9–4.—Slit-lamp appearance after polypropylene sutures are tied, showing 2 fixation sutures at iris midperiphery *(arrows)*. (Courtesy of Soong HK, Musch DC, Kowal V, et al: *Arch Ophthalmol* 107:660–665, May 1989.)

At 1 year, 45.1% of patients had 20/40 or better acuity whereas 24.4% had acuity of 20/200 or worse. At 2 years, 63.6% of patients had acuity of 20/40 or better and 18.2% had vision of 20/200 or worse. All but 3% of grafts were clear at last assessment. Cystoid macular edema (36.4%) and age-related macular degeneration (11.0%) were the most frequent causes of poor acuity. Endothelial cell loss in the grafts averaged 19% at 1 year.

Recent experience with Kelman-style 1-piece polymethylmethacrylate anterior chamber (AC) lenses with open-loop haptics and less anterior vaulting is favorable compared with the PC IOL iris-sutured group. Endothelial cell counts have been at least as good as with sutured PC lenses.

Although the overall results with iris-sutured PC IOLs are encouraging, it would be advisable to regard acapsular PC IOL implantation cautiously until 5- to 10-year results are known.

▶ How to manage the IOLs in pseudophakic bullous keratopathy remains controversial. Certainly, replacing bad AC and iris-fixated lenses is critical. Whether it is best to use an open-loop AC lens, an iris-sutured PC lens, or a PC lens sutured through the sclera is not clear. Perhaps all of these choices are viable for different indications. With all of these techniques, an anterior vitrectomy is necessary in most cases.

The PC IOL lens fixated to the iris by suturing from behind has had broad experience, but it is still not clear that this is the best way. A collaborative prospective study of these different techniques is now under way at several institutions in the United States.—P.R. Laibson, M.D.

The 50-Year Epidemic of Pseudophakic Corneal Edema
Waring GO III (Atlanta)
Arch Ophthalmol 107:657–659, May 1989   9–9

The advent of effective intraocular lenses for use in aphakic patients has been marred by an epidemic of pseudophakic corneal edema. From 5% to 10% of patients given certain types of intraocular lenses have had this problem. Multiple generations of cases of pseudophakic corneal edema have resulted from peaks of popularity of different lens styles (Fig 9–5). The mean "incubation time" from surgery to corneal edema is about 2 years.

Intense competition to develop a successful intraocular lens created an atmosphere in which premature claims of success overwhelmed both federal regulation and professional self-restraint. Pseudophakic corneal edema now is the leading indication for penetrating keratoplasty in this country.

It is fortunate that the epidemic now is subsiding; the incidence of pseudophakic corneal edema with current posterior chamber intraocular lenses is about 0.1%. Research, self-restraint, and close regulation are the keys to avoiding adverse efffects.

Current FDA rulings have gradually eliminated adjunct studies and

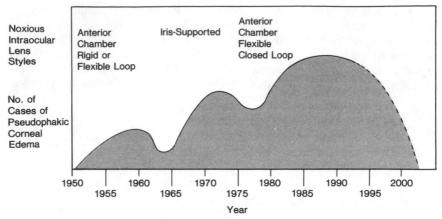

Fig 9–5.—Epidemic curve for pseudophakic corneal edema. The total cumulative number of cases is unknown. The curve shows only the relative number of cases that have occurred from 1950 to 1989. The *broken line* represents the hoped-for decline in the number of cases. The relative number varies regionally, depending on exposure. (Courtesy of Waring GO III: *Arch Ophthalmol* 107:657–659, May 1989.)

have limited the numbers of new styles of intraocular lenses made available. Some 625 lens styles are approved by the FDA for routine clinical use.

▶ This editorial describing an epidemic of pseudophakic bullous keratopathy reflects the opinion of most corneal surgeons that corneal transplantation for pseudophakic bullous keratopathy is the leading reason to do a corneal transplant in the United States today.

Why the situation developed is addressed by Waring in this editorial. It is interesting that in Switzerland only 3% of corneal transplants were done for pseudophakic bullous keratopathy, according to a recent study. Where science and technology as well as business have a hand in development of ophthalmic surgery, this kind of problem undoubtedly will occur.—P.R. Laibson, M.D.

Preliminary Computer Simulation of the Effects of Radial Keratotomy
Hanna KD, Jouve FE, Waring GO III (Emory Univ, Atlanta; Hôtel-Dieu Hosp, Paris)
Arch Ophthalmol 107:911–918, June 1989   9–10

A computerized mathematical model of the eye for simulating refractive surgery. The model is based on calculating stresses in the cornea and sclera, including the stress along a meridian that is perpendicular to the surface and that is tangent to the surface. Factors taken into account include the number of incisions, intraocular pressure, incision depth and length, baseline central corneal curvature, the effect of corneal power change on refraction, and the effect of Young's modulus.

Major changes in stress distribution occur at the paracentral and peripheral ends of the keratotomy incisions. The model predicted flattening of the central cornea with posterior displacement that increases with increased intraocular pressure. A change in incisional length of 0.5 mm significantly altered the correction. For clear zones of 3 to 4 mm, incisions of equal length produced comparable changes in refraction. Corneal radius of curvature had a negligible effect on the amount of refractive change.

Radial keratotomy alters stress distribution in the cornea and the anterior sclera back to about the 20-mm diameter zone but does not affect the equatorial or posterior sclera. A model that truly simulates the corneal response to refractive surgery will have to take into account the anisotropic nature of the cornea, viscoelastic tissue responses, and all the forces applied to the globe.

▶ To understand all the forces acting on and within the cornea is truly formidable. Add to that the effects of corneal refractive surgery and the task seems impossible.

If a computerized simulation of such effects were feasible, it would be of inestimable value to the corneal surgeon. Such pie-in-the-sky technology is attempted in this paper. Although it may take a Ph.D. to figure out these graphs, the minimal mathematical computations and the clinical applications make this paper one of the first that ophthalmologists can read and then perhaps begin to understand the technical difficulty and potential benefits that may be attainable by such computer models. This may be the wave of the future for understanding how the cornea functions.—P.R. Laibson, M.D.

Corneal Hydration Control in Fuchs' Dystrophy
Mandell RB, Polse KA, Brand RJ, Vastine D, Demartini D, Flom R (Univ of California, Berkeley)
Invest Ophthalmol Vis Sci 30:845–852, May 1989   9–11

Fuchs' dystrophy involves progressive endothelial guttata, stromal edema, epithelial edema, and corneal decompensation. A means of directly quantifying the functional state of the corneal endothelium would help in monitoring the progression of this and other corneal disorders. Corneal hydration control presumably depends to a substantial degree on endothelial function, and its assessment might provide guidelines for deciding whether to perform cataract extraction alone or corneal grafting or whether to remove an intraocular lens with a low endothelial cell count.

Corneal thickness was monitored after exposure to hypoxia or after overnight sleep. A modified optical pachometer was used, and the data were analyzed by a coupled exponential model. Twenty-two patients with Fuchs' dystrophy and 8 controls of similar age were tested; the mean recovery per hour was 25% and 34%, respectively, and the mean times to 95% of corneal thickness recovery were 10.2 and 7.1 hours, respectively. The mean open-eye steady-state thickness was 562 μm in

Fuchs' dystrophy and 537 μm in health persons. A recovery per hour of 17% is the minimum below which the cornea does not regain its open-eye steady state during the day and approaches decompensation.

This test may be a useful way of evaluating the state of the corneal endothelium in patients with Fuchs' dystrophy. Morning blur, though an indicator of abnormal corneal swelling, is too variable and subjective to be a reliable indicator of corneal status.

▶ A clinical test to evaluate the in vivo functioning of the human corneal endothelium would be invaluable in making decisions about corneal surgery. Direct assessment of endothelial function is impossible in the clinical setting, and only measuring corneal thickness gives us an idea of how well the endothelium functions. The 3 parameters of recovery from corneal swelling described here are not easy to do in the office because of the time consumed and the small variation from the normal, but they are a beginning step.—P.R. Laibson, M.D.

Toxic Ulcerative Keratopathy: An Unrecognized Problem
Schwab IR, Abbott RL (West Virginia Univ, Morgantown; Pacific Presbyterian Med Ctr, San Francisco)
Ophthalmology 96:1187–1193, August 1989   9–12

Nineteen patients with toxic ulcerative keratopathy were referred with other diagnoses, and were victims of overtreatment. Five of the patients had self-induced disease, which in 4 cases was factitious. The other 14 patients had iatrogenic toxic keratopathy.

Oval to round epithelial defects were present in the inferonasal quadrant, with coarse keratitis surrounding the defect (Fig 9–6). Intense ciliary flush and chemosis were noted. The epithelial defects had rolled margins. Both rose bengal and fluorescein stained the cornea. Upper tarsal smears showed activated epithelial cells, often containing toxic granules. Many of the patients with iatrogenic keratopathy had significant ocular surface disease such as keratoconjunctivitis sicca or a history of intraoc-

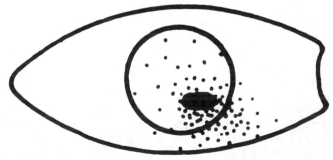

Fig 9–6.—Drawing of comet impact crater. Defects were usually horizontally oval with rolled edges. The keratitis, conjunctivitis, and chemosis were most intense just adjacent to the defect and were more intense in the inferior nasal quadrant than in the superior temporal quadrant. (Courtesy of Schwab IR, Abbott RL: *Ophthalmology* 96:1187–1193, August 1989.)

ular surgery. Apart from discontinuing the offending medication or preservative, treatment included patching, viscoelastic agents, and the use of contact lenses or goggles.

Keratopathy is seen with antiviral agents, antiglaucoma preparations, and antibiotics. The preservative frequently is the toxic part of an ophthalmic preparation. Benzalkonium appears to be a frequent offender. Close support and reassurance may be necessary for patients to stop using the medication in question. A preservative-free preparation often can be substituted to eliminate toxic effects. If the eye cannot be patched, a therapeutic contact lens or collagen shield may be effective. Tarsorrhaphy may sometimes be necessary.

▶ Self-induced external ocular disease is frequently difficult to diagnose and even harder to treat. A similar picture is seen in toxic ulcerative keratopathy or disease induced by sensitivity to medication or the preservative in medications. The authors described 19 patients with ulcerative keratopathy, and certain patterns of disease can be recognized. All ophthalmologists should consider toxic ulcerative keratopathy when continued superficial punctate keratitis and corneal ulceration does not get better despite vigorous therapy after presumed accurate diagnosis and application of appropriate medication. With long-term corneal surface disease, such as herpes simplex virus infection, the use of appropriate medications over long periods also may cause toxic ulcerative keratopathy. The point at which an antiviral, anti-inflammatory, or antibacterial no longer is effective but may cause toxic reaction is sometimes hard to discern, but must be considered by treating physicians.—P.R. Laibson, M.D.

Corneal Topography of Early Keratoconus
Maguire LJ, Bourne WM (Mayo Clinic, Rochester, Minn)
Am J Ophthalmol 108:107–112, August 1989   9–13

Seven patients in whom keratoconus was suspected were examined with a very sensitive computer-based corneal topography analysis system. These patients had normal keratometry readings and excellent spectacle-corrected visual acuity. They lacked slit lamp evidence of keratoconus. Cones were identified in 7 of the 9 eyes examined (Fig 9–7). Some of the patients had large amounts of corneal distortion despite the absence of substantial distortion of the keratometer mires. The cone apex was 1.3–2.5 mm from the visual axis in all cases. All cones were inferior to the visual axis. The degree of irregularity varied widely.

Very early stages of keratoconus may be detected with the Corneal Modeling System. One application is the testing of pilots at risk for visually disabling keratoconus before they begin their training. Normal slit lamp findings and normal keratometric and refractive data do not exclude early keratoconus. Screening by computer-based topographic analysis may help surgeons avoid performing refractive corneal surgery where there are unsuspected abnormalities of corneal curvature.

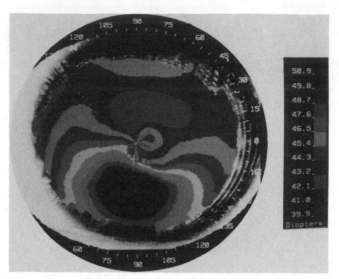

Fig 9–7.—Contour map of left eye. Cornea is more irregular. Each gradation represents a 1.1-D range of power. The overall range extends from 39.9 to more than 50.5 D. Location of the cone apex is readily apparent. Visual acuity was 20/20 with a spectacle correction of −2.50. (Courtesy of Maguire LJ, Bourne WM: *Am J Ophthalmol* 108:107–112, August 1989.)

▶ Incipient keratoconus is frequently hard to detect. The differentiation between a high irregular astigmatism and early keratoconus is difficult to make. Using a corneal topography analysis system, the authors were able to diagnose keratoconus in 9 eyes of 7 patients before slit lamp changes were seen. Corneal topographic analysis with expensive equipment such as the Corneal Modeling System are being used more and more frequently by corneal centers. It is still not worthwhile for a general ophthalmologist to purchase a $30,000 machine to diagnose early keratoconus, but as the price of these machines comes down and as more applications are found for their use, they may become helpful for the general ophthalmologist.—P.R. Laibson, M.D.

Anatomic Study of Transsclerally Sutured Intraocular Lens Implantation

Duffey RJ, Holland EJ, Agapitos PJ, Lindstrom RL (Univ of Minnesota, Minneapolis)

Am J Ophthalmol 108:300–309, September 1989   9–14

The procedure of ciliary sulcus-fixated intraocular lens implantation was investigated in 21 cadaver eyes. A transscleral suturing technique was used.

The sutures optimally exit the sclera less than 1 mm posterior to the corneoscleral limbus to achieve true ciliary sulcus fixation. The major arterial circle of the iris—located in the ciliary body—was avoided, as was the entire ciliary body. Excellent optic centration and haptic stabilization were achieved using a 1-piece, all-polymethylmethacrylate, 10-degree-vaulted, 13.5-mm haptic spread intraocular lens. The haptic suture is placed at the site of greatest haptic spread, making 1 transscleral suture pass per haptic.

Ciliary body erosion has been observed in eyes with ciliary sulcus-fixated posterior chamber lenses, but no resultant clinical problems are noted. Suturing at the point of greatest haptic spread allows more consistent total ciliary sulcus fixation of the haptic. This procedure is useful where capsular support is inadequate.

▶ Whether a secondary implant should be placed in the anterior chamber, sutured to the iris while resting behyind the iris, or transsclerally sutured via ciliary sulcus fixated sutures still is a subject of considerable discussion. These questions arise with patients who have pseudophakic bullous keratopathy and need intraocular lens exchange and vitrectomy, with patients who are aphakic and need a secondary implant, and occasionally with patients who have intraocular lenses in the anterior chamber and need these lenses to be exchanged. The authors have shown very nicely that, for the best transscleral fixation, sutures should exit the sclera approximately 1 mm from the posterior surgical limbus. Whether this placement of the intraocular lens in the posterior chamber is any better than anterior chamber lenses of good design has yet to be determined. Long-term follow-up studies of corneal clarity and visual acuity are still necessary to make this determination.—P.R. Laibson, M.D.

Contamination of K-Sol Corneal Storage Medium With *Propionibacterium acnes*
Sieck EA, Enzenauer RW, Cornell FM, Butler C (Fitzsimons Army Med Ctr, Aurora, Colo)
Arch Ophthalmol 107:1023–1024, July 1989   9–15

This is the first report of widespread contamination of K-Sol, a widely used corneal preservation medium, by *Propionibacterium acnes*. This organism can elude antibiotics and survive the storage process. *Propionibacterium acnes* was isolated from 5 K-Sol-stored donor rims in a 1-month period. Cultures of unopened bottles of K-Sol also yielded *P. acnes*.

Anaerobic bacteria resistant to gentamicin, such as *P. acnes*, can survive rigorous precautions, raising the question of whether gentamicin alone is adequate for subconjunctival postoperative use. The addition of another agent active against both aerobic and anaerobic organisms deserves consideration. All donor specimens should be cultured aerobically and anaerobically, and postoperative patients should be watched closely for delayed inflammation.

▶ The contamination of K-Sol with *P. acnes* in September 1988 was followed rapidly by the withdrawal of K-Sol from the marketplace. Fortunately, no cases of endophthalmitis occurred, and the laboratory at Fitzsimmons Army Medical Center kept the anaerobic cultures for a full 2 weeks. The slow-growing anaer-

/ Ophthalmology

obic, gram-positive rod was evident only after a considerable period. A lesson for the future may be that rim cultures should be taken routinely and kept in both aerobic and anaerobic media. The anaerobic media should be watched for 2 weeks. Dexsol now has replaced K-Sol, but this too contains only gentamicin, and the possibility of contamination persists.— P.R. Laibson, M.D.

Management Options for *Propionibacterium acnes* Endophthalmitis
Zambrano W, Flynn HW Jr, Pflugfelder SC, Roussel TJ, Culbertson WW, Holland S, Miller D (Univ of Miami)
Ophthalmology 96:1100–1105, July 1989   9–16

Nine patients with culture-proved *Propionibacterium acnes* endophthalmitis were seen an average of 4 months after extracapsular cataract extraction and posterior chamber lens implantation. Vitritis and a white plaque within the capsular bag were noted; the plaque sometimes enlarged. Four patients had granulomatous anterior uveitis, whereas 5 had nongranulomatous iridocyclitis. In 7 cases the onset of inflammation was delayed for longer than 2 weeks after surgery. Four patients were first seen with hypopyon, and 3 had beaded fibrin strands extending across the anterior chamber. Two patients had diffuse intraretinal hemorrhages consistent with hemorrhagic central vein occlusion.

Treatment included topical and intravenous antibiotics alone; intraocular and topical antibiotic therapy; pars plana vitrectomy with capsulectomy and intraocular antibiotic administration; and removal of capsular remnants with removal or exchange of the posterior chamber intraocular lens. Final acuity ranged from 20/20 to 20/60 in 6 eyes and from 20/200 to 20/400 in the other 3 eyes.

Propionibacterium acnes causes a wide range of ocular and periocular infections. If the presentation is relatively mild, intraocular culturing and intravitreal vancomycin are indicated. If conservative management fails, pars plana vitrectomy is recommended, with removal of the white intracapsular plaque and intraocular antibiotic injection. More aggressive initial treatment may be warranted if intense granulomatous iritis and vitritis are present. Endophthalitis caused by *P. acnes* should be confirmed using more than 1 anaerobic medium. Both the aqueous and the vitreous should be cultured.

▶ That 9 culture-proven cases of *P. acnes* were found retrospectively between 1984 and 1988 at 1 eye institute indicates that this type of mild delayed endophthalmitis is underdiagnosed. The authors have evolved an approach to management for the mild presentation and a more aggressive initial approach for advanced cases. Failure to consider *P. acnes* or other anaerobes as a cause of postoperative inflammation will delay the appropriate antibiotic or surgical treatment of this case and may cause permanent loss of vision.— P.R. Laibson, M.D.

The Changing Management and Improved Prognosis for Corneal Grafting in Herpes Simplex Keratitis

Ficker LA, Kirkness CM, Rice NSC, Steele ADM (Moorfields Eye Hosp, London)
Ophthalmology 96.1587–1590, November 1909   9 17

Improved microsurgery, topical antiviral therapy, and an understanding of the pathophysiology of corneal graft rejection and herpes simplex keratitis (HSK) recurrence have greatly affected the surgical management of HSK. Grafting inflamed eyes can be compromised by irreversible rejection or failure from recurrent HSK. Graft survival in a previously reported cohort recruited from 1967 to 1978 was reviewed and compared with that of a cohort recruited from 1979 to 1987.

The earlier cohort consisted of 91 patients, and the later one consisted of 54. The salient changes over time included transition from intracapsular to extracapsular cataract surgery and antiviral prophylaxis treatment of rejection episodes. Extracapsular cataract surgery was associated with a better graft survival, benefiting inflamed eyes that more often required concomitant surgery. Long-term survival of first grafts was 70%; the rate appeared to stabilize by 10 years. Antiviral prophylaxis improved rejection episodes and reduced the incidence of recurrent keratitis. The complete, prompt removal of loose sutures also improved graft survival (Fig 9–8). Postkeratoplasty glaucoma developed in 16 cases. Half were caused by the inflammatory sequelae of HSK, 5 had been treated with intracapsular cataract extraction, and synechiae developed in 3. Of these patients, 4 aphakic patients had vision losses.

Changes in the management of HSK have apparently resulted in im-

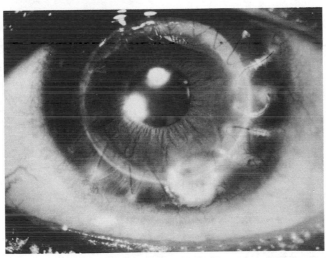

Fig 9–8.—Loose continuous graft suture with associated mucus and corneal infiltrates. (Courtesy of Ficker LA, Kirkness CM, Rice NSC, et al: *Ophthalmology* 96:1587–1596, November 1989.)

proved graft survival, especially in inflamed eyes. Interruped sutures and an extracapsular method for cataract extraction were recommended. Prompt attention should be given to loose sutures and other complications that threaten graft survival. Antiviral prophylaxis should be given for rejection during intensive steroid treatment. Acyclovir may be the drug of choice in the postoperative period.

▶ This very large series of patients with HSK who underwent keratoplasty at Moorfields Eye Hospital highlights the improved prognosis for grafting herpetic infections and the reasons for this success. Surgeons still have a better chance for graft survival if they operate on quiet eyes that do not have active herpetic keratitis. Emphasis is made that immediate access to emergency care must be provided so reactivation of herpetic keratitis in the graft can be managed quickly and such complications as loose sutures treated. Using topical steroids for control of inflammation, as well as antiviral prophylaxis during this steroid use, was important.—P.R. Laibson, M.D.

A Randomized Trial of Conjunctival Autografting for Pterygium in the Tropics

Lewallen S (Univ of California, San Francisco)
Ophthalmology 96:1612–1614, November 1989   9–18

The simplest method for removing pterygia—leaving the sclera bare and treating with lubricants or steroid drops—is associated with recurrence rates of 5% to 60%. A randomized prospective clinical trial comparing the conjunctival autografting technique with the bare sclera technique was done in the Caribbean, where the risk of pterygium recurrence is reportedly high.

Thirty-nine patients were enrolled in the study. Follow-up data on 34 were obtained. The patients were 21 women and 13 men with 35 pterygia. Sixteen were treated with the bare sclera technique, and 19 were grafted. The mean follow-up was 15 months. No surgical complications occurred. At follow-up, patients were classified as having no regrowth of pterygium or other symptoms; small, flat, avascular pterygium and other symptoms; or regrowth of pterygium to preoperative size or larger and other symptoms. In all cases of pterygium regrowth, patients reported the

Recurrence in Young (<37 Years) Patients by Procedure

	Conjunctival Autograft	Bare Sclera
	No. (%)	No. (%)
Recurrence*	3 (25)	8 (35)
No recurrence	9 (75)	11 (65)

*P > .1.
(Courtesy of Lewallen S: *Ophthalmology* 96:1612–1614, November 1989.)

occurrence within 6 to 8 weeks of surgery. Twenty-one percent of the grafted pterygia recurred, and 37% of those treated with bare sclera recurred in the first 2 groups, a difference that did not reach statistical significance (table).

The recurrence rate of grafted pterygia in this series was higher than that in other series, which may have been caused by differences in climate, patients' race, or patients' age. Patients younger than 37 years had a higher incidence of pterygium recurrence than those aged more than 37, and this was statistically significant. The conjunctival autograft group had 25% recurrence, but the bare sclera group had a 35% recurrence.

▶ Even though this study is small, the trend is clear that conjunctival transplants for pterygium have a high rate of pterygium recurrence in patients aged less than 37 years (25%). Nowhere else can these statistics be found, as the recurrence rate for pterygium removal with conjunctival transplant surgery is usually 10% or less. There was a trend toward statistical significance with a better prognosis for conjunctival transplants, but this study would have to have 4 times the number of patients to prove this trend. One good point from the study was that the prognosis for recurrent pterygium was better if the patient was aged more than 37.—P.R. Laibson, M.D.

Radial Keratotomy in Teenagers
I. A Practical Approach
O'Dell LW, Wyzinski P (Northwest Eye Ctr, Eugene, Ore)
II. A Dubious Idea
Smith RS (Albany Med Ctr, Albany, NY)
Refractive Corneal Surg 5:315–320, September–October 1989   9–19

More and more myopic teenagers are considering radial keratotomy. The pros and cons of doing this procedure in adolescents were discussed.

Twenty-seven teenagers had radial keratotomy in an 8-year period. Forty-one percent were male, 89% were white, and 60% wore contact lenses. Their ages ranged from 14 to 19 years. The average patient wore contact lenses for 4.25 D of myopia. Twelve other teenagers had radial keratotomy but were not included in the analysis because they had been followed up for less than 3 months. Myopia was reduced by a mean of 3.69 D, and cylindrical refractive error, by 0.08 D. Uncorrected binocular visual acuity was at least 20/60 in all patients. In 85%, it was 20/25 or better. There were no infections, ruptured globes, or lawsuits. Radial keratotomy was recommended for selected teenagers.

The major objections to using this approach in teenagers are its lack of predictability in individuals and that alternative methods for correcting ametropia are inherently safer. Many surgeons who perform radial keratotomy would disagree that this operation is appropriate for teenagers because of issues of informed consent, medical-legal questions, the rationalization of the need for surgery at an early age, problems related to eye maturity and wound healing, and changes in the stability of corneal and lenticular refraction and increases in axial length that occur in adolescence. These objections make radial keratotomy inadvisable in teenagers.

Two points of view on radial keratotomy in teenagers were presented. In one, it was argued that the procedure is appropriate for selected teenagers. In the other, significant objectives to this practice were raised.

▶ The arguments for and against radial keratotomy in teenagers are presented in this *opinion* article. As Dr. Richard Smith states, radial keratotomy in the teenager is "inadvisable." I would say it is a bad idea. There are too many unknowns when it comes to performing this surgery in the teenager, particularly that myopia still is progressing through these years. That contact lenses may cause their own problems, i.e., GPC, intolerance to lens wear, and even corneal infection, is no reason to perform an operation that will have lifelong effects for a condition that is still developing (myopia). This interesting, controversial article should be read in its entirety.—P.R. Laibson, M.D.

Corneal Changes Associated With Chronic UV Irradiation
Taylor HR, West SK, Rosenthal FS, Munoz B, Newland HS, Emmett EA
(Wilmer Inst, Johns Hopkins Univ, Baltimore)
Arch Ophthalmol 107:1481–1484, October 1989   9–20

Exposure to sunlight, specifically ultraviolet radiation (UVR), might be associated with a higher risk of several corneal disorderes. Pterygium occurs more often in tropical and sunny regions. The association between UVR exposure and corneal disease was explored in an epidemiologic study of an occupational group of men exposed to a range of UVR.

Eight hundred thirty-eight watermen working on the Chesapeake Bay were studied. A detailed occupational history was combined with laboratory and field measurements to calculate individual ocular exposure. Pterygium was found in 140 men; climatic droplet keratopathy, in 162; and pinguecula, in 642. According to logistic regression analysis, pterygium and climatic droplet keratopathy were associated significantly with a broad band of UVR exposure. The association with pinguecula was weaker.

Pterygium and climatic droplet keratopathy are induced by a wide band of UVR. Also, there is a dose-response relationship between UVR and both conditions. The etiologies of pterygium and pinguecula are probably different. Simple measures such as wearing a hat or glasses will protect eyes and may decrease the amount of pterygium and climatic droplet keratopathy attributable to UVR exposure.

▶ Why pterygium and pingueculum develop is not clearly understood. Are they different diseases, or is one a precursor of the other? Exposure to UV radiation frequently is stated as an etiologic factor, but good epidemiologic studies to determine this are rare. This study confirms our beliefs that exposure to sunlight and UVR well may be an important cause of pterygium formation but not necessarily pingueculum growth. Perhaps these are 2 different forms of anterior segment degeneration rather than a continuous spectrum of disease. In any case, protection of our eyes from sunlight is an important concept.—P.R. Laibson, M.D.

A Comparison of the Clinical Variations of the Iridocorneal Endothelial Syndrome

Wilson MC, Shields MB (Duke Univ Eye Ctr, Durham, NC)
Arch Ophthalmol 107:1465–1468, October 1989   9–21

The 3 major variations of iridocorneal endothelial syndrome are Chandler's syndrome, progressive iris atrophy, and the Cogan-Reese syndrome. The presentation and course of patients in each of these subgroups were studied to better understand the clinical significance of this classification.

The medical records of 37 consecutive patients from 1 practice were reviewed. Twenty-one had Chandler's syndrome; 8, Cogan-Reese syndrome; and 8, progressive iris atrophy. None of the patients had bilateral disease, although 2 with Cogan-Reese syndrome and 1 with progressive iris atrophy had endothelial anomalies in the fellow eye. These abnormalities consisted of asymptomatic islands of beaten-silver appearance to the endothelium. Corneal endothelial anomalies typically consisted of a hammered-silver appearance of the posterior corneal surface and were noted in 87% of the patients. The remaining 6 had significant corneal edema that obscured visualization of subtle posterior corneal details.

The endothelial anomaly was focal in 12 cases and diffuse in 19. Stro-

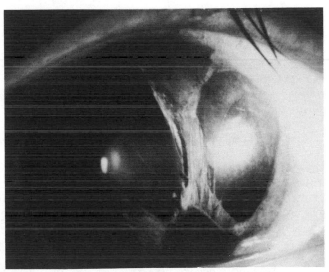

Fig 9–9.—Marked inferior corectopia and iris atrophy with multiple iris holes in a patient with progressive iris atrophy. (Courtesy of Wilson MC, Shields MB: *Arch Ophthalmol* 107:1465–1468, October 1989.)

mal iris atrophy was noted in 12 patients. Twenty-seven had corectopia, which was mild to moderate in Chandler's syndrome and moderate to severe in progressive iris atrophy and Cogan-Reese syndrome (Fig 9–9). Thirty-four patients had peripheral anterior synechiae. Nineteen patients were available for follow-up for 1 to 12 years. Fifty percent of patients with the Cogan-Reese syndrome, 75% with progressive iris atrophy, and only 40% of those with Chandler's syndrome needed filtering surgery.

The intraocular pressure was controlled successfully in 9 of 10 patients with either surgery alone or surgical and drug treatment. Four of 5 patients needing corneal transplantation had Chandler's syndrome, and the fifth had Cogan-Reese syndrome. Corneal edema had persisted despite adequate intraocular pressure control in 3 of these patients.

Chandler's syndrome was the most common clinical variant in this series. Patients with this syndrome had more severe corneal edema than those with the other 2 variants. Patients with progressive iris atrophy or the Coagan-Reese syndrome had worse secondary glaucoma.

▶ The iridocorneal endothelial syndrome is not as uncommon as many ophthalmologists think. This study from just 1 center reviews 37 consecutive patients with this problem. Unfortunately, only 19 of these patients were followed up for 1 to 12 years. Chandler's syndrome was the most common problem requiring a corneal transplant, as patients with this are more likely to have corneal edema than patients with Cogan-Reese syndrome or progressive iris atrophy. The significant corneal decompensation in Chandler's syndrome probably indicates that there is more endothelial abnormality in this disease. This is an excellent, up-to-date review of this very interesting, but not rare, anterior segment problem.— P.R. Laibson, M.D.

Intraocular Lens Implants for Uniocular Cataracts in Childhood
Burke JP, Willshaw HE, Young JDH (Ninewells Hosp and Med School, Dundee, Scotland; Children's Hosp, Birmingham, England)
Br J Ophthalmol 73:860–864, 1989   9–22

Successful management of monocular congenital cataracts in children is difficult, time-consuming, and dependent on patient compliance. The generally accepted treatment is a contact lens, which often is given up or associated with complications. A selected series of children with unilateral aphakia in whom posterior chamber and flexible 1-piece anterior chamber lenses were implanted was described. Complications from an intraocular lens were thought to be less significant than the inevitable severe amblyopia of inadequately treated patients.

Of 20 children aged 0.3 to 15.1 years, 6 had anterior and 14 had posterior chamber implants. Mean follow-up was 2.4 years. After surgery, 10 children had transient fibrinous uveitis, 4 needed lens repositioning, 1 needed lens removal, and 8 needed posterior capsulotomy. The complications necessitating further surgery occurred mostly in eyes with posterior chamber implants. Eight of 16 patients cooperated satisfactorily with conventional amblyopia treatment. After surgery, 9 of 18 children had peripheral fusion, and 4 regained visual acuity of better than 6/9. Visual acuity did not improve beyond 3/60 in 6 patients. In 19 eyes, the optical pathway to the retina was clear and the implants stable without signs of persisting inflammation.

In this series, the visual results were encouraging. Intraocular lenses were generally well tolerated and were anatomically stable, with no signs of persisting inflammation in 19 eyes. The preferred treatment for an infant with compliant parents is lensectomy or lens aspiration plus capsulotomy, contact lens wear, and intensive occlusion treatment.

▶ Whether to place an intraocular lens in a child at the time of uniocular cataract surgery is controversial. There are too few long-term reports in the ophthalmic literature to justify intraocular lens use in infants and children. Even this report has a mean follow-up of only 2.4 years, and 25% of 20 patients needed either lens repositioning (4) or removal (1). That is far too high a complication rate, compared with the adult, to routinely recommend intraocular lenses in children. Contact lenses are still the standby for uniocular cataract surgery in infants and children; however, that does not help the surgeon who must decide whether to put in an intraocular lens at the time of uniocular cataract surgery. Perhaps a trial of a contact lens before the surgery to see whether it can be tolerated would be worthwhile. Epikeratoplasty is a fallback operation if an aphakic child cannot wear a contact lens.— P.R. Laibson, M.D.

India-US Case-Control Study of Age-Related Cataracts

Mohan M, Sperduto HD, Angra SK, Milton HC, Mathur HL, Underwood DA, Jaffery N, Pandya CB, Chhabra VK, Vajpayee RB, Kalra VK, Sharma YR, India–US Case-Control Study Group (All India Inst of Med Sciences, New Delhi; Natl Eye Inst, Bethesda, Md; Natl Inst of Occupational Health, Ahmedabad, India)
Arch Ophthalmol 107:670–676, May 1989   9–23

It is estimated that if the development of cataract were delayed 10 years, the number of operations required would decline by 45%. A hospital-based case-control study of 1,441 patients with age-related cataract and 549 controls was undertaken to identify risk factors.

The risk of cataract was increased with lower educational achievement, decreased cloud cover at the site of residence, and (for posterior subcapsular and mixed cataracts) the use of aspirin less often than once per month. Diets low in selected nutrients were variably implicated, as were higher blood pressure and a lower body mass index. Another risk factor was a lower antioxidant index based on red blood cell levels of glutathione peroxidase and glucose-6-phosphate dehydrogenase and plasma levels of ascorbic acid and vitamin E. Most of these factors were associated with certain types of cataract only.

Socioeconomic factors may explain the association between cataract and limited education as well as a possible relationship with the use of less expensive cooking fuels such as wood and cow dung. Increased blood pressure may relate to nuclear and mixed cataracts. Aspirin more than once monthly may protect against posterior subcapsular and mixed types of cataract.

▶ The cause of most cataracts remains obscure and usually is relegated to an aging process. Well-planned, large-scale screening studies testing many different aspects in the patients' environment, such as food intake and exposure to sunlight, are few. This study identifies an interesting and variable mix of associations for specific cataract types in India. Once more, the bottom line is that age-related cataract development is a complex multifactorial process. The study does not solve the controversy over aspirin protecting against cataracts but only adds a little fuel to the fire of those taking such a position.—P.R. Laibson, M.D.

Adherence of *Staphylococcus epidermidis* to Intraocular Lenses
Griffiths PG, Elliot TSJ, McTaggart L (Newcastle Gen Hosp, Newcastle Upon Tyne; Queen Elizabeth Hosp, Birmingham, England)
Br J Ophthalmol 73:402–406, June 1989   9–24

   Staphylcococcus epidermidis is the most frequent cause of endophthalmitis and also the most common cause of infected joint replacements and other prostheses. Studies of animals have produced evidence that intraocular lenses can have a role in the development of intraocular infection after cataract surgery. When *Propionibacterium acnes* was placed in the anterior chamber after cataract surgery, the presence of an intraocular lens increased susceptibility to infection.

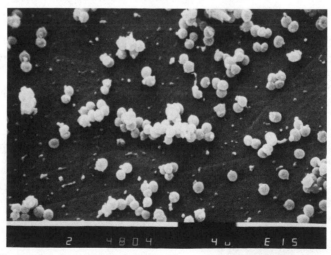

Fig 9–10.—*Staphylococcus epidermidis* (E004) adherent to the surface of an intraocular lens after 4 hours' incubation. The fluffy material on the surface of some organisms represents the early stages of polysaccharide glycocalyx production. Black space bar =4 μm. (Courtesy of Griffiths PG, Elliot TS, McTaggart L: *Br J Ophthalmol* 73:402–406, June 1989.)

Studies with an in vitro model showed that *S. epidermidis* can colonize intraocular lenses (Fig 9—10). Bacterial adherence was associated with production of a polysaccharide glycocalyx. The adherent organisms resisted apparently bactericidal concentrations of antibiotics.

Subconjunctival injection of 20 mg of gentamicin may not suffice to kill organisms that adhere to the lens surface. Colonizing *S. epidermidis* may cross the posterior capsule and multiply in the vitreous. Adherence to the lens may explain localized endophthalmitis as well as late-presenting cases and recurrences after apparently successful treatment with steroids and antibiotics. Adherence might be minimized by using different methods to surface finish lenses as well as by avoiding contact with the conjunctiva during surgery.

▶ Late-onset endophthalmitis is a particularly difficult complication of cataract and intraocular surgery to diagnose. The differential diagnosis between noninfective uveitis and viritis and infectious endophthalmitis is hard to make, usually only time and appropriate removal of lens remnants and the intraocular lens provide the proper diagnosis in the pathology laboratory. A good case is made for adherence and colonization of *S. epidermidis* to the intraocular lens in this paper.

Keeping the intraocular lens away from the conjunctiva, irrigating the lens with saline before insertion, and possibly using materials other than polymethylmethacrylate may help to avoid this complication.—P.R. Laibson, M.D.

10 Retina

Advances in the Treatment of Retinopathy of Prematurity

WILLIAM E. BENSON, M.D.
Wills Eye Hospital, Philadelphia, Pennsylvania

J. ARCHIBALD MCNAMARA, M.D., FRCSC
Retina Service, Wills Eye Hospital, Philadelphia, Pennsylvania

Retinopathy of Prematurity Is an Increasingly Important National Health Problem

Because the best predictors for the development of retinopathy of prematurity (ROP) are birth weight and duration in oxygen, it is easy to understand why the incidence of ROP is increasing rapidly in the United States. First, many premature infants are being born by drug-abusing women who have little or no prenatal care. Second, quantum leaps in neonatal medicine are saving many prematurely born children who formerly would not have survived. Third, oxygen is being used more often. After many excellent clinical and experimental studies in the 1950s showed that it played an important role in the development of ROP, oxygen was used more sparingly. Unfortunately, as the incidence of ROP dropped, the incidence of death and brain damage was increased (1). As a consequence of these factors, we have smaller and smaller neonates spending more and more time in oxygen. Both a relative and an absolute increase in the incidence of ROP has occurred (2).

Treatment of Active Retinopathy of Prematurity

Successful treatment for ROP by cryotherapy (3–7) and photocoagulation (8) was reported by several investigators in the 1970s, but because of the small numbers of patients in their studies and because approximately 80% of affected neonates show spontaneous regression (9), not all authorities were convinced that such treatment was indicated. The currently accepted "International Classification of Retinopathy of Prematurity" (ICROP) (10) helped to spur the institution of the controlled, randomized studies by the Cryotherapy for Retinopathy of Prematurity Cooperative Group (CRYO-ROP). (The updated data from this group were chosen for one of the KEY articles for this year.) Threshold disease is defined as at least 5 contiguous or 8 cumulative clock hours of extraretinal fibrovascular proliferation (stage 3) in zones I or II, which basically encompass all of the fundus except for the temporal retina anterior to the equator.

The accepted treatment strategy is to place contiguous single spots of cryotherapy to the avascular retina, but the fibrovascular ridge itself should not be treated because of the possibility of inducing a hemorrhage. The new pediatric cryoprobe makes cryotherapy easier, but it is still difficult to perform well, because of the tiny orbit and frequently small pupil.

The goal of the CRYO-ROP study was to prevent an unfavorable outcome, which was defined as (1) a retinal fold involving the macula, (2) a retinal detachment involving the posterior pole (zone 2), or (3) the proliferation of retrolental tissue that obscured the view of the posterior pole. Unfavorable outcomes occurred in 51% of the control eyes versus only 31% of the eyes that received cryotherapy (11). The difference was statistically significant ($P < .00001$) and proved beyond doubt that eyes with threshold disease should have treatment. When the disease was confined to zone 2, an unfavorable outcome occurred in 49% of the control eyes versus only 23% of the treated eyes. The current feeling of the CRYO-ROP group is "that it is premature to recommend unconditionally performing bilateral cryotherapy at a single treatment session for all bilateral threshold cases, since the long-term incidence of undesirable side effects is not yet known and since 47% of the control group experienced spontaneously favorable outcomes." Our personal recommendation is to treat all eyes that have reached threshold. If both eyes have reached threshold, then we treat the more advanced disease first. If that eye begins to respond to treatment within a few days, we treat the disease in the second eye.

Eyes with zone 1 fibrovascularization with plus disease (Rush disease) have an especially poor prognosis. In this group, 94% of the control eyes had unfavorable outcomes versus 78% of the treated eyes. For such patients, the CRYO-ROP group recommends cryotherapy for both eyes within a brief time.

Laser Photocoagulation of Retinopathy of Prematurity

As mentioned above, it is difficult technically to apply cryotherapy to affected patients. Further, severe bradycardia or arrhythmia developed in 9% of the neonates in the CRYO-ROP study. At the Wills Eye Hospital, we now are comparing, in a randomized, prospective study, laser photocoagulation by the newly developed binocular indirect ophthalmoscopic delivery systems with cryotherapy. It is too early to predict the results, but we hope that they will be good because laser treatment causes less pain and thereby requires less anesthesia. So far, it looks like bradycardia and arrhythmia are less common.

Retinal Detachment in Retinopathy of Prematurity

The management of retinal detachment in active retinopathy of prematurity is somewhat controversial. In some cases, treatment is not necessary. It is well recognized that retinal detachment anterior to the fibrovascular ridge often resolves spontaneously as normal retinal vessels cross the ridge to vascularize the anterior hypoxic retina. In such cases, cryotherapy alone may be sufficient treatment. Scleral buckling procedures should not be considered until the detachment has progressed well posterior to the equator. The technique used at the Wills Eye Hospital is to treat the avascular zone of retina with cryotherapy, drain the subretinal fluid, and encircle the globe (12). The best results are achieved in cases with shallow subretinal fluid. Approximately 60% to 75% of shallowly detached retinas can be reattached (12, 13). Patients with total detachment and a dense membrane in the retrolental space need vitrectomy. Schepens and Hirose (14) pioneered the subtotal open sky technique, which currently is favored at Wills (15). The main advantage of this technique is that the surgeon can remove the anterior membrane most completely. Charles (16), de Juan and Machemer (17), and Trese (18) advocate a closed approach. Both techniques report reattachment in approximately one third of cases.

References

1. Cross KW: Cost of preventing retrolental fibroplasia? *Lancet* 2:954–956, 1973.
2. Phelps DL: Vision loss due to retinopathy of prematurity. *Lancet* 1:606, 1981.
3. Yamashita Y: Studies on retinopathy of prematurity: III. Cryocautery for retinopathy of prematurity. *Jpn J Clin Ophthalmol* 26:385–393, 1972.
4. Payne JW, Patz A: Treatment of acute proliferative retrolental fibroplasia. *Trans Am Acad Ophthalmol Otolaryngol* 76:1234–1241, 1972.
5. Sasaki K, Yamashita Y, Maekawa T, et al: Treatment of retinopathy of prematurity in active stage by cryocautery. *Jpn J Ophthalmol* 20:384–395, 1976.
6. Takagi I: Treatment of acute retrolental fibroplasia. *Nippon Ganka Gakkai Zasshi* 82:323–330, 1978.
7. Kingham JD: Acute retrolental fibroplasia: Treatment by cryosurgery. *Arch Ophthalmol* 96:2049–2053, 1978.
8. Majima A, Takahashi M, Hibino Y: Clinical observations of photocoagulation on retinopathy of prematurity. *Jpn J Clin Ophthalmol* 30:93–97, 1976.
9. Kalina RE, Karr DJ: Retrolental fibroplasia: Experience over two decades in one institution. *Ophthalmology* 89:91–95, 1982.
10. The Committee for the Classification of Retinopathy of Prematurity: An international classification of retinopathy of prematurity. *Arch Ophthalmol* 102:1130–1134, 1984.
11. Cryotherapy for Retinopathy of Prematurity Cooperative Group: Multicenter trial of cryotherapy for retinopathy of prematurity: Three-month outcome. *Arch Ophthalmol* 108:195–204, 1990.
12. Greven CM, Tasman W: Scleral buckling in stages 4b and 5 retinopathy of prematurity. Presented at the annual meeting of the American Academy of Ophthalmology, New Orleans, 1989.
13. McPherson AR, Hittner HM, Lemos R: Retinal detachment in young premature infants with acute retrolental fibroplasia. Thirty-two cases. *Ophthalmology* 89:160–169, 1982.
14. Hirose T, Schepens CL, Katsumi O, et al: Open sky vitrectomy in stage 5 ROP: Anatomical and visual results. Presented at the annual meeting of the American Academy of Ophthalmology, New Orleans, 1989.
15. Tasman W, Borrone RN, Bolling J: Open sky vitrectomy for total retinal detachment in retinopathy of prematurity. *Ophthalmology* 94:449–452, 1987.
16. Charles S: Vitrectomy for stage 5 retinopathy of prematurity. Presented at the annual meeting of the American Academy of Ophthalmology, New Orleans, 1989.
17. de Juan Jr E, Machemer R: Retinopathy of prematurity: Surgical technique. *Retina* 7:63–69, 1987.
18. Trese MT: Surgical results of stage V retrolental fibroplasia and timing of surgical repair. *Ophthalmology* 91:461–466, 1984.

Results of a Temporary Balloon Buckle in the Treatment of 500 Retinal Detachments and a Comparison With Pneumatic Retinopexy

Kreissig I, Failer J, Lincoff H, Ferrari F (Universitäts-Augenklinik Tübingen, West Germany; New York Hosp–Cornell Med Ctr, New York)
Am J Ophthalmol 107:381–389, April 1989   10–1

The results of treating 500 detachments with a parabulbar balloon and cryopexy in 1980 to 1986 were reviewed. The patients had either a single break or a group of breaks close together, subtending less than 6 to 8 mm for about 1 clock hour at the equator. Follow-up ranged from 6 to 91 months.

With the balloon procedure, retinas in 93% of treated eyes were reattached successfully (Fig 10–1). Retinas in 2.4% of eyes became redetached after withdrawal of the balloon; another break was responsible in

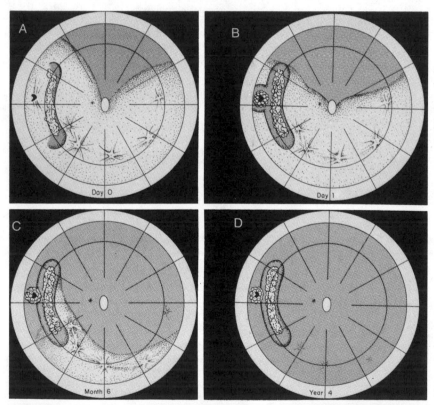

Fig 10–1.—A, 3-quadrant detachment with proliferative vitreoretinopathy and star folds in 2 quadrants in an eye with a previous buckle operation and diathermy, the balloon being used as reoperation. **B,** 1 day after balloon was inserted under the horseshoe tear at the 9 o'clock meridian, the tear has attached to the balloon buckle and has been surrounded by laser applications. **C,** 6 months later, the residual tractional detachment persists. **D,** 4 years after the balloon operation, the traction detachment has flattened. Remnants of star folds are visible. Visual acuity is 20/40. (Courtesy of Kreissig I, Failer J, Lincoff H, et al: *Am J Ophthalmol* 107:381–389, April 1989.)

7 instances. A second operation was done in 8.4% of eyes. Usually a segmental sponge buckle was placed without drainage of subretinal fluid. Thirty-six eyes had attachment after the second operation. In all, 99% of eyes eventually had complete attachment and 2 eyes had partial attachment. Superficial erosion resulted from improper tube placement in 25 eyes. One of 184 patients having a balloon left in place beneath the temporal rectus muscle for 12 days had diplopia.

A comparable attachment rate is achieved using an intraocular gas bubble. However, complications, including proliferative vitreoretinopathy are more frequent and more serious.

▶ Doctors Kreissig and Lincoff are great innovators in retinal detachment surgery. There is no doubt that the results obtained by the balloon technique are excellent. The reason all retinal surgeons currently do not use this technique is that with standard techniques the success rates are 95% or better with one operation and 99% for final reattachment. In addition, wearing the balloon involves some inconvenience for the period required to keep the retinal break sealed. For similar reasons the newly introduced technique of pneumatic retinopexy also will require years to be established by all physicians.—W.E. Benson, M.D.

Factors Associated With Visual Outcome After Photocoagulation for Diabetic Retinopathy: Diabetic Retinopathy Study Report #13
Kaufman SC, Ferris FL III, Seigel DG, Davis MD, DeMets DL, DRS Research Group (Natl Eye Inst, Bethesda, Md; Univ of Wisconsin–Madison)
Invest Ophthalmol Vis Sci 30:23 28, January 1989   10 2

Risk factors for marked visual loss were sought in patients in the Diabetic Retinopathy Study who were followed up for 5 years after panretinal photocoagulation. Neovascularization on and around the optic disk was the chief risk factor. The risk of marked visual loss also increased with hemorrhages/microaneurysms, retinal elevation, proteinuria, and hyperglycemia. Increasing "treatment density" was associated with a lower risk of severe visual loss.

These results are similar to previous findings for untreated eyes. The findings support the common practice of repeating photocoagulation when initial treatment fails to stabilize or reduce retinal neovascularization. Neovascularization is the most prominent factor in the time until severe visual loss occurs.

▶ This study confirms that neovascularization on or around the optic disk is the chief risk factor for severe visual loss from diabetic retinopathy. The important new finding from this study is that eyes that received denser treatment had a lower rate of severe visual loss than eyes with less dense treatment. It is important to remember, however, that although this difference was statistically significant, the clinical significance is less striking. Seven percent of the eyes with 51% to 92% coverage of the area just beyond the arcades had severe visual loss compared with 15% of those who had less than 35% coverage of the same area. In other words, although those with "tighter" treatment did 100% better, the risk even for those with less treatment is still quite low. Furthermore, those with the tighter treatment would be expected to have more side effects, such as visual field loss.—W.E. Benson, M.D.

Persistent and Recurrent Neovascularization After Krypton Laser Photocoagulation for Neovascular Lesions of Ocular Histoplasmosis
Macular Photocoagulation Study Group (Emory Eye Ctr, Atlanta; Johns Hopkins Univ; St Lukes Hosp, Cleveland; Texas Retina Assocs, Dallas; Ingalls Mem Hosp, Harvey, Ill, and Chicago; et al)
Arch Ophthalmol 107:344–352, March 1989   10–3

Treatment of 144 eyes with krypton red laser photocoagulation was done with retrobulbar anesthesia, and angiograms were obtained within 3 days before photocoagulation. The goal was to treat an entire area of neovascularization to produce uniform whitening of the overlying retina. A treatment standard was used to ensure adequate energy delivery (Fig 10–2). Treatment extended 100 μm beyond hyperfluorescent areas on the border away from the fovea and 100 μm into any blood on the foveal side if hyperfluorescence was 100 μm or farther from the foveal center.

Neovascularization persisted in 23% of eyes and recurred in 8%. Five eyes had a new independent area of neovascularization during follow-up. Nearly half the 23 patients with high blood pressure had persistent neovascularization. Another risk factor was neovascularization within 200 μm of the foveal center. Treatment of the entire area of neovascularization on the foveal side tended to prevent persistent disease.

Nearly a third of eyes given krypton laser photocoagulation for choroidal neovascularization secondary to ocular histoplasmosis will have

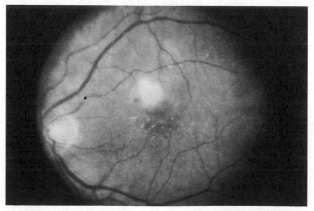

Fig 10–2.—Treatment intensity standard. Treatment protocol specified a uniform, white burn at least as intense as the treatment standard. (Courtesy of the Macular Photocoagulation Study Group: *Arch Ophthalmol* 107:344–352, March 1989.)

persistent or recurrent disease within 5 years. Persistence and recurrence both have a negative effect on visual acuity. Fluorescein leakage from the center of a treatment scar at 6 weeks is not related to an increased risk of recurrence. Initial treatment is an important factor in the subsequent course. Nevertheless, excessive treatment of parafoveal disease must be avoided.

▶ It is interesting that high blood pressure is a risk factor for ocular histoplasmosis. The reasons for this are not clear. The most important finding from this study, however, is that treatment of the choroidal neovascular membrane must be complete and extend onto the foveal side of the lesion to prevent recurrent disease. Those who treat ocular histoplasmosis must be confident enough in recognition of macular details to provide complete treatment without directly damaging the foveola.—W.E. Benson, M.D.

Dextromethorphan Protects Retina Against Ischemic Injury In Vivo
Yoon YH, Marmor MF (Stanford Univ)
Arch Ophthalmol 107:409–411, March 1989   10–4

Dextromethorphan, a potent NMDA (N-methyl-D-aspartate) receptor antagonist, reportedly protects against hypoxic-ischemic damage in animal models of brain injury. Dextromethorphan now is shown to protect against retinal ischema in intact rabbits. The retina was used as a model because excitatory amino acid receptors are prevalent at this site, and function may be monitored electroretinographically.

Retinal ischemia was induced by increasing the intraocular pressure above systolic pressure for 60 or 75 minutes. Pretreatment with intravenous dextromethorphan greatly improved the postischemic recovery of electroretinogram b-wave amplitude. Several animals treated with dextromethorphan before 45 minutes of ischemia had minimal or no damage 2 hours later. Control animals, in contrast, had substantial damage including disrupted photoreceptor outer segments and cell loss in the nuclear layer.

Pretreatment with dextromethorphan protects retinal tissue from ischemic damage in vivo. The findings implicate neuroexcitation at the NMDA receptor in ischemic retinal damage in the clinical setting. If NMDA receptor antagonists can slow retinal-cell loss, they might mitigate the effects of some of the prime causes of blindness, such as diabetic retinopathy.

▶ This study opens up an exciting area in retinal diseases. Current management for central retinal artery obstruction is not satisfactory, although in our clinic we have been able to show some improvement in visual acuity for 35% of patients who have had vigorous anterior chamber paracentesis and inhalation of 95% oxygen and 5% carbon dioxide. It will be interesting to see whether the addition of dextromethorphan to this regimen helps to improve visual acuity. The authors also speculate that dextromethorphan may protect eyes from other forms of ischemic damage, such as is seen in diabetic retinopathy. This should be amenable to a prospective clinical trial. It is hoped that results will be positive.—W.E. Benson, M.D.

Cataract Surgery and Intraocular Lens Implantation in Patients With Uveitis
Foster CS, Fong LP, Singh G (Massachusetts Eye and Ear Infirmary; Harvard Med School, Boston)
Ophthalmology 96:281–288, March 1989   10–5

Cataract is a frequent complication of chronic uveitis, and surgery for cataract is complicated by uveitic changes. Intracapsular lens removal usually is advocated. The results of extracapsular extraction in 44 of 38 patients with uveitis were reviewed. Thirty-two eyes received posterior chamber lens implants. Surgery was undertaken no less than 3 months after inflammation was eliminated. Immunosuppression to suppress inflammation was used perioperatively.

Eighty-seven percent of eyes given posterior chamber implants achieved stable acuity of 20/40 or better, as did 67% of 12 eyes not given implants. The results strongly support deferral of cataract surgery until inflammation is eliminated. Three eyes in the present series needed laser capsulotomy. Intraocular lens placement carries no added risk in selected uveitic eyes subjected to extracapsular cataract extraction. An all-polymethylmethacrylate lens should be placed within the capsular bag.

▶ Years ago, patients with severe uveitis underwent cataract surgery only as a last resort. More recent reports have shown that lensectomy combined with vitrectomy is a useful procedure in that the eye survives the procedure without severe inflammation. However, ocular rehabilitation is best with placement of an intraocular lens. This article shows that implants can be given to carefully selected patients with uveitis that is properly managed with careful surgery. Clearly such patients are better off with this regimen.—W.E. Benson, M.D.

Exposure to Sunlight and Other Risk Factors for Age-Related Macular Degeneration
West SK, Rosenthal FS, Bressler NM, Bressler SB, Munoz B, Fine SL, Taylor HR (Johns Hopkins Hosp, Baltimore; Univ of Massachusetts, Worcester)
Arch Ophthalmol 107:875–879, June 1989   10–6

There is growing concern that long-term exposure to ultraviolet (UV) radiation may increase the risk of age-related macular degeneration. The authors surveyed 838 Maryland watermen (none of them aphakic), 93% of whom had stereoscopic fundus photos available to assess macular degeneration. A personal ocular UV exposure index was determined based on interview data and laboratory and field measurements.

Neither cumulative UV-A exposure nor UV-B exposure was related to macular degeneration, within age groups or after adjusting for age. Both age and nuclear opacity were associated independently with a raised risk of macular degeneration.

The risk of age-related macular degeneration is not increased in phakic subjects exposed heavily to UV light. The results of studies relating experimental light exposure to photoreceptor damage and retinal pigment epithelial atrophy cannot necessarily be taken to indicate that light is an important cause of macular degeneration.

▶ I am delighted with the results of this excellent epidemiologic study. Some investigators have made the leap from experimental evidence that excessive UV light can be toxic to the retina to the conclusion that exposure to UV light in the environment is a risk factor in age-related macular degeneration. This study provides strong evidence that persons with extensive exposure to UV light do not have an increased incidence of significant macular degeneration. Now with increased confidence we can tell our patients not to be frightened by the scare tactics of sunglass manufacturers.—W.E. Benson, M.D.

The Care of Diabetic Patients by Ophthalmologists in New York State
Olsen CL, Kassoff A, Gerber T (New York State Dept of Health, Albany; Albany Med College)
Ophthalmology 96:739–745, June 1989   10–7

A survey of 1,655 ophthalmologists in New York state was intended to delineate methods of ocular care of diabetic patients. More than 90% of the respondents recommended at least annual retinal examinations.

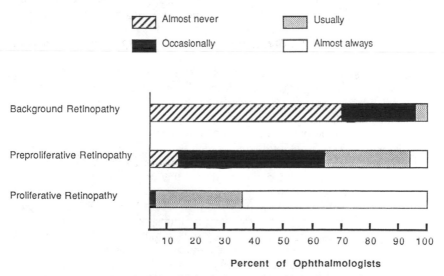

Fig 10–3.—Frequency with which ophthalmologists recommend laser photocoagulation for diabetic retinopathy. (Courtesy of Olsen CL, Kassoff A, Gerber T: *Ophthalmology* 96:739–745, June 1989.)

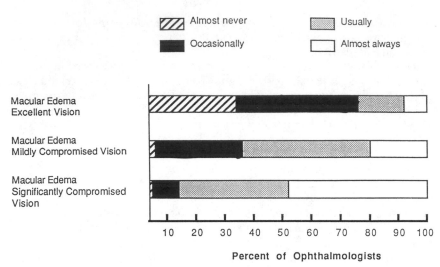

Fig 10–4.—Frequency with which ophthalmologists recommend laser photocoagulation for macular edema. (Courtesy of Olsen CL, Kassoff A, Gerber T: *Ophthalmology* 96:739–745, June 1989.)

About one third usually recommends and nearly two thirds almost always recommend laser treatment for proliferative retinopathy (Fig 10–3). Decisions on treating macular edema depended closely on the quality of vision. Although one fourth of respondents usually recommend laser treatment when vision is excellent, nearly two thirds do so when vision is mildly compromised, and nearly three fourths do so when vision is significantly compromised (Fig 10–4).

Most ophthalmologists in New York state appear to be well informed about the epidemiology of diabetic retinopathy and guidelines for treatment. However, the present findings are based on hypothetical patients, and further information on recommendations for real patients is needed.

▶ The results of this study are somewhat shocking. Although the Diabetic Retinopathy Study clearly proved a strong treatment benefit for panretinal photocoagulation, 6% of the ophthalmologists in New York state only occasionally or almost never recommend panretinal photocoagulation. These physicians are clearly depriving their patients of a chance for maintaining excellent visual acuity. Second, only 63% recommend laser treatment for macular edema even when visual acuity is mildly compromised, although the Early Treatment Diabetic Retinopathy Study has demonstrated clearly that the rate of visual deterioration is slowed significantly by focal macular treatment. A third surprising finding is that up to 51% of ophthalmologists recommend examinations every 6 months for diabetic patients who have no retinal disease. Such a frequency for follow-up examinations undoubtedly results in many unnecessary and costly patient encounters. It seems that ophthalmology has a big job to do in making the findings from significant studies known to all practitioners in our specialty.—W.E. Benson, M.D.

Pneumatic Retinopexy: A Multicenter Randomized Controlled Clinical Trial Comparing Pneumatic Retinopexy With Scleral Buckling

Tornambe PE, Hilton GF, Retinal Detachment Study Group (Univ of California, San Diego; Univ of California. San Franciso; Rush Univ, Chicago; Univ of Medicine and Dentistry of New Jersey, East Brunswick; Univ of South Florida, Tampa; et al)

Ophthalmology 96:772–784, June 1989   10–8

Pneumatic retinopexy and scleral buckling were compared in a 7-center randomized clinical trial of 198 patients with retinal detachment. Retinal breaks no greater than 1 clock hour in size were present in the superior two thirds of the fundus, and significant proliferative vitreoretinopathy was absent. Patients were followed for 6 months or longer.

Scleral buckling led to reattachment in a single procedure in 82% of cases, and pneumatic retinopexy, in 73%. The rates of reattachment with postoperative laser therapy or cryotherapy were 84% and 81%, respectively. Final acuity of 20/50 or better was achieved in 56% of eyes having preoperative macular detachment for 2 weeks or less after scleral buckling and in 80% after pneumatic retinopexy. Rates of proliferative vitreoretinopathy were 5% and 3%, respectively. New retinal breaks occurred in 13% of the scleral buckling group and in 23% of the pneumatic retinopexy group. Complications were similar in the 2 groups.

The anatomical results of the 2 operations were comparable, but pneumatic retinopexy had less morbidity and provided better postoperative vision. One patient had *Staphylococcus epidermidis* endophthalmitis after pneumatic retinopexy. Pneumatic retinopexy now is recommended in appropriate cases.

▶ The controversy over pneumatic retinopexy continues. Randomized controlled clinical trials are frequently the best way to evaluate a clinical question. Although randomization is supposed to eliminate physician bias, randomization errors still can occur. For example, in this study, 12 of 95 eyes randomized to scleral buckling procedures had their maculae detached for more than 14 days vs. only 1 of 103 eyes being treated with pneumatic retinopexy. As the authors point out, this is a statistically significant difference that may well bias the results of the study, which indicated that patients with pneumatic retinopexy had better visual acuities than patients who had scleral buckling procedures. Other problems with this study include the low rate of success after 1 operation in the patients who underwent scleral buckling procedures. Only 82% had repair after 1 operation. This seems to be very low for the group under consideration.

In one of the largest centers in this multicenter trial, the primary success rate was only 74%. This study may demonstrate a benefit for pneumatic retinopexy, but it is not clear that the results from primary scleral buckling procedures are those obtained by most retinal surgeons across the country. The final word on pneumatic retinopexy has yet to be written.—W.E. Benson, M.D.

Clinicopathologic Study of Organic Dye: Laser in the Human Fundus

Brooks HL Jr, Eagle RC Jr, Schroeder RP, Annesley WH, Shields JA, Augsburger JJ (Wills Eye Hosp, Philadelphia)
Ophthalmology 96:822–834, June 1989   10–9

Four patients scheduled for enucleation because of choroidal melanoma agreed to experimental laser photocoagulation to compare the histologic appearance of acute chorioretinal lesions produced by different dye laser wavelengths with krypton red and argon green laser controls. Three patients received simulated "light" and "heavy" treatment of an extrafoveal choroidal neovascular membrane with wavelengths 577 nm (yellow), 595 nm (orange), and 600 nm (orange). One had simulated panretinal photocoagulation with 4 different dye laser wavelengths.

All dye laser wavelengths as well as the krypton red and argon green controls produced full-thickness retinal damage during simulated heavy treatment in areas of attached retina. The most marked inner retinal damage was from 600-nm orange. The longer wavelengths produced deeper choroidal penetration during heavy extrafoveal treatment. During simulated extrafoveal light treatment, all dye laser and both control wavelengths spared the inner retina and produced similar patterns of outer retinal and pigment epithelial damage. Here, too, choroidal uptake varied with the wavelength, the longest wavelengths producing deeper involvement.

These findings indicate that caution is in order when treating heavily extrafoveally with 590 and 600 nm. Decreased choroidal penetration by shorter wavelengths may result from increased hemoglobin absorption by the choriocapillaris or from increased scatter.

▶ This well-conceived study clearly demonstrates that all wavelengths of light can cause full-thickness retinal damage when heavy treatment is given. We are all familiar with the retinal absorption curves that were extensively published when the krypton laser was introduced, which purported to show that the krypton laser would result in less intraretinal damage than the argon green and blue-green lasers. These diagrams clearly do not correlate with the clinical situation. This study also confirms other studies that have shown severe retinal damage caused by the orange (590- to 600-nm) spectrum.

I agree with the authors' conclusion that the absorption of light in conversion to thermal energy by the melanin in the retinal pigment epithelium and choroidal melanocytes far outweighs the absorption by xanthophyll pigment or by hemoglobin.

In the peripheral lesions, the study confirms the conclusions of others that the amount of choroidal damage is increased with increasing wavelengths. Although this may not be significant in the long-term survival of the eye, it seems that argon green should be used to minimize it. We are awaiting the results of the krypton argon retinal neovascularization study.—W.E. Benson, M.D.

Retinal Detachment After Neodymium:YAG Laser Posterior Capsulotomy
Rickman-Barger L, Florine CW, Larson RS, Lindstrom RL (Univ of Minnesota, Minneapolis)
Am J Ophthalmol 107:531–536, May 1989   10–10

The records of 397 patients who had posterior capsulotomy with Nd:YAG laser in 1983 to 1988 were reviewed. The series included 366 eyes that were followed up for 3 months or longer.

Retinal detachment developed in 13 eyes (3.6%) after capsulotomy, 11 within 1 year of surgery. Significant risk factors for detachment included male sex with an axial length of 25 mm or greater, a history of lattice degeneration, and a history of retinal detachment in the fellow eye. Of men with axial lengths of 25 mm or more, retinal detachment developed in 17.6%.

Postoperative ophthalmoscopy is critically important in the first year after posterior capsulotomy.

▶ Although the Nd:YAG laser avoids the necessity of entering the eye to surgically open an opaque posterior capsule, it appears that the laser may well be associated with retinal detachment. One question that this study does not answer, however, is, How many patients who get retinal detachment after Nd:YAG capsulotomy had preexisting tears that went on to cause detachment? I have had the good fortune of examining a few patients before Nd:YAG capsulotomy in whom I found retinal breaks that then were treated successfully with cryotherapy. These patients subsequently did not have retinal detachment. The point is that before Nd:YAG capsulotomy, a careful retinal examination is essential.

All patients should be examined carefully at regular intervals after Nd:YAG capsulotomy, and if the results of this study are confirmed by others, patients who are male, highly myopic, or both need to be followed up especially carefully.—W.E. Benson, M.D.

Long-Term Natural History of Lattice Degeneration of the Retina
Byer NE (Univ of California, Los Angeles)
Ophthalmology 96:1396–1402, September 1989   10–11

Lattice degeneration remains the most important primary peripheral retinal lesion associated with the later development of retinal detachment (RD). Prophylactic treatment of lattice degeneration has been favored for many years, even in patients without RD or tractional tears. However, no data have confirmed the appropriateness of prophylactic treatment. Between 1962 and 1969, an initial series of patients undergoing complete routine ophthalmologic examination in whom lattice degeneration of the retina was found was enrolled in a continuing, prospective long-term follow-up study. All patients were left untreated to define the natural course of this retinal abnormality. The findings for 423 eyes in 276 untreated patients are reported. The average follow-up was 10.8 years (range, 1–25 years).

By the end of the follow-up period, 120 of the 276 patients had atrophic retinal holes involving 150 eyes. Of these 150 eyes, 66 had 1 or more holes in the superior half of the retina, and 106 had 1 or more holes in the inferior retina. Of 261 atrophic holes, 100 were in the upper part of the retina and 161 were in the lower part. Twenty-eight of 150 eyes with atrophic retinal holes were in patients aged less than 30 years and 122 were in patients aged more than 30 years. Subclinical RDS, defined as detachments with subretinal fluid extending at least 1 disk diameter (DD) from the retinal break but not more than 2 DD posterior to the equator, occurred in 10 of the 150 eyes, involving 9 of the 120 patients with atrophic retinal holes. Tractional retinal tears were seen in 8 eyes involving 8 patients. One of these led to a clinical RD.

In addition, clinical RD or progressive subclinical RD developed in 3 of the 423 eyes with lattice degeneration. Two of the 3 eyes were associated with atrophic retinal holes. Both had successful reattachment of their retinas. The third clinical RD was associated with a symptomatic tractional tear. This patient had successful treatment with a buckling procedure. Thus, a total of 4 (0.94%) of 423 untreated eyes or 4 (1.4%) of 276 patients with lattice degeneration went to clinical RD. Subclinical RD was seen in 10 eyes with atrophic holes involving 9 patients, but it remained localized over many years or progressed very slowly.

In view of the extremely low risk for lattice degeneration to progress to clinical RD, the recommendation to treat all atrophic holes in lattice degeneration should be abandoned, even in myopic eyes. The data show that a myopic refractive eye does not increase the likelihood of having atrophic retinal holes in lattice degeneration.

▶ Norman Byer, M.D., has more experience in the follow-up and management of peripheral lesions that predispose to retinal detachment than any other ophthalmologist. This latest update of his ongoing studies conclusively proves that prophylactic treatment of lattice degeneration, with or without holes, is a procedure with very low yield. One would have to treat more than 100 eyes to prevent 1 retinal detachment; even then, there would be no guarantee that treatment of any given eye would prevent detachment in that eye because tears in the retina can occur in areas of retina devoid of lattice. In many cases, subclinical detachments caused by lattice with holes can be followed without treatment, for they usually progress very slowly. In summary, there is little justification for treating asymptomatic lattice degeneration.—W.E. Benson, M.D.

Acetazolamide for Treatment of Chronic Macular Edema in Retinitis Pigmentosa
Fishman GA, Gilbert LD, Fiscella RG, Kimura AE, Jampol LM (Univ of Illinois, Chicago; Univ of Iowa, Iowa City; Northwestern Univ, Chicago)
Arch Ophthalmol 107:1445–1452, October 1989   10–12

A recent study reported that treatment of chronic macular edema with acetazolamide yielded a partial or complete resolution of edema and improvement in visual acuity in 16 of 41 patients. A masked, crossover study was done to further assess the efficacy of acetazolamide in patients with retinitis pigmentosa and chronic macular edema.

Included in the study were 12 patients with visual acuities ranging from 20/20 to 20/400 in at least 1 eye and angiographic leakage primarily from retinal or choroidal capillaries through the retinal pigment epithelium. Patients were assigned randomly to 2-week treatment periods of either acetazolamide in doses of 250 mg per day or 500 mg per day, or placebo.

Ten patients given acetazolamide reported subjective improvement in visual acuity. None taking placebo thought that they had had improvement. One patient who was first given acetazolamide believed he had some residual effect during the 2-week placebo period. All 10 patients also had objective improvement on visual acuity testing. Seven of the 10 patients showed an improvement of 1 line in at least 1 eye; the other 3 patients showed improvement of 2 lines in at least 1 eye. Six of the 12 treated patients also had angiographic improvement in both eyes, which mainly resulted from less detectable leakage from retinal capillaries rather than from choroidal capillaries. The 500-mg-per-day dose of acetazolamide was more effective than the 250-mg-per-day dose.

The results of this study are encouraging, but because of potential side effects, caution is indicated when using carbonic anhydrase inhibitors in the treatment of macular edema in retinitis pigmentosa.

▶ In 1988, a breakthrough report by Cox, Hay, and Bird (1) showed that acetazolamide (Diamox) actually could decrease cystoid macular edema (CME) and improve visual acuity in many patients with ocular conditions in which the primary abnormality was in the retinal pigment epithelium such as aphakic CME, CME from pars planitis, and CME associated with retinitis pigmentosa. No benefit was found for retinal conditions such as diabetic macular edema or macular edema from retinal venous occlusive disease. Fishman and colleagues now present confirmatory evidence. With a majority of patients with retinitis pigmentosa, they too showed decreased leakage on fluorescein angiography and improved visual acuity. It is true that the improvement in Snellen visual acuity was not enormous, but in these unfortunate patients any improvement is helpful, and their subjective improvement was frequently large. The next step is to develop more effective drugs to treat these conditions.—W.E. Benson, M.D.

Reference

1. Cox et al: *Arch Ophthalmol* 106:1190, 1988.

A New Culture Method for Infectious Endophthalmitis

Joondeph BC, Flynn HW Jr, Miller D, Joondeph HC (Univ of Miami, Fla; Wayne State Univ, Detroit)
Arch Ophthalmol 107:1334–1337, September 1989   10–13

The identification of organisms responsible for infectious endophthalmitis often has been accomplished with a membrane filter system (MFS). This method, which processes large-volume aspirates obtained during vitrectomy, produces a high yield of positive cultures but is technically difficult and time-consuming. Researchers describe a simple alternative to MFS: direct inoculation of blood culture bottles (BCBs) with vitreous specimens.

Eighty-three cases of infectious endophthalmitis were retrospectively reviewed in a pilot study of the BCB system. The infection had occurred postoperatively in most cases (91%). Positive cultures were obtained for 77 patients (93%), often within 1 to 3 days (table). A laboratory study compared MFS, direct media inoculation, and 3 BCB systems. At least 1 BCB system became positive at the same time as the MFS for each of the 9 tested organisms.

Fourteen patients with endophthalmitis took part in a prospective clinical comparison of the MFS and BCB. Of 10 cases that were culture positive, growth was noted first with MFS in 4, first with BCB in 2, and at

Pilot Series: 80 Culture-Positive Isolates	
Organism	No. (%)
Gram–positive	
Staphylococcus epidermidis	38
Staphylococcus aureus	13
Streptococcus species	13
Propionibacterium acnes	4
Bacillus species	2
Clostridium perfringens	1
Total	71 (89)
Gram–negative	
Pseudomonas species	3
Morganella species	1
Proteus mirabilis	1
Serratia rubidaea	1
Total	6 (8)
Fungi	
Candida albicans	1
Aspergillus fumigatus	1
Rhodotorula rubra	1
Total	3 (4)

(Courtesy of Joondeph BC, Flynn HW Jr, Miller D, et al: *Arch Ophthalmol* 107:1334–1337, September 1989.)

the same time in 5. Results thus confirmed the laboratory findings and the value of direct inoculation of BCBs.

The BCB system is particularly useful when a hospital does not have facilities for MFS or when a specimen is obtained while the hospital microbiology laboratory is closed. Although MSF is slightly more sensitive than either BCB systems or direct cultures, the direct inoculation of BCBs is a valuable adjunct or alternative culture method.

▶ It is my clinical impression that the majority of vitrectomies for endophthalmitis are done at night. This is not surprising, because endophthalmitis usually is diagnosed by a referring ophthalmologist during office hours and by the time a patient can be made ready for surgery, it is late in the day. In some hospitals, microbiology laboratories have 24-hour coverage and anterior chamber and vitreous aspirates can be processed immediately, to the patient's obvious benefit. In many other hospitals, such support is not available. Specimens often are not processed correctly and the opportunity to identify causative organisms is lost. For ophthalmologists who practice in these hospitals, the article by Joondeph and colleagues is valuable because the identification rate was practically identical to the rate achieved by the most sophisticated system available.—W.E. Benson, M.D.

Surgical Management of Vitreomacular Traction Syndromes
Margherio RR, Trese MT, Margherio AR, Cartright K (William Beaumont Hosp, Royal Oak, Mich)
Ophthalmology 96:1437–1445, September 1989   10–14

Vitreomacular traction can result in a number of ocular conditions, including the development of idiopathic macular holes. Surgery was performed on a series of 106 consecutively seen eyes that had undergone rapid change in vision associated with vitreous traction of the macular region.

The clinical appearance of the foveal area of these eyes was consistent with 1 or more of a variety of conditions such as macular cyst, lamellar macular hole, loss of foveal reflex, involutional macular thinning, and glistening light reflex. Visual acquities in 99% of the affected eyes were 20/50 or worse. In most eyes, the distance between the retinal vasculature and its underlying shadow was increased, suggesting retinal elevation (Fig 10–5).

After surgery, vision improved in 89% of the eyes, 7% were unchanged, and 4% worsened. In approximately half (45%), visual acuity improved to 20/50 or better. Nuclear sclerosis was a surgical complication in 16 eyes; retinal detachment, macular pucker, and macular holes occurred in 2%. Postoperative macular holes did not develop in patients for whom the can opener technique was used. To avoid this complication, the cortical vitreous or glial membrane should not be removed from the fovea.

One study found that 89% of eyes with macular cysts and vision less

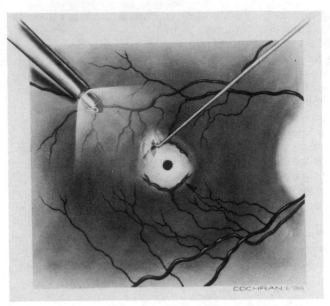

Fig 10–5.—Opening created in preretinal membrane using 23-gauge bent needle. Dissection done over retinal vessel to guard against forming retinal hole. *Arrow* shows the vascular shadowing that helps confirm the presence of the membrane by noting the distance between the elevated neurosensory retina and the underlying retinal pigment epithelium. (Courtesy of Margherio RR, Trese MT, Margherio AR, et al: *Ophthalmology* 96:1437–1445, September 1989.)

than 20/50 progressed to macular holes and loss of vision. Surgical intervention should be considered in patients with deteriorating vision and a history of full-thickness macular holes. Furthermore, surgery should be considered urgent in these cases. The traction present on the foveal region should be removed in a way that will not disrupt the integrity of the fovea.

▶ The number of conditions formerly thought to be untreatable continues to decrease. We used to be forced to tell a patient with a macular hole in 1 eye and who was losing vision in the other eye that "there is nothing we can do." Now, several surgeons have proven conclusively that a timely vitrectomy with removal of preretinal membranes can preserve vision. Obviously, the surgery is difficult and exacting and should be undertaken only by experienced surgeons.—W.E. Benson, M.D.

New and Previously Unidentified Retinal Breaks in Eyes With Recurrent Retinal Detachment With Proliferative Vitreoretinopathy
Moisseiev J, Glaser BM (Johns Hopkins Hosp, Baltimore)
Arch Ophthalmol 107:1152–1154, August 1989   10–15

In the preoperative examination of patients with recurrent retinal detachment (RRD) and proliferative vitreoretinopathy (PVR), little atten-

tion has been paid to the location or cause of new or previously uniden-
tified retinal breaks. This question was examined in 72 such breaks found
in 41 eyes. All patients had undergone previous retinal reattachment procedures.

These breaks were located primarily (65.3%) on the buckle; 16
(22.2%) were posterior to the buckle, and only 8 (11.1%) were found in
an area distant from the buckle. Thirty-one of the 47 breaks on the
buckle were on the posterior slope; 13, on its crest; and 3, on the anterior slope.

Many (40.2%) of these tears were adjacent to a cryopexy-induced
chorioretinal scar and were thought to be stretch tears. Such a high percentage appears significant and suggests that the borders of these scars
are subject to tearing by traction forces brought about by the proliferative process. The part of the retina that borders chorioretinal scars is vul-
nerable to new tears, especially when the edge of the scar falls on the posterior slope of the buckle. In patients with RRD and PVR, this scar area
should be watched carefully for retinal breaks.

▶ In the 1920s, Jules Gonin, the father of retinal detachment surgery, established the necessary step for curing detachments: (1) find all breaks and (2)
treat all breaks. Despite the remarkable technical progress (vitrectomy, membrane peeling, retinotomies, long-lasting gases, silicone oil, retinal tacks, retinal
glues, etc.) made in recent years, Gonin's principles are still valid. It is true that
a small undetected break in an eye filled with silicone oil or a small undetected
break fortuitously placed on a scleral buckle may not lead to redetachment, but
it is certain that the surgeon who finds all the breaks is most likely to have the
highest cure rate. This article confirms that new breaks can occur on the scleral
buckle. An old rule of finding retinal breaks is that a break usually is found
within 1 clock hour of the most superior location where subretinal fluid crosses
the buckle. Also, the article warns us to look closely near areas of previous
cryotherapy because 40% of the breaks were found there.—W.E. Benson,
M.D.

Intravenous Fluorescein Interference With Clinical Laboratory Tests
Bloom JN, Herman DC, Elin RJ, Sliva CA, Ruddel ME, Nussenblatt RB, Pales-
tine AG (Natl Eye Inst; Warren G Magnuson Clinical Ctr, NIH, Bethesda, Md)
Am J Ophthalmol 108:375–379, October 1989   10–16

As many as 650,000 fluorescein angiograms may have been done in
this country in 1984. The possibility that subsequent laboratory test results may be erroneous because of interference by intravenously administered fluorescein was examined in 4 adults. Studies were done 5 minutes
and 3, 6, and 12 hours after fluorescein injection. Serum and urine chem-
istry tests were performed on 7 commonly used instruments.

All 4 tests (cortisol, digoxin, quinitine, thyroxine) done with the TDx
instrument indicated interference by fluorescein, which was present up to
12 hours after its administration. Interference was not evident 24 hours

after fluorescein injection. Serum creatinine values and total protein estimates also were affected, but results of urine tests were not.

These findings corroborate several clinical reports of interference with
laboratory tests by intravenously administered fluorescein. Patients
should be advised accordingly, and the referring physician notified. Renal
insufficiency might prolong the time during which an uncontaminated
blood sample cannot be obtained. Interference is method specific, so that
it may be possible to obtain correct estimates using selected techniques.

▶ It is becoming more and more difficult to keep up with the rapidly increasing
number of new drugs being introduced to medicine each year. Even though
ophthalmologists do not prescribe most of these drugs, it is incumbent on us
to be aware of their more important side effects and their interactions with the
drugs we do prescribe. Similarly, we now must remember that intravenous fluorescein angiography can interfere with certain laboratory tests, especially if
the patient has renal insufficiency. Patients must be warned to alert their other
physicians that fluorescein has been given.—W.E. Benson, M.D.

Retinal Detachment and Its Relation to Cataract Surgery
Gray RH, Evans AR, Constable IJ, McAllister IL (Lions Eye Inst, Perth, Australia)
Br J Ophthalmol 73:775–780, 1989   10–17

Microsurgical techniques and extracapsular cataract surgery may have
lowered the risk of retinal detachment (RD), but posterior capsulotomy is
known to increase the risk. Of 1,044 patients having 1,089 eyes operated
on during 1976–1987 for primary rhegmatogenous retinal detachment
with causes other than penetrating injury, nearly three fourths of eyes in
the series were phakic. Intracapsular extraction was done in a decreasing
proportion of patients during the review period.

The average frequency of RD was 6.7 per 100,000 population per
year. It was 4.8 for phakic patients and 1.9 for aphakic–pseudophakic
patients. The incidence in the latter patients fell to 0.7 in 1983 but subsequently increased. When the annual number of RD procedures done on
aphakic–pseudophakic eyes were compared with the number of cataract
operations in the previous year, the average risk of RD was 1.75% in
1976–1982 and fell to 0.9% in 1983–1987.

The incidence of aphakic–pseudophakic RD has risen by 55% from
1976 to 1987, whereas the number of cataract operations has risen by
245% in the same period. At least some of the risk reduction is attributable to better microsurgical techniques, especially the avoidance of vitreous loss. The increasing use of extracapsular surgery also is a factor.

▶ Aphakic retinal detachments used to account for approximately one third of
all retinal detachments. Now pseudophakic detachments do. This may appear
strange because several studies have shown that the advent of extracapsular
cataract extraction with the placement of posterior chamber lenses has reduced the incidence of retinal detachment after cataract surgery by about 75%.

However, in Western Australia, and probably in the United States, because of the dramatic increase in the total number of cataract operations being performed, the total number of retinal detachments after cataract surgery actually is increasing.—W.E. Benson, M.D.

Early Retinal Adhesion From Laser Photocoagulation

Folk JC, Sneed SR, Folberg R, Coonan P, Pulido JS (Univ of Iowa, Iowa City)
Ophthalmology 96:1523–1525, October 1989   10–18

Argon laser photocoagulation often is used to create a chorioretinal

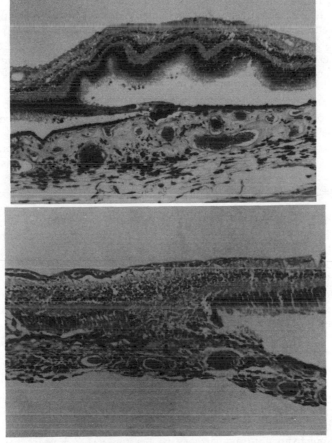

Fig 10–6.—Pathology of 2 argon blue-green laser endophotocoagulation burns placed in the eye of a diabetic patient 20 hours before death. The retina remained attached at the sites of laser burns despite adjacent detachment. A physiologic adhesion occurred between the neurosensory retina and the retinal pigment epithelium as evidenced by the traction on the photoreceptor layers. Hematoxylin-eosin: original magnifications: top, ×7; bottom, ×16. (Courtesy of Folk JC, Sneed SR, Folberg R, et al: *Ophthalmology* 96:1523–1525, October 1989.)

adhesion about retinal breaks. Endophotocoagulation may be used at the end of vitrectomy surgery for detachment with proliferative vitreoretinopathy to produce a broad zone of adhesion. Cryopexy produces more breakdown of the blood-ocular barrier and more dispersion of pigment epithelial cells into the vitreous. With the laser, access to the retina overlying previously buckled areas can be achieved without exposing or moving the explant, which is required for transscleral cryopexy.

Eight monkeys received argon blue-green and krypton red laser photocoagulation to various areas of their retinas. In addition, a diabetic patient had vitrectomy surgery with argon blue-green laser endophotocoagulation for a macular traction detachment. The monkey retinas remained firmly attached at areas of laser treatment 24 hours before, regardless of which instrument was used or of whether burns were placed in normal or bleeding retina (Fig 10–6). In the patient also, the retina was detached post mortem in many areas but remained attached at laser-treated sites.

The neurosensory retina and retinal pigment epithelium are joined by adhesion 24 hours after laser application. Early and increasing adhesion after laser photocoagulation is useful in treating recently reattached retinas, and also in treating retinal breaks without detachment.

▶ When performing vitrectomy for retinal detachments complicated by proliferative vitreoretinopathy, it is essential to release as much traction as possible so that retinal breaks are flat at the end of surgery. If they are not, or even if they are, the operation may fail because residual traction opens them or holds them open. This article confirms the clinical impression of many surgeons that the rapid adhesion created by laser photocoagulation helps to cure many of these difficult cases.—W.E. Benson, M.D.

Loss of Human Photoreceptor Sensitivity Associated With Chronic Exposure to Ultraviolet Radiation
Werner JS, Steele VG, Pfoff DS (Univ of Colorado, Boulder)
Ophthalmology 96:1552–1558, October 1989   10–19

The lens of the eye absorbs most incident ultraviolet (UV) radiation but, when it is removed, radiation can reach the photoreceptors. There is evidence that cystoid macular edema is more likely in pseudophakic patients with an intraocular lens that transmits UV radiation than in those with a UV-absorbing lens. This study of 8 pseudophakic patients with posterior chamber lenses was designed to assess the effects of UV exposure on cone receptor sensitivity through psychophysical measurements. The intraocular lens in 1 eye contained UV-absorbing chromophores; the other lens did not.

The time from cataract surgery to testing was 2.3 years for patients having UV-PMMA lenses and 5 years for those with clear PMMA lenses. For about 5 years, the eyes of each patient differed in UV exposure by about 86:1. Exposure to ambient UV radiation was associated with a selective loss of sensitivity of the short-wave cone photoreceptors. Short-wave cones in exposed eyes were 1.7 times less sensitive than those in unexposed eyes. The loss of sensitivity increased over time, but not to a statistically significant degree.

It is possible that UV radiation accelerates the normal aging of short-wave cones. The findings lend urgency to the need to protect the eye from UV radiation. The aging of the population, increasing time spent outdoors, and reduced UV filtering by the ozone layer make this issue especially important.

▶ When ultraviolet-absorbing chromophores are incorporated into intraocular lenses, there is an 86-fold reduction in the retina's exposure to ultraviolet light. Such intraocular lenses (IOLs) reduce the incidence of fluorescein angiographically detectable cystoid macular edema, and prevent a 0.23 log unit loss of sensitivity in the short-wave length photoreceptors. However, eyes with such IOLs do not have better visual acuity or statistically significantly better color vision. Should all IOLs contain these chromophores? In my opinion, until longer-term studies have been completed, it remains to be proven.—W.E. Benson, M.D.

11 Visual Physiology

The Treatable Forms of Nystagmus

ROBERT D. REINECKE, M.D.
Foerderer Eye Movement Center for Children, Wills Eye Hospital, Philadelphia, Pennsylvania

The following words are intended to call attention to the necessity of carefully examining all patients with nystagmus to find those who will benefit from treatment. Today the state of the art suggests that eye movement recordings should be considered for most patients with nystagmus to find those for whom treatment may be helpful. The following suggests a few examples of such treatments.

By recording the eye movements of various forms of nystagmus, certain distinguishing features are emerging that characterize the nystagmus. Several types of nystagmus show encouraging responses to specific treatments. The following nystagmus patients currently seem to merit consideration of selective intervention.

Infantile Nystagmus

DISTINGUISHING CHARACTERISTICS

Large-amplitude slow nystagmus appearing at birth to 3 months of age may have caused consideration of a diagnosis of blindness. The large amplitude nystagmus gradually converts to smaller-amplitude, fine, faster pendular nystagmus, which at about 9 months converts to jerk nystagmus with increasing velocity of the slow phase. Between 9 months and 2 years of age a null point usually develops.

ASSOCIATED FINDINGS

High astigmatism, strabismus, and various degrees of albinism are associated findings. Family history often reveals that the parents' irides transilluminate to various degrees, some mild nystagmus may be present in one or both parents, and one or both parents were towheaded until puberty and started tanning at puberty.

TREATMENT

Careful refraction with attention for large astigmatism, which should be corrected, is the treatment. If the null point is eccentric a Kestenbaum surgical procedure should be considered and can be done any time before age 8. If there is a large amount of astigmatism and an eccentric null point, the null point should be centralized as soon as the glasses are given. For null points that are central some early encouraging results are being reported with bilateral recessions combined with Fadens of all four recti muscles. We suggest periodic recordings of the eye movements even if no treatment is offered.

Early vision can be estimated with sweep visual evoked potential recordings using horizontal stripes if the nystagmus is horizontal. The overall prognosis of such patients is excellent; in most cases vision is better than 20/60 and even better for close work.

INHERITANCE

Inheritance is usually recessive, but may be X-linked. If X-linked and the family history is good—particularly if the family is accessible—these children and families must be seen because they eventually will lead us to the genetic markers for this condition and the subsequent localization of the involved gene.

Manifest Latent Nystagmus

DISTINGUISHING CHARACTERISTICS

Recordings of such patients show a jerk nystagmus with the fast phase toward the fixing eye. The slow phase has a distinguishing decreasing velocity. The nystagmus is symmetric but often changes in amplitude and frequency depending on which eye is fixing.

ASSOCIATED FINDINGS

The underlying consideration is that the patient is not binocular if this form of nystagmus is present and that making the patient binocular should eliminate the nystagmus. There may be one field of gaze from which binocularity is absent such as an A or V pattern. Restoration of binocularity should convert the manifest latent nystagmus to latent nystagmus. Amblyopia or strabismus are frequent causes of this nystagmus, but accommodative esotropia is another cause.

TREATMENT

Treatment of the cause of the lack of binocularity is urgent because this nystagmus should disappear if the patient can be made binocular. Amblyopia should be treated with patching. Constant patching is necessary because short-term patching will not allow the nystagmus to lessen as it will with long-term patching. If strabismus is the cause, it should be treated with glasses or surgery. Any anisometropia should be treated with appropriate glasses. Unilateral ptosis should be treated as well as any other impediment to binocularity.

Nystagmus Causing Oscillopsia in a Monocular Patient

Occasionally nystagmus may develop in an adult. Often such patients have oscillopsia that may be disabling. A condition such as multiple sclerosis most typically will be the cause.

DISTINGUISHING CHARACTERISTICS

The nystagmus may be downbeat, horizontal, pendular, or jerk. For consideration of this treatment the patient must either have poor vision in the other eye or be willing to patch the other eye, because it is unlikely that an induced paralysis of both eyes will result in parallel visual axes that can be fixated with head movements.

TREATMENT

Although rare, this type of patient seems to benefit greatly by the injection of botulinum toxin to paralyze the movement of the eye. The patient moves the head for fixation and is typically not aware that the eye is not moving. With the potential availability of botulinum antitoxin, which may allow successful prevention of the frequent ptosis, this treatment offers some hope for more frequent intervention with these patients.

Downbeat or Upbeat Nystagmus With Poor Head Position

A variety of conditions can cause downbeat or upbeat nystagmus, such as platybasia, multiple sclerosis, or any posterior fossa lesion. The patient typically will have a position of least nystagmus, such as up gaze.

ASSOCIATED FINDINGS

Because the cause of the nystagmus is the midbrain posterior fossa lesion, a patient may have cerebellar symptoms and long tract signs, depending on the severity of the condition. The associated ocular findings tyupically include worsening of the nystagmus when the patient looks to either side. The nystagmus often becomes torsional in addition to vertical on lateral gaze.

TREATMENT

The nystagmus itself is typically permanent after the underlying cause, such as platybasia, is treated. If the cause is multiple sclerosis, the condition may subside, but if present for 6 months or more the nystagmus tends to be permanent. Treatment options include only the injection of botulinum toxin and the occlusion of the other eye, or the vertical repositioning of the null point such that patients can engage in their usual vocations. If the null point is superior and the patient needs a reading area below, the null point is moved with vertical recti muscle repositioning in the Kestenbaum fashion. In such a case the superior recti would be recessed and the inferior recti resected. Such repositioning of the null point is semipermanent, lasting 6 to 10 years, in my experience.

Eye Disease in a Geriatric Nursing Home Population
Whitmore WG (New York Hosp–Cornell Univ Med Ctr, New York)
Ophthalmology 96:393–398, March 1989   11–1

All 225 residents of a New York City nursing home—more than three fourths of them female—had eye examinations within 1 year. Their average age was 85 years. Of the testable subjects, 44% had visual acuity of 20/40 or better in at least 1 eye, whereas 30% had acuity of 20/200 or less in both eyes.

The prevalence of senile cataract, including aphakia and pseudophakia, was 81%. Prevalence rates of age-related macular degeneration, open-angle glaucoma, and diabetic retinopathy were 37%, 11%, and 2.1%, respectively. The prevalence of both cataract and macular degeneration was highest in patients aged 85 years and more. A majority of the legally blind persons had cataract, and half of them had age-related macular degeneration.

This study, in which all subjects were examined by 1 ophthalmologist, emphasizes the prevalence of eye disease in geriatric patients. Nursing home patients in general seem to have higher rates of cataract, age-related macular degeneration, and open-angle glaucoma than geriatric persons outside nursing homes. These patients must not be overlooked by those who provide ophthalmologic care.

▶ Although abundant eye disease is demonstrated to be present in a nursing home, the authors fail to point out criteria that must be used to selectively offer treatment for such patients. Patients in nursing homes certainly deserve to have their eye needs evaluated carefully. Some can be helped dramatically.— R.D. Reinecke, M.D.

Effect of Monocular Visual Loss Upon Stability of Gaze

Leigh RJ, Thurston SE, Tomsak RL, Grossman GE, Lanska DJ (Case Western Reserve Univ, Cleveland; Geisinger Med Ctr, Danville, Pa)
Invest Ophthalmol Vis Sci 30:288–292, February 1989   11–2

Visual input from 1 eye normally can stabilize the line of sight of both eyes, but prolonged lack of vision in 1 eye can lead to drifting of that eye. The eye coil/magnetic field method was used to measure eye movements in 4 patients with monocular visual loss and clinical vertical gaze instability as they attempted steady binocular fixation of a visual target. Two normal subjects also were studied as they fixed on a target monocularly. A patient with bilateral congenital blindness also was evaluated.

In the patients with monocular visual loss, gaze instability was greater in the blind eye, both vertically and horizontally. Low-amplitude bidirectional drifts were more prominent vertically, and unidirectional drifts with nystagmus were more prominent in the horizontal plane. The congenitally blind subject had nystagmus with horizontal and vertical components and a wandering null point. Gaze-evoked nystagmus was not apparent in the monocularly blind subjects.

Gaze instability in monocular blindness may indicate disruption of a monocular vision stabilizing system, disordered vergence mechanisms, or both. Abnormal neural integration is more likely in bilateral congenital blindness.

▶ The article points out the instability of gaze if reduced vision is present in 1 eye, and even covering 1 eye of a normally sighted person produces some abnormal gaze problems. If the 2 eyes are blind, the eyes move in such a manner that diagnostically important patterns of eye movement are difficult to interpret.—R.D. Reinecke, M.D.

Visual Pathway Abnormalities in Albinism and Infantile Nystagmus: VECPs and Stereoacuity Measurements

Guo S, Reinecke RD, Fendick M, Calhoun JH (Wills Eye Hosp, Philadelphia)
J Pediatr Ophthalmol Strabismus 26:97–104, March–April 1989   11–3

In albinos, an abnormal decussation of optic nerve fiber with increased contralateral projection leads to hemispheric asymmetry of monocular vi-

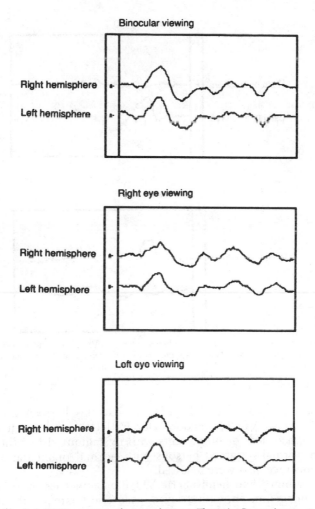

Fig 11–1.—The flash VECP responses of a normal person. The major P wave is seen symmetrically in both binocular and monocular stimulations. The negative direction is down. (Courtesy of Guo S, Reinecke RD, Fendick M, et al: *J Pediatr Ophthalmol Strabismus* 26:97–104, March–April 1989.)

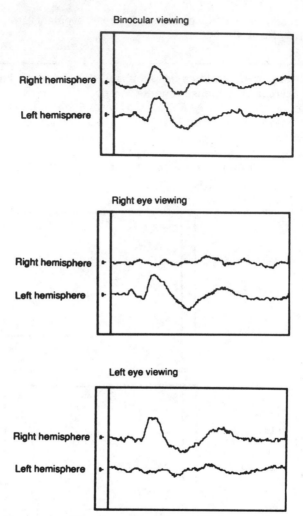

Fig 11–2.—The responses of binocular and monocular flash VECPs of an albino nystagmus patient. The responses on binocular stimulation are symmetric, but the monocular P wave shows a significantly reduced amplitude over the hemisphere ipsilateral to the eye stimulated. (Courtesy of Guo S, Reinecke RD, Fedick M, et al: *J Pediatr Ophthalmol Strabismus* 26:97–104, March–April 1989.)

sual evoked cortical potentials (VECPs) that may be related to a lack of stereopsis. Flash VECP, Random Dot E (RDE), and Titmus stereotest data were recorded for 40 patients with nystagmus, 19 of them albinos. Nineteen normally sighted persons with normal pigmentation matched for age and race also were assessed.

All the albinos had hemispheric VECP asymmetries more than 2 SDs from the normal mean, with delayed ipsilateral P latency, reduced ipsilateral P amplitude, or both (Figs 11–1 and 11–2). Only 1 albinotic subject had positive RDE and stereofly findings. A large majority of normally pigmented nystagmic patients passed the stereofly test, and a majority had positive RDE results.

Albinism is not always easy to diagnose, and VECP asymmetry may help in making the diagnosis. Albinotic persons with nystagmus have abnormal visual pathways and impaired or absent binocular vision. In contrast, patients with infantile nystagmus but normal pigmentation do not have marked abnormalities of optic nerve decussation.

▶ Determining when a patient with infantile esotropia should have surgical intervention is a common problem. All data support intervention to surgically align the eyes by age 2 years. This article points out that, if the patient is found to have albinism, the lack of potential for stereopsis makes the surgical intervention less compelling at an early age, and waiting would carry few disadvantages for such patients.—R.D. Reinecke, M.D.

Comparison of the Effects of Atropine and Cyclopentolate on Myopia
Yen M-Y, Liu J-H, Kao S-C, Shiao C-H (Yang-Ming Med College, Taipei, Taiwan)
Ann Ophthalmol 21:180–187, May 1989   11–4

Excessive close work long has been thought to be an important cause of myopia, and cycloplegics have been used to control myopic progression. Myopia is associated with higher degrees and intensity of schooling.

One percent atropine eye drops every other night, 1% cyclopentolate drops each night, and normal saline drops each night were compared in 96 children with simple myopia who were followed for 1 year. Mean myopic progression was −0.219 D in the atropine recipients, −0.578 D in patients given cyclopentolate, and −0.914 D in those given saline. Both drugs were significantly effective in slowing myopic progression, and atropine was more effective than cyclopentolate.

Atropine delays the progress of myopia but does not halt the tendency toward progression in susceptible subjects. Both atropine and cyclopentolate can produce serious ocular and systemic side effects and must be carefully prescribed. Side effects are less marked with cyclopentolate.

▶ The authors give us 1 more document suggesting that cycloplegic drugs do work in myopia. This is such an important subject that it is unfortunate that a large-scale project cannot nail down the exact benefits of this therapy for myopia.—R.D. Reinecke, M.D.

Visual Sensory Disorders in Congenital Nystagmus
Weiss AH, Biersdorf WR (Univ of South Florida, Tampa)
Ophthalmology 96:517–523, April 1989   11–5

Most patients with congenital nystagmus (CN) appear to have an underlying disorder of the visual sensory system. Data for 81 patients seen from 1981 to 1987 with CN and normal-appearing eyes were reviewed.

Conjugate bilateral ocular oscillations of symmetric amplitude and frequency were detected before age 6 months. Seventy-four patients (91%) had disorders of the visual sensory system. Albinism and congenital or early-onset disorder of the retinal photoreceptors were most frequent. The remaining 7 patients had motor CN.

Patients presenting with CN should be carefully evaluated for underlying disorder of the visual sensory system. Albinism was the most prevalent sensory disorder in the present series. Macular hypoplasia is a reliable sign of albinism. Disorders of photoreceptor function also are frequent. Twenty-four of the present patients had achromatopsia, a nonprogressive disorder. Thirteen patients had disorders involving both rod and cone photoreceptors. Three patients in the series had optic nerve abnormalities.

▶ The authors correctly point out that the cause of nystagmus usually can be found, and in unselected patients a variety of ocular disorders may accompany nystagmus. In an institution like Wills Eye Hospital, where we see about 5 new cases of nystagmus per week and the various specialty clinics often see the patients first, the number of cases without ocular pathology is much greater than in this paper. Nevertheless, we are well advised to expect to find clinical abnormalities of the visual system when nystagmus is seen. I would add that it seems helpful to obtain an electro-oculogram for most patients because manifest latent nystagmus may be found, which often can be treated, and thus the nystagmus changed to latent with the resultant improvement in nystagmus and vision.— R.D. Reinecke, M.D.

Lithium-Induced Downbeat Nystagmus
Halmagyi GM, Lessell I, Curthoys IS, Lessell S, Hoyt WF (Royal Prince Alfred Hosp, Sydney, Australia; Lahey Clinic, Burlington, Mass; Univ of Sydney; Massachusetts Eye & Ear Infirmary, Boston; Univ of California, San Francisco)
Am J Ophthalmol 107:664–670, June 1989   11–6

A variety of adverse neurologic side effects of lithium therapy has been recognized. Of 6 patients in whom blurring or oscillopsia developed from downbeat nystagmus while they were receiving lithium carbonate and 6 previously reported patients, downbeat nystagmus developed insidiously as an isolated disorder in all but 2 despite satisfactory therapeutic control. There was no clinical or biochemical evidence of acute lithium intoxication. The nystagmus lessened or remitted in only 2 of 6 patients who were able to reduce or stop lithium.

Cerebellar signs, including nystagmus, are noted in patients acutely intoxicated with lithium. Visual complaints are frequent in patients with any type of downbeat nystagmus. Rather than movement, "blurred vision" may be described. Some patients may retain good visual acuity. Several of these patients failed to have improvement when lithium was reduced or withdrawn. In addition, patients who continued on lithium therapy or resumed treatment did not have marked deterioration.

▶ The authors point out the presence of this drug-induced downbeat nystagmus. Because some patients are loath to admit being on this drug for depression, the clinician should be well aware of it as a cause of the nystagmus to avoid unnecessary testing It is noteworthy that all of the patients I have seen mirror the authors' patients in not wishing to stop the drug in spite of the visual disability because they have found the drug so effective.—R.D. Reinecke, M.D.

Electro-Oculographic Detection of Microsymptoms: Inherited Versus Spontaneous Cases of Congenital Nystagmus
Shallo-Hoffmann J, Watermeier D, Petersen J, Mühlendyck H (Univ of Göttingen, West Germany)
Am Orthoptic J 39:125–133, 1989   11–7

Inheritance of congenital nystagmus (CN) has been verified only by the presence of more than 1 affected person in a family. Electro-oculographic (EOG) studies of 10 families with CN were undertaken to learn whether abnormal involuntary eye movements are a sign of hereditary transmission in seemingly unaffected family members. It was hypothesized that inherited CN is not rare and that micromanifestations might radily be overlooked at clinical work-up.

Abnormal eye movements were recorded in at least 1 member of 6 of the 10 families studied. Higher than normal intensity scores were found under 3 test conditions. Slow-phase instabilities were found in 2 families, and fast-phase instabilities, in 4. A total of 20 relatives were examined.

Congenital nystagmus is inherited more often than was previously realized. More than half of these cases thought to be "spontaneous" had clinically unaffected relatives with evidence of abnormal eye movements. Inherited CN can readily be missed on clinical examination. The most frequent abnormality is an increased rate of saccadic intrusions.

▶ As more and more parents wish genetic counseling, we need tools for guiding the transmission of ocular disorders. The EOGs of relatives of patients with infantile or congenital nystagmus and the finding of subclinical eye movement disorders may aid us in this search. We are coming to the point that eye movement recordings for eye movement disorders will become the norm.—R.D. Reinecke, M.D.

Results After Surgery for Null Point Nystagmus With Abnormal Head Position
Biglan AW, Hiles DA, Ying-Fen Z, Kortvelesy JS, Pettapiece MC (Univ of Pittsburgh; First Teaching Hosp of Beijing)
Am Orthoptic J 39:134–142, 1989   11–8

Most workers have described immediate improvement of the head turn after surgical repositioning of the eyes in patients having nystagmus associated with an eccentric null point, but the long-term results are uncertain. Forty-six patients with null point nystagmus and abnormal head position were followed up after the Kestenbaum operation or one of its modifications. Thirty-four were followed up for 2 years or longer; the mean period was 6.5 years.

Visual acuity was improved in 56% of the patients. Nearly half the patients had improved stereoacuity at follow-up. Peripheral and central fusion was unchanged. Forty-one percent of patients met criteria for a second operation during follow-up, most often because of an abnormal head position. Visual acuity is diminished by nystagmus in these patients, and a compensatory head posture therefore is assumed to allow optimal vision. The present patients all had surgery on both eyes at once. If coexisting strabismus was present it was corrected along with the nystagmus.

The Kestenbaum procedure improves abnormal head posture and also benefits visual acuity and stereoacuity; it is not a purely cosmetic operation. If a residual head posture is present shortly after surgery, it probably results from inadequate initial surgery rather than a drift of the null point toward its original site.

▶ The surprising success of Kestenbaum surgery to improve the visual acuity of patients over and above their best acuity at their preoperative null point continues to surprise all. The authors appropriately point out that if the results are not what you expect, further surgery is indicated at that point and waiting for further change is not justified. Articles such as this eventually will give us rigorous criteria for time and type of surgery.— R.D. Reinecke, M.D.

Effect of Spectacle Use and Accommodation on Myopic Progression: Final Results of a Three-Year Randomized Clinical Trial Among Schoolchildren

Pärssinen O, Hemminki E, Klemetti A (Central Hosp of Central Finland, Jyväskylä; Univ of Helsinki)
Br J Ophthalmol 73:547–551, 1989   11–9

Some believe that accommodation increases myopic progression and recommend spectacles for distant vision only, whereas others believe that spectacles should be worn continuously. Three-year results now are available from a randomized trial comparing 3 different styles of correcting myopia in schoolchildren. The children used fully correcting lenses continuously for distant use only, or bifocals with +1.75 D addition. A total of 240 mildly myopic children aged 9 to 11 years participated in the study.

Differences in the increases in spherical equivalent at 3 years were not significantly different in the right eye. In the left, however, the change in the distant-use group, −1.87 D, significantly exceeded that in the continuous-use group (−1.46 D). The groups did not differ in school achievement, number of accidents, or satisfaction with glasses. Myopia progressed faster as more daily close work was done in all groups. Progression was correlated with a shorter average reading distance at follow-up but not with accommodation.

Progression of myopia in children appears related to frequent reading and close work and to a short reading distance. Progression cannot, however, be limited by decreasing accommodation with bifocals or by reading without spectacles. Continuous use of fully corrected spectacles therefore can be recommended for myopic children, but this does not necessarily apply to myopic adults.

► This article gives assurance that the use of bifocals to minimize the progression of myopia is worthless and verifies the clinical impression that one should give these children the full minus to minimize the adverse side effects of myopia. We continue to need such a definitive study on the controversial use of atropine for myopic control.— R.D. Reinecke, M.D.

Expenditure Targets Not Included in Energy and Commerce Committee's Physician Payment Reform Proposal
Foreman J
Arch Ophthalmol 107:1284, September 1989   11–10

Expenditure targets (ETs) are physician payment allocations determined by a congressional committee. If the ET for the total amount allocated to pay all physicians or a group of physicians is exceeded, the allocation would be decreased the next year. The American Medical Association has objected strongly to ETs. A new Medicare fee schedule established by the Energy and Commerce proposal would be based on another controversial issue, the Harvard Resource-Based Relative Value Scale (RBRVS)

Ophthalmic services comprise a fairly large portion of total fees charged to Medicare for operative procedures. Ophthalmic surgery made up 18.7% of the $9.4 billion of all total charges submitted to Medicare in 1985.

Both reform packages under consideration must be approved by the House. The Senate Finance Committee, which also oversees Medicare, has not yet started to review physician payment reforms. The final version of the Medicare reform legislation is therefore far from completed.

House Committee Endorses Expenditure Targets
Foreman J
Arch Ophthalmol 107:1125, August 1989   11–11

The House Ways and Means Committee recently approved a proposal limiting total Medicare payments to physicians, but the proposal met with strong reactions from physicians and other legislatures.

The president of the Academy of Ophthalmology, in presenting the Academy's proposals for physician payment reform, recommended opposing any further cuts in cataract surgery; developing criteria to require surgeons to document their preoperative and postoperative care arrangements; considering the possibility of random second opinions; prohibiting the unbundling of the global fee for cataract surgery; and including primary eye care office visits in the current list of primary care visit services. The AMA strongly objected to expenditure targets, arguing that they would lead to rationing because the plan would force physicians to limit care on a case-by-case basis. In addition, the AMA suggested practice parameters as an alternative to expenditure targets, and proposed that the subcommittee elicit the help of the AMA and specialty societies in developing a more effective use review system. The AMA recommended establishing professional liability reforms by controlling rising nonphysician services in part B Medicare payments.

▶ The changes proposed by our Congress may have far-reaching effects on the manner of funding and ultimately the practice of ophthalmology. These may be the first winds of the rationing of ophthalmologic care.—R.D. Reinecke, M.D.

Reproducibility of Refraction and Visual Acuity Measurement Under a Standard Protocol

Blackhurst DW, Maguire MG, Macular Photocoagulation Study Group (Johns Hopkins Med Institutions, Baltimore)
Retina 9:163–169, October 1989   11–12

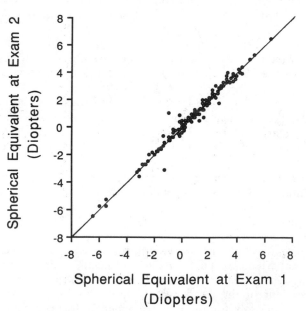

Fig 11–3.—Comparison of spherical equivalent of corrections (diopters) obtained by subjective refraction by 2 examiners. *Solid diagonal line* indicates the line of equality. (Courtesy of Blackhurst DW, Maguire MG: *Retina* 9:163–169, October 1989.)

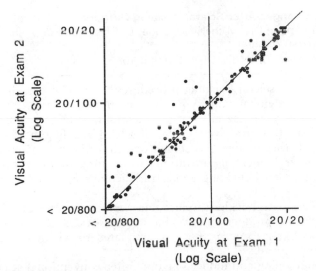

Fig 11–4. Comparison of best-corrected visual acuity measurements made by 2 examiners. *Solid diagonal line* indicates the line of equality. *Solid vertical line* at 20/100 divides observations into good and poor visual acuity. (Courtesy of Blackhurst DW, Maguire MG: *Retina* 9:163–169, October 1989.)

Certified examiners in the Macular Photocoagulation Study, a set of multicenter randomized clinical trials of laser photocoagulation for choroidal neovascular membranes, performed independent replicate refractions and acuity measurements on patients with acuities of 20/20 to 20/800. Eighty-two patients with neovascular age-related macular degeneration, ocular histoplasmosis, and idiopathic neovascularization were included in the study.

The median spherical equivalent was 1.0 D, with spherical equivalents ranging from −6.5 to +6.5 (Fig 11–3). Visual acuity scores showed greater discrepancy between examiners for eyes with poor vision than did the refraction data (Fig 11–4). The mean difference for eyes with poor acuity was −0.39. The standard deviation of visual acuity scores in this group was 1.05, compared with 0.57 for persons having good vision.

Refraction and visual acuity measurements made with a standard protocol are highly reliable. If a standard procedure is used in testing, clinicians may be able to distinguish between true changes and measurement error, even in low-acuity patients with age-related macular degeneration. Acuity changes of 2 or more lines are very likely to reflect true deterioration in vision and the possible onset of increased pathologic conditions.

▶ Often we ask ourselves, Is the change in visual acuity due to refraction changes? Here is one of the few studies I know of that systematically revealed that refractive errors found by different examiners are not significantly different if reasonably similar paradigms of refraction are done. Visual acuity on the other hand does vary among examiners, especially in the poorer acuity ranges.—R.D. Reinecke, M.D.

Refractive Changes After Scleral Buckling Surgery

Smiddy WE, Loupe DN, Michels RG, Enger C, Glaser BM, deBustros S (Johns Hopkins Univ, Baltimore)
Arch Ophthalmol 107:1469–1471, October 1989   11–13

Conventional scleral buckling procedures for retinal detachment alter the shape of the globe and may produce an altered refractive state. Pneumatic retinopexy has the advantage of avoiding such changes. In a prospective study, the refractive sequelae of scleral buckling in 75 eyes of 69 patients with rhegmatogenous retinal detachments was examined. Conventional scleral buckling operations were done in these cases, using sponges for radial hbuckling and hard silicone elements to encircle the globe.

Encircling scleral buckles produced an average increase of 0.99 mm in axial length and produced an average myopia of 2.75 D. Induced astigmatism was likely to occur, but was unrelated to whether a radial element was employed.

Axial lengthening and induced myopia after conventional scleral buckling surgery are associated chiefly with the use of encircling elements, or segmental elements combined with an encircling band. A radial buckle carries a low risk of significant refractive change, but induced astigmatism remains a possibility.

▶ The necessity of carefully refracting the patients after retina surgery is documented here. The average change of −3.00 D after scleral bucklings is certainly significant.—R.D. Reinecke, M.D.

Tinted Lenses and Dyslexics: A Controlled Study

Tinted Lenses Study Group, SPELD Inc (Kensington, Australia)
Aust NZ J Ophthalmol 17:137–141, 1989   11–14

Do tinted lenses influence the reading ability of dyslexic children? This prospective trial included 24 nonasthmatic dyslexic children, aged 9 to 12 years, whose reading ability was assessed with the Neale Analysis of Reading. Thirteen of the children received glasses containing tinted lenses. The 11 controls were matched for age and sex; they were fitted with tinted lenses after 1 school term and were followed up for 2 further terms.

No significant difference in changes in reading age were found between the treated and control groups after 1 school term. After 2 terms in about 6 months, only 44% of children still wore their glasses.

Experience with more than 1,200 children fitted with tinted lenses suggests that some do derive considerable benefit. Because many asthmatic children were kept out of the present study to avoid medication effects on cerebral function, children who would have responded favorably to tinted lenses may have been excluded.

▸ Although the study is somewhat limited in its number of patients, the use of tinted lenses in this study showed no improvement. Some proponents of the use of the tint in the United Stages and Australia seem to be taking advantage of the desperate feelings of the parents of dyslexic children. Those critics of this system such as myself welcome this impartial evaluation of the problem.—R.D. Reinecke, M.D.

AMA Looks Toward a Cure for U.S. Health Care
Foreman J
Arch Ophthalmol 107:1433, October 1989   11–15

The American Medical Association (AMA) Board of Trustees recently discussed how to provide comprehensive cost-effective access to health care in a way that builds on the present pluralistic system, and how to rememdy existing gaps in coverage while maintaining the many benefits available to a large proportion of Americans. Other goals are to lower the burden of complex governmental and private insurance paperwork and the cost of the current professional liability system.

All the poor must receive medical care, not just the 40% who presently receive care. Health care insurance should be expanded to all employed Americans. A Medicare commission is recommended to develop ways of ensuring continued financial access by older persons. It is hoped that the current pay-as-you-go system will be replaced by a prefunded, actuarially sound system allowing all of the elderly to purchase the health insurance of their choice through qualified plans. Long-term care financing arrangements should encourage public and private partnerships.

A multifaceted provision system is a cost-effective means of maintaining choice in health care. A reduction in the administrative burdens of government and other third-party payers is mandatory. Until financial barriers to mainstream care for all are removed, physicians should be encouraged to reaffirm their tradition of providing free care to patients who cannot afford to pay.

▸ The AMA wants to expand the Medicare system. I suspect it is playing into the hands of those favoring the Canadian system. Only time will tell.—R.D. Reinecke, M.D.

Subject Index

Neuropathy
optic
dysthyroid, methylprednisolone pulse
therapy in, 106
ischemic, bilateral anterior, and optic
disc drusen and systemic
hypotension, 92
ischemic, progressive nonarteritic,
optic nerve decompression for, 90
sinusitis of intranasal cocaine abuse
and, 83
Newborn
ocular prophylaxis for prevention of
chlamydial and gonococcal
conjunctivitis, 24
pupils of, 165
shaken baby syndrome, retinal
hemorrhage predictive of
neurologic injury in, 92
Nonsteroidal anti-inflammatory drugs
effect on maintenance of mydriasis
during cataract surgery, 14
Null point
nystagmus with abnormal head
position, results after surgery, 235
Nursing home
population, geriatric, eye disease in,
229
Nystagmus
congenital
electro-oculographic detection of
microsymptoms in, 235
visual sensory disorders in, 233
downbeat, 229
associated findings, 229
lithium-induced, 234
treatment, 229
infantile, 227–228
associated findings, 227
distinguishing characteristics, 227
inheritance of, 228
treatment, 227–228
visual pathway abnormalities in, 231
manifest latent, 228
associated findings, 228
distinguishing characteristics, 228
treatment, 228
null point, with abnormal head
position, results after surgery, 235
oscillopsia in monocular patient due to,
228–229
distinguishing characteristics,
228–229
treatment, 229
treatable forms of, 227–229
upbeat, 229
associated findings, 229
treatment, 229

O

Oblique muscle (*see* Inferior oblique)
Ocular
(*See also* Eye)
adnexal hemorrhage, infantile, eyelid
depigmentation after corticosteroid
injection for, 100
herpes simplex, epidemiology of, 40
histoplasmosis, persistent and recurrent
neovascularization after krypton
laser photocoagulation for, 208
hypertensives, testing of, 59
infarction and amaurosis fugax, in
adolescents and young adults, 88
intraocular (*see* Intraocular)
manifestations of AIDS, 146
in children, 166
melanoma, and female hormones, 127
motor paresis, transient, and internal
carotid artery occlusion, 81
pemphigoid, cicatricial,
immunophenotypic analysis of
inflammatory infiltrate in, 137
periocular (*see* Periocular)
prophylaxis, neonatal, for prevention of
chlamydial and gonococcal
conjunctivitis, 24
reticulum cell sarcoma, primary, 121
surface, effect of ophthalmic solutions
on (in rabbit), 34
Ophthalmic
manifestations of leukemia, 120
pathology, immunohistochemistry in,
133–136
solutions, effect on ocular surface (in
rabbit), 34
viscoelastic agents, drug binding of,
26
Ophthalmologist
average, and axial length, 11
diabetic care by, 211
Ophthalmopathy
Graves' (*see* Graves' opthalmopathy)
Optic
disc (*see* Disc)
nerve
decompression for progressive
nonarteritic ischemic optic
neuropathy, 90
disease in HIV infection, 85
glioma, orbital, in adult, 149
hypoplasia, superior segmental, as
sign of maternal diabetes, 86
involvement in retinoblastoma,
138
neuropathy (*see* Neuropathy, optic)

Author Index

A

Abbott RL, 188
Abelson MB, 11
Abrams DA, 62
Abramson DH, 138
Adams RE, 1
Agapitos PJ, 178, 190
Alavai A, 86
Albert DM, 138
Alfarano R, 101
Allara RD, 180
Alward WLM, 63
Amendola BE, 122
Anderson RL, 104, 107
Angra SK, 199
Annesley WH, 214
Apple DJ, 10
Arentsen JJ, 28, 39
Arrigg CA, 69
Arthur BW, 170
Arzeno G, 69
Augsburger JJ, 115, 120, 127, 128, 214
Avram D, 113

B

Bailey TM, 30
Baringer JR, 77
Barnes D, 149
Bartalena L, 89
Bartlett JG, 146
Bartley GB, 104
Batenhorst RL, 58
Baylis HI, 99, 109
Bazin R, 183
Beck RW, 13
Becker BB, 98
Behrens M, 92
Bellows AR, 69, 71
Beniz J, 136
Bennett SR, 63
Benson WE, 203
Berghout A, 90
Bergin DJ, 149
Berlin AJ, 108
Bernard P-M, 183
Bernardino VB, 144
Bernier J, 183
Berry FD, 98
Bickler-Bluth M, 59
Biersdorf WR, 233
Biglan AW, 96, 169, 235
Binder PS, 182
Biswas J, 136
Björklund H, 18
Blackhurst DW, 238
Blankenship GW, 43
Bloom JN, 221
Bogazzi F, 89

Boisjoly HM, 183
Bosley TM, 86, 87, 90
Bosworth JL, 125
Bott AD, 81
Bourne WM, 32, 181, 189
Bowden FW III, 28
Boyer D, 136
Boyle DL, 70
Brady LW, 120, 122
Brady SE, 39
Brancato R, 101
Branch DW, 77
Brand RJ, 187
Bremer DL, 173
Bressler NM, 210
Bressler SB, 210
Briley DP, 79
Bron AM, 64
Brooks DE, 70
Brooks IIL Jr, 211
Brown BZ, 112
Brunner Forbor FL, 64
Buckman G, 105, 148
Burk LL, 41
Burke JP, 198
Burke PJ, 120
Burnstine RA, 169
Butler C, 191
Byer NE, 215

C

Caldwell DR, 62
Calhoun JH, 231
Capoferri C, 101
Carter CJ, 70
Cartright K, 219
Causey D, 136
Chan C-C, 27
Char D, 99
Chauhan BC, 59
Chawluk J, 86
Chen HS-L, 68
Chhabra VK, 199
Clorfeine GS, 7
Coffey R, 163
Cogen MS, 100
Cohen EJ, 21, 28, 39
Cohen MS, 90
Constable IJ, 222
Coonan P, 223
Cooper DG, 59
Corbett JJ, 88
Cornell FM, 191
Coull BM, 79
Cowan GM, 142
Crandall AS, 62
Cravy TV, 8
Crawford JB, 148
Creighton JB, 13
Cruysberg JRM, 112, 159
Culbertson WW, 192

Cummings C, 24
Curthoys IS, 234

D

Dalton J, 121
Dang Y, 165
Datiles MB, 144
Daun ME, 10
Davis MD, 207
deBustros S, 240
Deichman CB, 9
de la Cruz Z, 140
de la Monte SM, 142
Delke I, 24
Demartini D, 187
DeMets DL, 207
Dennehy PJ, 166
Deupree DM, 96
Digre KB, 77
Donnenfeld E, 137
Donoso L, 123
Donovan JP, 106
Donzis PB, 38
Douglas GR, 59
Drance SM, 55, 59, 70
Dubé I, 183
Duffey RJ, 190
Duinkerke-Eerola KU, 159
Dunkelberger GR, 60
Dunn JP Jr, 38
Durcan FJ, 77

E

Eagle RC Jr, 123, 133, 214
Edelhauser HF, 26
Edelstein DJ, 67
Edsell TD, 16
Edwards PA, 144
Egan KM, 126, 130
Eldridge R, 144
Elin RJ, 221
Elliot TSJ, 200
Elliott JH, 17
Ellsworth RM, 138
Elsas FJ, 100
Emmett EA, 196
Enger C, 140, 240
Engstrom RE Jr, 41
Enzenauer RW, 191
Epstein DL, 67
Evans AR, 222

F

Fagerholm P, 18
Fagien S, 106
Failer J, 206